Safe Motherhood Initiative
A Silent Revolution

FEDERATION OF OBSTETRIC GYNAECOLOGICAL SOCIETIES OF INDIA
FOGSI

SAFE MOTHERHOOD COMMITTEE - FOGSI
SAVE MOTHER & CHILD

Safe Motherhood Initiative
A Silent Revolution

Editor
Sadhana Gupta
MS (Obs and Gyne) MNAMS FICOG FICMU FICMCH
Chairman, Safe Motherhood Committee FOGSI (2011–2013)
Past President, Gorakhpur Obstetric and Gynecological Society
Senior Consultant
Department of Obstetrics and Gynecology
Jeevan Jyoti Hospital and Medical Research Center
Gorakhpur, Uttar Pradesh, India

Forewords
Sabaratnam Arulkumaran
Hema Divakar

Under the aegis of
Safe Motherhood Committee (2011–2013)
Federation of Obstetric and
Gynaecological Societies of India

JAYPEE BROTHERS MEDICAL PUBLISHERS (P) LTD

New Delhi • London • Philadelphia • Panama

Jaypee Brothers Medical Publishers (P) Ltd.

Headquarters
Jaypee Brothers Medical Publishers (P) Ltd.
4838/24, Ansari Road, Daryaganj
New Delhi 110 002, India
Phone: +91-11-43574357
Fax: +91-11-43574314
Email: jaypee@jaypeebrothers.com

Overseas Offices

J.P. Medical Ltd.
83, Victoria Street, London
SW1H 0HW (UK)
Phone: +44-2031708910
Fax: +02-03-0086180
Email: info@jpmedpub.com

Jaypee-Highlights Medical Publishers Inc.
City of Knowledge, Bld. 237, Clayton
Panama City, Panama
Phone: + 507-301-0496
Fax: + 507-301-0499
Email: cservice@jphmedical.com

Jaypee Medical Inc.
The Bourse
111, South Independence Mall East
Suite 835, Philadelphia, PA 19106, USA
Phone: + 267-519-9789
Email: jpmed.us@gmail.com

Jaypee Brothers Medical Publishers (P) Ltd.
17/1-B, Babar Road, Block-B, Shaymali
Mohammadpur, Dhaka-1207
Bangladesh
Mobile: +08801912003485
Email: jaypeedhaka@gmail.com

Jaypee Brothers Medical Publishers (P) Ltd.
Bhotahity, Kathmandu, Nepal
Phone: +977-9741283608
Email: Kathmandu@jaypeebrothers.com

Website: www.jaypeebrothers.com
Website: www.jaypeedigital.com

Inquiries for bulk sales may be solicited at: jaypee@jaypeebrothers.com

Safe Motherhood Initiative—A Silent Revolution

First Edition: **2014**

ISBN: 978-93-5152-182-2

Printed at Rajkamal Electric Press, Plot No. 2, Phase-IV, Kundli, Haryana.

Dedicated to

All positive efforts for safe motherhood

Contributors

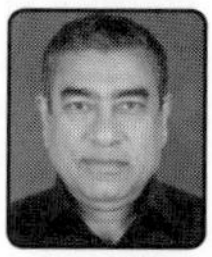

Abu Jamil Faisel
President, Voluntary
Health Science Society
Country Representative
Endanger Health Project
Bangladesh

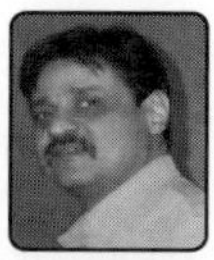

Ajey Bhardwaj
National Coordinator
EmOC Program

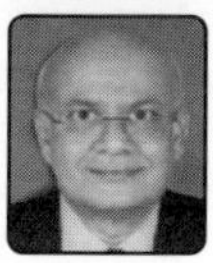

AK Debdas
Past Vice President
Federation of Obstetric
and Gynaecological
Societies of India (FOGSI)
Past Chairman
Indian College of Obstetricians and
Gynecologists (ICOG)
Rajkumari Foundation
Jamshedpur, Jharkhand, India

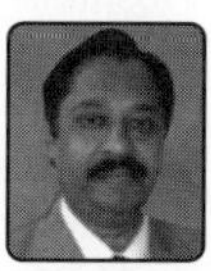

Alpesh Gandhi
Vice President
FOGSI 2013
Past Chairman
Practical Obstetric
Committee FOGSI
Ahmedabad, Gujarat, India

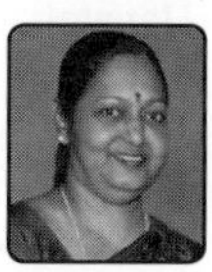

Arulmozhi Ramarajan
Head
Department of Obstetrics
and Gynecology
Church of South India
Hospital
Bengaluru, Karnataka, India
Past President Bengaluru Society of
Obstetrics and Gynecology
Bengaluru, Karnataka, India

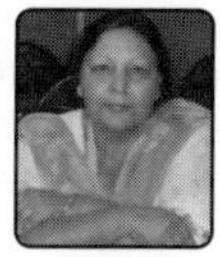

Ashma Rana
Unit Chief
Department of Obstetrics
and Gynecology
Tribhuvan University
Kathmandu
President
Nepal Society of Obstetricians
and Gynecologists
Kathmandu, Nepal

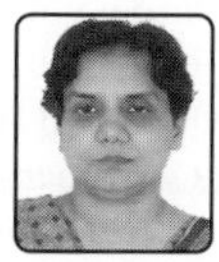

Asmita Rathore
Director-Professor
Department of Obstetrics
and Gynecology
Maulana Azad Medical
College
New Delhi, India

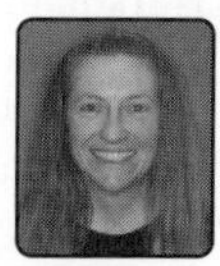

Coffey Patricia
Group Leader
Health Technologies for
Women and Children
Technology Solutions
Program and Research Coordinator
Program for Appropriate Technology
in Health (PATH) Foundation
Atlanta

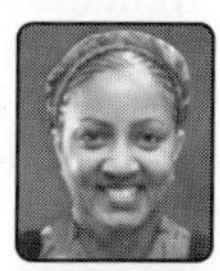

Denise Lionetti
Program and Research
Coordinator
PATH Foundation
Atlanta

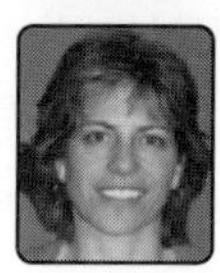

Elizabeth Abu-Haydar
Public Health Specialist
Technology Solutions
Program and Research
Coordinator
PATH Foundation
Atlanta

Fatema Shabnam
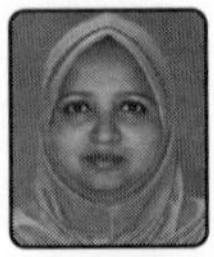
Program Manager
Mayer Hashi Project
Engender Health Project
Bangladesh

Ferdousi Begum
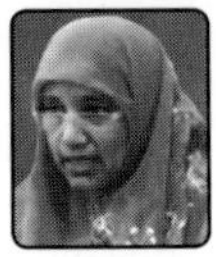
Associate Professor
Department of Obstetrics
and Gynecology
Institute of Child and
Mother Health
Dhaka, Bangladesh

Girija Wagh
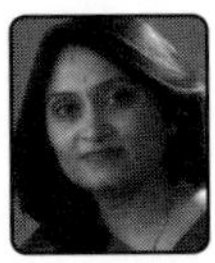
Professor and Head
Department of Obstetrics
and Gynecology
Bharati Vidyapeeth
Deemed University Medical
College and Hospital
Pune, Maharashtra
India

Harshalal R Seneviratne
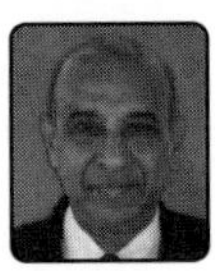
Past President
Sri Lanka College of
Obstetricians and
Gynecologists
Convenor
UNFPA-SAFOG Workshop
Sri Lanka

Hemantha Parera
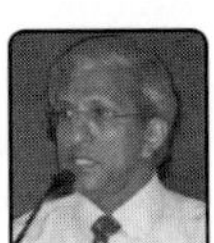
Consultant
Sri Jaywardenepura
General Hospital
Sri Lanka
President
Sri Lanka College of Obstetricians and
Gynecologists
President
Menopause Society of Sri Lanka
Sri Lanka

Hema Divakar
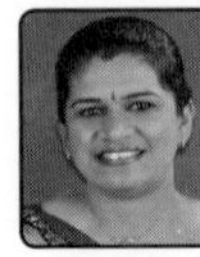
President, FOGSI, 2013
Senior Consultant
Divakar's Specialty
Hospital, Bengaluru
Karnataka, India

Hema J Shobhane
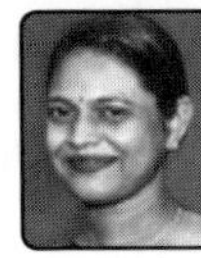
Assistant Professor and
Head,
Maharani Laxmi Bai
Medical College
Jhansi, Uttar Pradesh, India
Coordinator
Safe Motherhood Committee, FOGSI

KS Prashanth
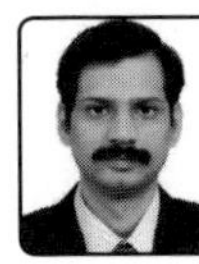
Senior Consultant
Public Health
Administration
National Health System
Resource Center
National Rural Health Mission
Government of India

Leila Fahel
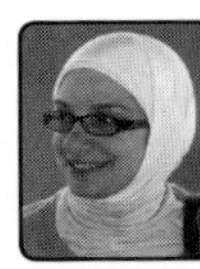
Senior Trainee
Obstetrics and Gynecology
Bradford Teaching
Hospitals
Yorkshire and Humber, UK

Lubna Hassan
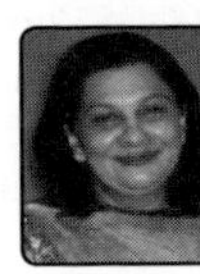
Consultant, Obstetrician
and Gynecologist
Chief Executive
The Woman's Hospital
Hayatabad, Peshawar, Pakistan

Meenal A Chidgupkar
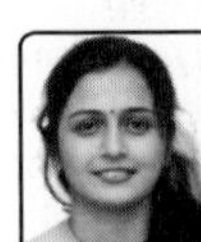
Consultant, Obstetrician
and Gynecologist
Dr Chidgupkar Hospital
Pvt Ltd
Solapur, Maharashtra, India

Milind R Shah
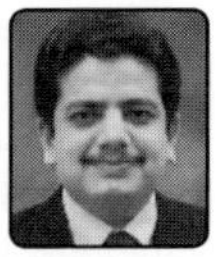
Professor and Head
Department of Obstetrics and Gynecology
Gandhi Natha Rangji Homeopathic Medical College
Solapur, Maharashtra, India
Past Vice President FOGSI (2011)
Past Chairman
Rural Obstetrics Committee of FOGSI (2004–08)
Past President
Solapur Obstetrics and Gynecologcal Society (2001–2002)
Solapur, Maharashtra, India

MK Valsan
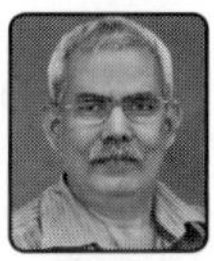
Professor and Head
Department of Obstetrics and Gynecology
MES Medical College
Perinthalmanna, Kerala
Director
Dr Valsan's Infertility Center
Calicut, Kerala, India

Nitya Nand Deepak
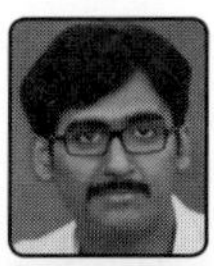
Program Coordinator
Oxytocin Initiative
PATH Foundation, Atlanta

Noah Perin
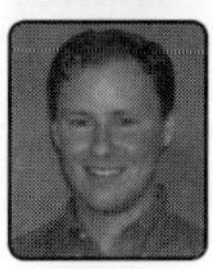
Commercial Officer I
Health Innovation Portfolio
Technology Solutions
PATH Foundation, Atlanta

Padma Munjuluri
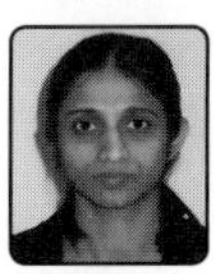
Consultant
Department of Obstetrics and Gynecology
Bradford Teaching Hospitals NHS Trust, United Kingdom
Deputy Training Programme Director (West Locality)
Health Education, Yorkshire and Humber, UK

PK Sekharan
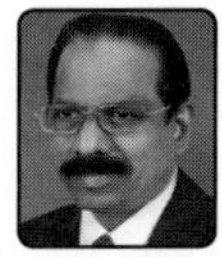
Senior Consultant
PVS Hospital
Calicut, Kerala, India
Past Vice President
FOGSI, 2010

Prakash Bhatt
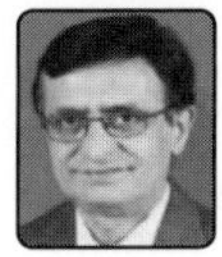
National Technical Consultant
EmOC-FOGSI Project
Vice President
FOGSI, 2005
Chairman FOGSI
Rural Obstetrics Committee (1999–2003)

Pratap Kumar
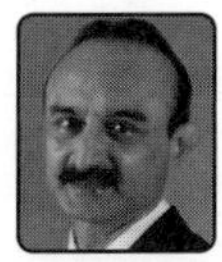
Professor
Department of Obstetrics and Gynecology
Kasturba Medical College
Manipal University
Manipal, Karnataka, India

Sabaratnam Arulkumaran
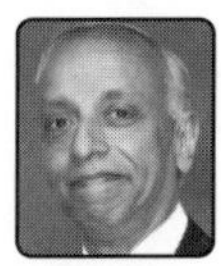
Professor Emeritus
Department of Obstetrics and Gynecology
St. George's Hospital and University of London, London, UK
President, FIGO (2012–2015)

Sadhana Desai
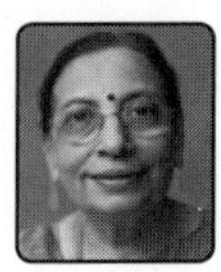
Director, Fertility Clinic, Mumbai
Chairman, FOGSI
Infertility Committee (1998–2002)
Emeritus Professor
Department of Obstetric and Gynecology
Hospital Institute of Medical Sciences
Mumbai, Maharashtra, India
Convener RCH—FOGSI
President—FOGSI, 2003

Sadhana Gupta
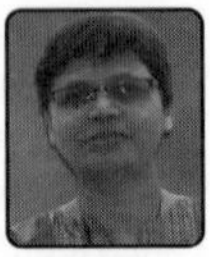
Chairman, Safe Motherhood Committee
FOGSI (2011-2013)
Past President, Gorakhpur Obstetric and Gynecological Society
Senior Consultant
Department of Obstetrics and Gynecology
Jeevan Jyoti Hospital and Medical Research Center
Gorakhpur, Uttar Pradesh, India

Sanjay Gupte
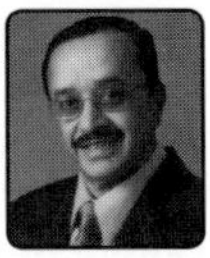
Director
Gupte Hospital
Postgraduate Institution and Center of Research in Reproduction
Pune, Maharashtra, India
President—FOGSI, 2010

Terek Meguid
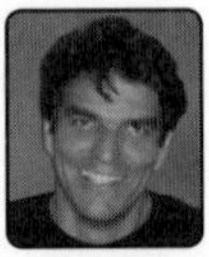
Department of Obstetrics and Gynecology
Mnazi M Hospital
Zanzibar, Tanzania

Vikram Sinai Talaulikar
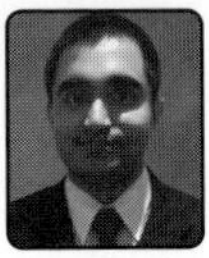
Clinical Fellow
Reproductive Medicine Unit
University College London Hospital, London, UK

W Sita Shankar
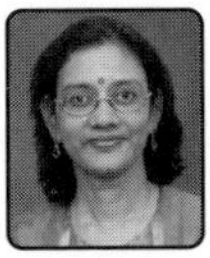
Director
Department of Maternal and Child Health/ Nutrition, India
PATH Foundation
Atlanta

Foreword

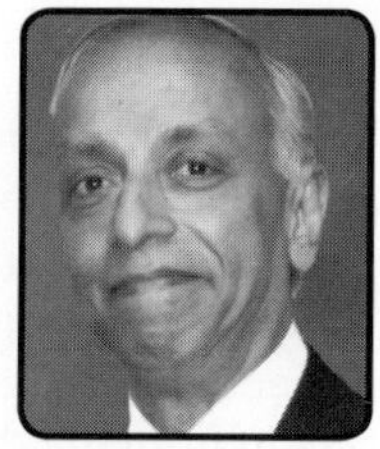

Twelve years ago, the world united around Millennium Development Goal 5 (MDG 5) and committed to improving maternal health and reducing maternal mortality by 2015 to a level just 25 percent of the 1990 level. The basis for this initiative, recognized by country leaders, is that the health of nations rests upon the health of mothers. Moreover, saving a mother's life is not only intrinsically valuable but also the impact extends to her family, her community and her country as a whole. Recognizing this important task, the Safe Motherhood Committee of the Federation of Obstetric and Gynaecological Societies of India (FOGSI) has been working very hard all over India to improve provision of emergency obstetric services, safe abortion care and contraception. In 2014, it is releasing the book *Safe Motherhood Initiative—A Silent Revolution* to encapsulate their experience and that of other countries.

Since the launch of MDG 5, dramatic progress has been made in saving women's lives. By 2010, maternal mortality had declined by 47 percent from the 1990 baseline. This success reflects the extraordinary dedication shown by numerous stakeholders within countries, from grassroots, non-governmental organizations (NGOs) to professional associations and from international donors to political leaders. However, even with this remarkable improvement, more than 780 women around the world still die every day from pregnancy or childbirth-related complications, even though more than 80 percent of these deaths are preventable. While admiring the great progress made so far, we have to recognize that the current pace of improvement is insufficient. If it continues unchanged, nearly 90 percent of countries will fail to meet.

Millennium Development Goal 5 on time and more than half will probably still fall short in 2040.

Maternal mortality remains one of the most unbalanced health indicators in the world, with 99 percent of deaths occurring in low- and middle-income countries. But the good news is that the handful of countries that have really transformed their record are drawn from every region of the world and every stage of economic development. In fact, almost half of the countries on track to meet MDG 5 have a per capita GDP below $1,000. Of course, their impressive improvement is often due in part to their starting point of very high maternal mortality, but their achievement still shows that a low level of economic development does not represent an insurmountable barrier to saving women's lives.

The success of individual countries gives us cause for hope and these are described as country experience in this book. By reading the book, one could argue that all countries have the ability—as well as the responsibility—to make real and lasting improvements to maternal health.

The information provided in the book will be applicable to countries at all stages of the journey to meet MDG 5—from countries that are just starting to gather momentum for change to countries that are in the "final mile" of optimizing maternal health. I congratulate the Editor, Dr Sadhana Gupta, contributors and FOGSI for undertaking this valuable task in bringing the information to all concerned to save mothers' lives and improve women's health

Sabaratnam Arulkumaran
President
Federation of Gynaecology and Obstetrics (FIGO)
Professor Emeritus
Department of Obstetrics and Gynecology
St George's Hospital and University of London
London, UK

Foreword

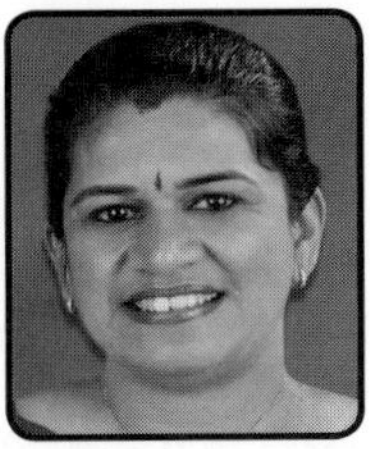

According to the United Nations, “Maternal mortality is not just a personal tragedy. It is not just a development, humanitarian and health issue. Maternal mortality is a human rights issue.” The most pressing need of the hour is to save the mothers. What has been achieved is indeed commendable, but considering the sheer size of our country, what still needs to be done presents a huge challenge. The time has now come for effective implementation of innovative methods suited for our country’s needs.

An emphasis on making emergency obstetric care available to all women who develop complications is central to reducing maternal mortality. Postpartum hemorrhage (PPH) and pre-eclampsia, eclampsia (PE/E) continue to remain the two major causes of maternal mortality. The fast track initiative program by FOGSI was aimed to broadly achieve our objectives "Helping Mothers Survive (HMS)”. The program witnessed leaders in FOGSI and Champions of FOGSI in the form of Dr Sadhana Gupta and team, working tirelessly and passionately—with great dedication and commitment, offering focused training and capacity building of frontline health care providers to handle PPH and PE/E. We have recognized the magnitude of the problem, formulated what should be done and now we need to act so as to impact the change.“Keep Educating Yourself (KEY)”: KEY initiative with the mantra of ‘Each one teach one’ included Pan India CME programs sensitizing the obs-gyne towards standard protocols and the need for adherence to uniform protocols. The fields of medicine and science never stop moving forward—and neither should physicians. “YUVA-Towards Tomorrow (YTT)” Medicine changes rapidly with new scientific information and technology. Albert Einstein said, ‘Learn from yesterday, live for today and hope for tomorrow.’ Programs for technical skill development and to prepare the young doctors for future challenges and create the youth leaders of tomorrow to relentlessly carry forward the mission of doing their best for women’s healthcare.

Congratulations to Dr Sadhana Gupta to put the chapters together to bring our focus to act on priority to ensure safe motherhood. The book is our strength and will be the catalyst for the change we want to see in women's health care in developing countries. I invite all of you to be a part of "Silent revolution"—time to stop talking and start acting !

Hema Divakar
President, FOGSI 2013
Senior Consultant
Divakar's Specialty Hospital
Bengaluru, Karnataka, India

Preface

It is a moment of great contentment and joy for me while I write this preface and address to reader at the occasion of release of the book entitled *Safe Motherhood Initiative—A Silent Revolution.*

Its name itself is complete saying. Revolution is not destruction; it is neither radical nor violent. Revolutions always start in silence of heart, warmth of home and life. They are not to be talked in loud voice; they are seen and felt in form of happiness, peace and growth.

How and when motherhood became gradually unsafe for human race, it is hard to perceive. However, people from a few groups like midwife or birth attendant, doctors and women itself always tried the methods to make it safe. The boom of scientific development and technology in medicine really made childbirth safe for women, society and nations who have ways and means to access good quality health care. Western world and developed countries reduced the risk of death and disease in mothers and newborn to marked extent. Unfortunately, the earth planet has been coldly and cruelly, acceptably divided in three world—developed, developing and poor countries. More unfortunately, the people of these worlds are held responsible for it, knowingly ignoring the political, economical, social exploitation and active as well passive extortion. Today, in each country or even state and town, we can see these three parts of world.

Mothers and children are nature's boon and gift to pursue the life, medical science is to protect and preserve life, how come the fruits of technology are not being shared by all uniformly. Did the poor and developing world not contribute most to development of research by providing those human, material and natural resources? Then, why good quality universal essential and emergency care is not available for a greater part of world?

The disparity in maternal mortality statistics in three worlds is widest among all health statistics.

It is a conscience pricking question for all who believe in equality and equanimity. Maternal death is preventable by simple priority interventions and does not require expansive, cumbersome hi-technology. India is the second most populous country of the world, mothers and children constitute the major portion of its population and we have maternal mortality rate ranging from 89 to 380/100,000 live birth. The neighboring countries, such as Pakistan, Bangladesh, Nepal and Bhutan, share not only boundaries but also the historical and cultural, and political environment. We also have our light post-Kerala and Sri Lanka, where despite many adversities the mothers and children were cared well with very good health statistics.

This book is a humble attempt to put together all the positive efforts done at global and national levels in the field of safe motherhood.

We are fortunate enough to have chapters from the learned and experienced galaxy of contributors.

In the book, there are four sections—First is international—In this section Professor Sir Sabaratnam Arulkumaran, a strong advocate and incessant worker for safe motherhood, has illustrated the global historical perspective of initiation of safe motherhood in political, economic and professional organization. It is interesting to note that cruciality and tragedy of maternal death drew attention only in recent past, but at the same time, grew very rapidly in the main stream and frame of millennium development goals.

Dr Lubna Hassan has in-depth analyzed the situation of maternal health and politico-economic constraints in Pakistan with will to go miles with determination. Dr Fatema Shabnam, Dr Abu Jamil Faisal and Dr Ferdousi Begum have given details of many safe motherhood initiatives in Bangladesh which are giving fruitful results in the form of rapidly improving maternal health indices. Dr Ashma Rana tells vividly about many innovative steps taken in breathtakingly beautiful yet geographically difficult country Nepal. Sri Lanka is truly shining pearl of Asia, where despite facing terrorism for a decade, health statistics is matching the developed world. Political will and determination of medical personnel is the key to change. Dr Hemantha Parera's chapter will be a learning lesson to many of us. Dr Harshalal R Seneviratne emphasizes the significance of task shifting and sharing in obstetric care in this region and initiative taken by various organizations and associations. Dr Terek Meguid shares his experience and painful observation on maternal health care in Africa and compels us to introspect ourselves as people responsible for maternal health. On the other hand, Dr Padma Munjuluri has elaborated the situation and concern of developed world from her experience in the UK.

The book is published under the aegis of Safe Motherhood Committee of Federation of Obstetric and Gynaecological Societies of India (FOGSI), and rightly India has been given total one section. India is a unique country for its diversity, its population density, vastness and rich democratic values. It poses many challenges in building as well delivering health programs all over country. Despite that India has given and materialized the universal health care to a marked extent, essential and emergency obstetric care to one and all. Chapters by Dr PK Sekharan and Dr Asmita Rathore gives statistics methodology, need and complexity of maternal death audit. While Dr Sanjay Gupte and Dr Girija Wagh share experience of FOGSI eclampsia registry and its outcome in the form of medical education program for adherence to evidence-based practice. Dr Sadhana Desai and Dr Prakash Bhatt have given review of FOGSI Emergency Obstetric Care Program for nonspecialist doctors.

Dr Arulmozhi Ramarajan has emphasized on data collection and lesson learning from cases of severe acute maternal morbidity or near-miss maternal mortality.

National Rural Health Mission and Janani Surakhsa Yojna (JSY) are pro-people innovative program of central Government of India and created real ripples and waves in Indian Rural Area by identifying a huge cadre of community link health worker, rightly named ASHA—(Hope literally, Accredited Social Health Activist) and cash payment for user and helper both. Dr KS Prashanth tells about hopes and impacts of the program in India.

Dr Milind R Shah elaborates role of safe abortion services for the cause of safe motherhood and national and international issues and projects to make abortion safe.

Dr Pratap Kumar shares experience and statistics of his teaching institute—Manipal University, who works beyond the boundaries and domain of hospital. His experience is learning points for all teaching institution. Dr Hema Divakar, a visionary leader of FOGSI, is a right contributor to look for very important yet a little underutilized potential of professional bodies in delivering safe obstetric services and ensures quality of care by their members.

Kerala is really God's own country where women are empowered, educated and healthy. Dr MK Valson gives interplay of all societal, political and medical factors which make Kerala a shining example of safe motherhood in this continent.

I myself along with co-author and dear friend Dr Hema J Shobhane have plunged into history of maternal health initiative and hopefully have come out with a few pearls.

The third section of book entails "Innovations for Safe Motherhood" in this, PATH foundation has been liberal enough to give details of all simple technological tools which either available can be used by middle and lower levels of health care providers and has potential to affect obstetric health delivery system in positive ways. Dr AK Debdas has been one of the innovative minds in FOGSI and we are proud to present details of his innovation like PPH bag, growth tape and descentometer. For women who become critically ill, critical care is required at nearby place; Role of High Dependency Obstetric Unit for saving maternal life is highlighted by Dr Alpesh Gandhi. Dr Hema Divakar shares innovative approach to teaching and learning by organizing series of Helping Mother Survive (HMS) Programs all over country. In the fourth section myself Dr Sadhana Gupta, conclude the book by sharing observation and thoughts of multidimensional change in order of world scenario and their direct and clandestine relationship with issue of Safe Motherhood for all.

Safe motherhood is basic right of every woman and family. The book is a humble and introspective observation of all the happenings for the cause of ensuring safe journey of women and newborn in the process of childbirth. It has to be under the backdrop of sociopolitical, economic, and cultural environment. World is not fragmented, nor the human soul. Happiness and sorrow is same for one and all.

Please go through the book, reciprocate back for sharing and suggestion.

Devote your time, treasure and talent for mothers and children.

Keep walking for happy and healthy world.

Sadhana Gupta

Acknowledgments

It is deep sense of gratitude and thanks to all persons, places; thoughts and events which incepted the seed of idea of this book entitled *Safe Motherhood Initiative—A Silent Revolution.*

First and foremost, I bow my head before God Almighty, who is source of all inspiration and action of Universe. I thank him for his blessing conferred on me to accomplish this work.

I owe my special thanks to Sir Dr Sabaratnam Arulkumaran who has kindly accepted to write foreword as well author one of the most difficult chapters of the book "Global and Historical Perspective of Safe Motherhood Initiative: A Small Beginning and a Long Journey". His prompt acceptance and thorough and throughout interest in all activities of Safe Motherhood Committee has been source of inspiration.

I acknowledge with deep respect and warm affection Dr Hema Divakar, President FOGSI 2013, whom I first shared the idea of the book. Her enthusiasm and encouragement for the book gave me the courage and confidence to go ahead. Her prompt responses and communication despite very busy schedule of her presidential post kept me going and working hard for the book.

My immense thanks to all learned and experienced authors and co-authors for their valuable contribution. The overwhelming response from all contributors at first communication gave moral boost when it was needed most. All authors contributed in time despite their holding important organizational and professional post. It only made possible the timely publication and aesthetic formating of the book. I thank all the authors and contributors for their dedicated effort and class chapters for the book from core of my heart. Their time and talent is invaluable and words fail to express my gratitude.

I thank FOGSI Managing Committee to permit me to release the book under the aegis of Safe Motherhood Committee. I also thank zonal coordinators, members of Safe Motherhood Committee, who throughout my tenure remained with me for various academic, social and organizational works for issue of Safe Motherhood. I also thank executives and all members of FOGSI, for their cooperation, love and appreciation for me and my work. Without which this mammoth task could not have been possible.

My special thanks to M/s Jaypee Brothers Medical Publishers (P) Ltd, Shri Jitendar P Vij (Group Chairman), Mr Ankit Vij (Managing Director), Mr Tarun Duneja (Director-Publishing), Mr KK Raman (Production Manager) and his team for gracious acceptance for publication of the book. I am thankful for the whole team of Jaypee Brothers Medical Publishers (P) Ltd., New Delhi, India, for their hard work and cooperation, so that the book could take this present shape.

I thank my family members, close friends, as they stood by me in good as well as difficult times and for being always understanding.

Lastly, I owe thanks to our patients—mother and women, who take the responsibility to bring forth the new life to the world by risking their own life. With this book, I pray in silence for their glooming health and happiness for them in every corner of the world.

Contents

Section I—International

Section II—India

Section III—Innovations for Safe Motherhood

Plate 1

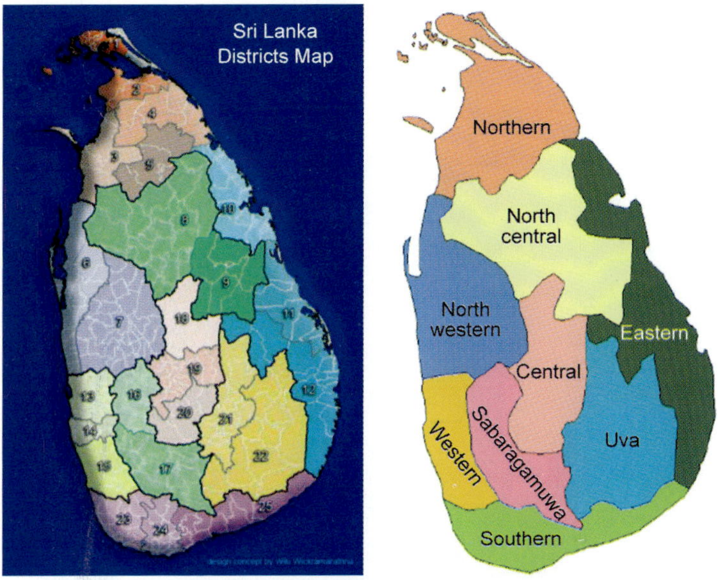

Fig 2 Political demography of Sri Lanka

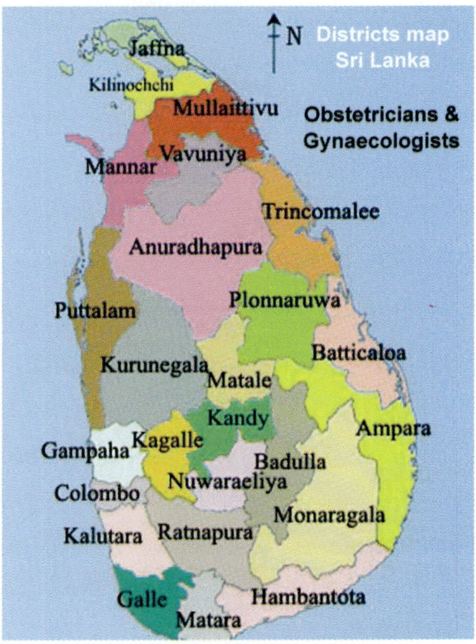

Fig 4 Specialist care centers in Sri Lanka

Plate 2

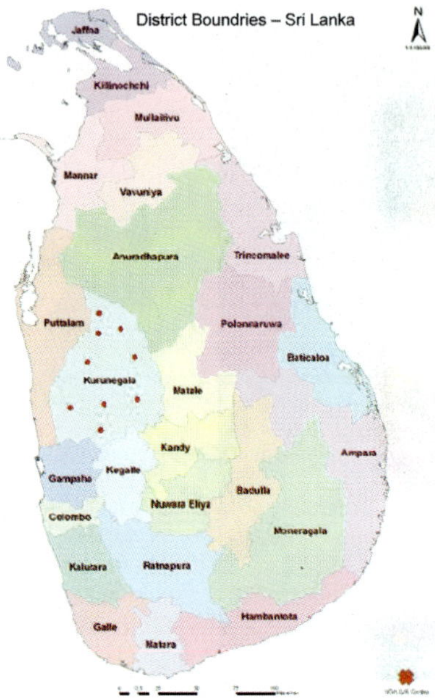

Fig 5 District-wise peripheral units in Sri Lanka

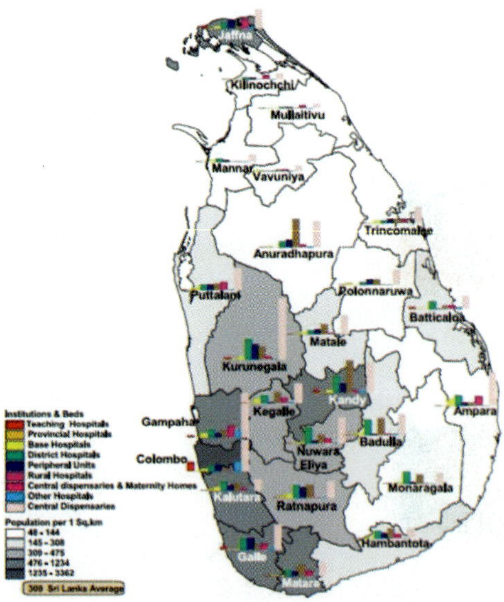

Fig 6 Health institutions in Sri Lanka

Plate 3

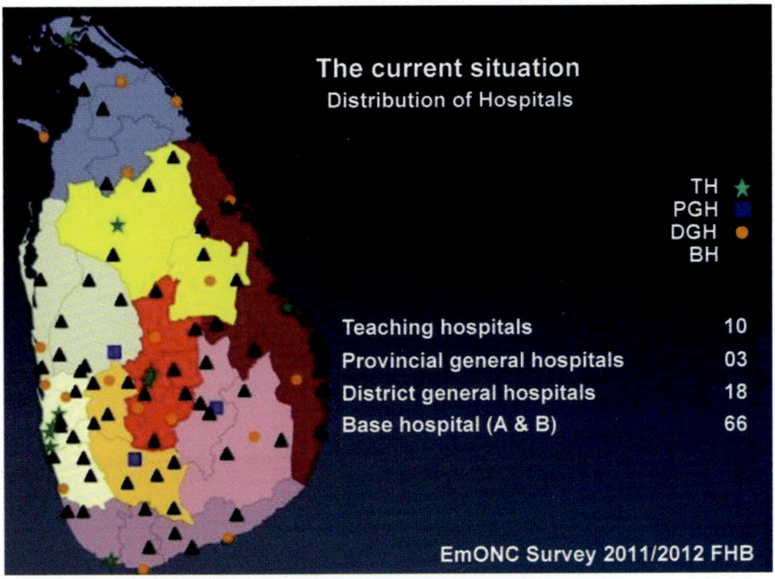

Fig 7 Current distribution of hospitals in Sri Lanka

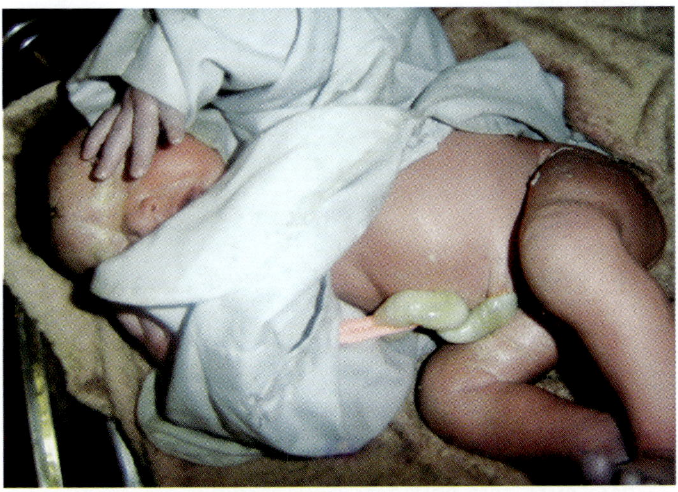

Fig. 1 The first institutional delivery done at Rural Health Center at Dobair during the flood of 2010

Plate 4

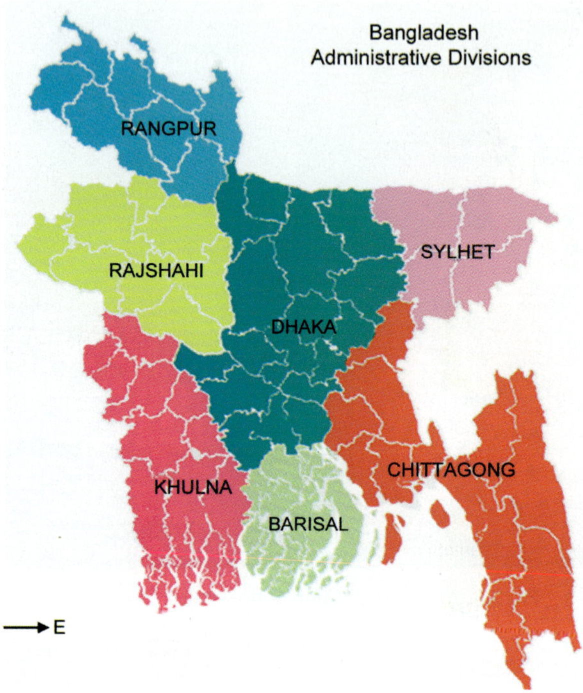

Demographics

- Area: 147,570 sq km
- Population: 150 million
- Population density: 1000/sq km
- Overall literacy rate: 50 percent
- Per capita income: US$ 600
- Life expectancy: 66.7 years
- Maternal morality ratio: 194/100000 LB
- Contraceptive prevalence rate: 62 percent
- Total fertility rate: 2.3
- Unmet need for family planning: 12 percent
- Antenatal care coverage (At least 1 visit): 67.7 percent
- Antenatal care coverage (At least 4 visit): 25.5 percent
- Delivery in health facility: 28.8 percent
- Delivery by medically trained person: 31.7 percent
- Postnatal care coverage (Within 2 days): 27 percent
- Met need (%) of Obst care in EmOC facilities: 70 percent
- Caesarean section (%) in the EmOC facilities: 12 percent
- Case fatality rate: 0.7 percent

Census 2011, BMMS 2010, BDHS 2011, DGHS 2012.

Fig. 1 Demographic characteristic of Bangladesh

Plate 5

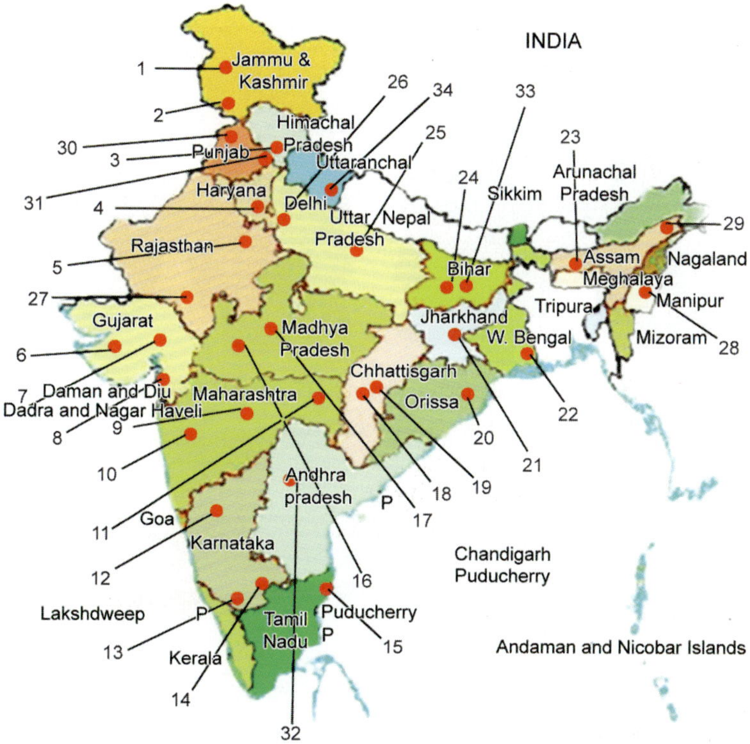

Fig 3 Marking of tertiary training centers by 2013 for EmOC program

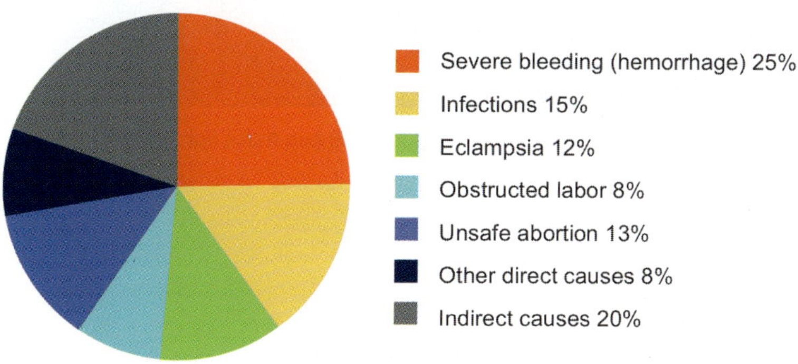

Fig. 1: Causes of meternal death in Kerala

Plate 6

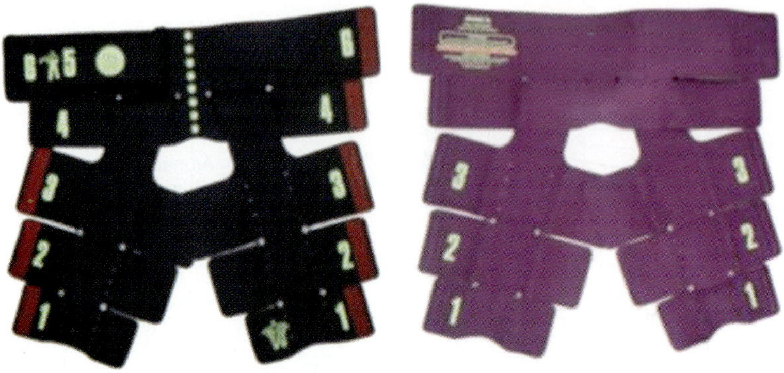

Fig. 6 NASG manufactured in India (*Source:* PATH/VISCO)

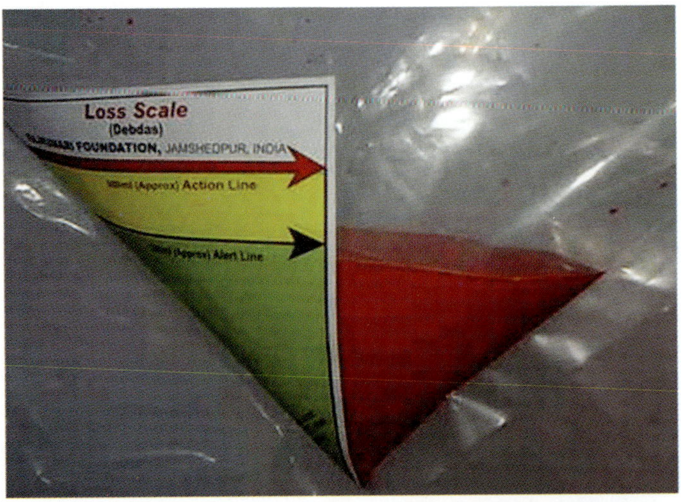

Fig. 8 Postpartum hemorrhage (PPH) bag traffic light model

Section I

International

*"When you change your mind about you,
everything and everyone changes with you"*

Chapters

1

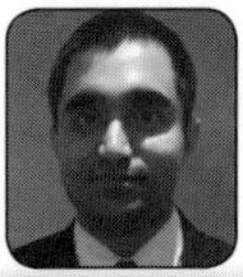

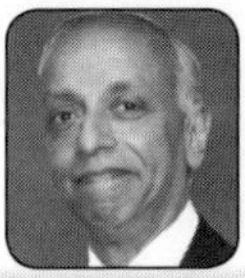

Global and Historical Perspective of Safe Motherhood Initiative: A Small Beginning and a Long Journey

Vikram Sinai Talaulikar, Sabaratnam Arulkumaran

INTRODUCTION

Traditionally, labor has been considered as one of the most hazardous journeys a fetus ever undertakes. However, this holds true not just for the fetus but also for the mother. The process of labor and delivery are fraught with a number of risks which can lead to maternal morbidity and mortality.

There were times in history when the ordeals of labor and delivery were considered a rebirth for the woman; because of the dangers of prolonged labor, obstructed labor, bleeding and infections invariably leading to maternal death. We have certainly moved on from those times—the progress in technology and advances in medical science have achieved spectacular results and ensured safe motherhood to majority of women all over the world.

However, there is still lot to be achieved. Every two minutes, somewhere in the world a woman dies from complications of pregnancy or childbirth, yet more than 80 percent of these deaths are preventable.[1] While the health care professionals, scientists, politicians from across the world have been putting in untiring efforts to make birthing safer, new challenges have emerged. This chapter looks at the history of safe motherhood movement and its progress over the years; and describes some of the challenges with their potential solutions that lie ahead.

HISTORY OF SAFE MOTHERHOOD INITIATIVE

In 1987, the World Bank, in collaboration with World Health Organization (WHO) and United Nations Population Fund (UNFPA), sponsored the Safe Motherhood Conference in Nairobi, Kenya. The launch of the safe motherhood initiative (SMI) was seen as a major milestone in the race to reduce the global burden of maternal mortality, particularly in the developing countries. It issued a call to action to reduce maternal mortality and morbidity by one half by the year 2000 and also gave birth to the Inter-Agency Group (IAG) for safe motherhood. The IAG included the three sponsors of the conference plus United Nations International Children's Emergency Fund (UNICEF), United Nations Development Programme (UNDP), and two international nongovernmental organizations, International Planned Parenthood Federation (IPPF) and the Population Council. This initiative led to a series of regional and national conferences that made safe motherhood an accepted and understood term in the public health world. All events that make pregnancy unsafe, irrespective of the gestation or outcome, are part and parcel of safe motherhood. Subsequent work on safe motherhood by the IAG and others outlined clear strategies and specified interventions for the reduction of maternal morbidity and mortality, often referred to as the 'Pillars of Safe Motherhood' (Fig. 1).

Since the launch of SMI, many countries have been able to improve the health and well-being of mothers and newborns over the last 2 decades.

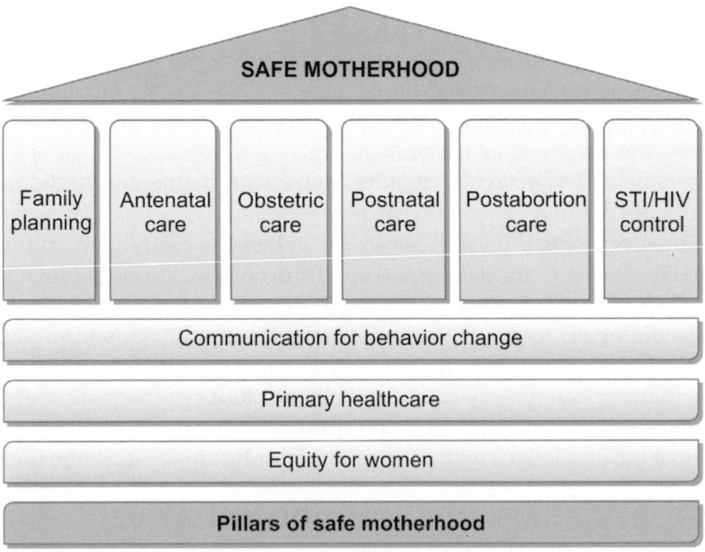

Fig. 1 Pillars of safe motherhood—adapted from world bank safe motherhood initiative (http://web.worldbank.org/WBSITE/EXTERNAL/TOPICS/EXT HEALTH NUTRITION AND POPULATION/EXTPRH/0,,contentMDK:20200213~menuPK:548457~pagePK:148956~piPK:216618~theSitePK:376855,00.html)

However, countries with the highest burdens of mortality and illness have made the least progress, and inequalities between countries are still a major challenge. At the Nairobi conference, Dr Fred Sai stressed on the need to improve women's status, educate communities, and strengthen and expand core elements of maternal health-antenatal care, delivery care, and postpartum care at the community and referral levels.[2] Although all goals set by the initiative were not achieved, important lessons were learnt which shaped the future of safe motherhood programs.

Challenges Facing the Safe Motherhood Services

Even today, the maternal mortality is unacceptably high. About 800 women die from pregnancy or childbirth related complications around the world every day.[3,4] In 2010, 287,000 women died during and following pregnancy and childbirth. Almost all of these deaths occurred in low-resource settings, and most could have been prevented. The major challenge today is the inequality of maternal care in highly developed verses resource limited countries. While maternal deaths have plunged to extremely low levels in the developed nations, the care still continues to be far below the desired standards in the poorest countries of the world. In many places, inequalities within countries are increasing between those who live in better conditions and have access to care, and those who for a variety of reasons are excluded (Fig. 2).

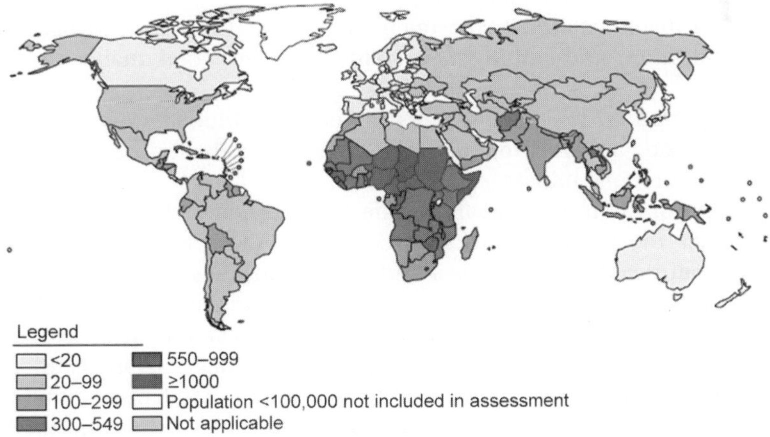

Fig. 2 Map with countries by category according to their maternal mortality ratio (MMR), death per 100,000 live births, 2010 adapted from WHO (World Health Organization)[6]

The second challenge has been the emergence of complex high-risk modern obstetric patients. Due to advances in healthcare and epidemics of chronic diseases such as diabetes and obesity—obstetricians all over the world have to care for women with complex health issues which place them at high-risk of complications.

While most pregnant women in developing countries visit antenatal care services at least once, what is lacking is the provision of professional childbirth care, either institutional or at home, and of emergency obstetric and newborn care services. Postpartum follow-up care is also very rarely available. Very few developing countries have accurate data on maternal and newborn deaths and morbidities, and less than one developing country in three reports national data on postpartum care. There is lack of evidence based information and quality monitoring data to inform policy decisions and program implementation.

Other challenges are deteriorating infrastructures, maintenance of stocks of drugs, supplies and equipment despite increasing demand, lack of transport, ineffective referral services and inadequate availability of emergency obstetric care services.

Safe Motherhood at Ten and Further Progress

It has been realized that maternal deaths are not just the result of substandard or inaccessible medical care, but a result of a long chain of problems—lack of education for girls, early marriage, lack of access to contraception, poor nutrition and women's low social, economic, and legal status.[3] These factors contribute to women's poor health before and during pregnancy, increasing their vulnerability to life-threatening complications and limiting their ability to receive good quality health care.

During 1997 to 98, the IAG developed an ambitious two-year "Safe Motherhood at Ten" programme to mark the tenth anniversary of the safe motherhood initiative.

One of the primary goals of Safe Motherhood at Ten was to pull together the growing body of research on the impact of different maternal health interventions, and identify the "lessons learned" for program planners working in a wide range of circumstances. The Safe Motherhood at Ten programme focused on articulating these lessons and sharing them with country-level partners, so that program planners could draw on them to design effective safe motherhood interventions.

The Safe Motherhood at Ten programme included two key events:

1. Safe Motherhood Technical Consultation in Colombo, Sri Lanka in October 1997. A meeting of national and international programmers,

policy-makers and technical experts identified the most effective strategies for making motherhood safer.

2. World Health Day, April 7, 1998. An international Call to Action was put out for key decision-makers (governments, donors, technical assistance agencies) at World Bank Headquarters in Washington DC; and a campaign to encourage national and local efforts to raise awareness about safe motherhood and launch new programs.

The key messages on reducing maternal mortality from the Safe Motherhood technical consultation in Colombo included:

- Recognizing that every pregnancy faces risks.
- Increasing access to family planning services.
- Improving the quality of antenatal and postpartum care.
- Ensuring access to essential obstetric care (including postabortion care)
- Expanding access to midwifery care in the community.
- Training and deploying appropriate skilled health personnel (such as midwives).
- Ensuring a continuum of care connected by effective referral links and supported by adequate supplies, equipment, drugs and transportation.
- Reforming laws to expand women's access to health services and to promote women's health interests.

In 1999, using the lessons learned since 1987, WHO, UNFPA, UNICEF and the World Bank issued a 'joint statement' that is now the basis of the consensus on:

- Prevention and management of unwanted pregnancy and unsafe abortions
- The need for every woman to have skilled care in pregnancy and childbirth, and
- The importance of access to referral care when complications arise.

The safe motherhood initiative is in its third decade. By now, we mostly know what needs to be done to save the lives of mothers and newborns. The real challenge is how to deliver services and scale up interventions, particularly to those who are vulnerable, hard to reach, marginalized and excluded. Political will at national and district level is the key to achieving the desired targets.

MDG 5: The World Recognizes the Need for Action

At the turn of the millennium, world leaders met to discuss priorities for making the world a better place to live in. Eight millennium development goals (MDGs) were proposed. MDG 5 deals with maternal mortality—

deaths of women during pregnancy or within 42 days of the end of that pregnancy.[5] It specifies that by 2015, the level of maternal mortality should fall to just 25 percent of the 1990 level. In sub-Saharan Africa, a number of countries have halved their levels of maternal mortality since 1990. In other regions, including Asia and North Africa, even greater headway has been made. However, between 1990 and 2010, the global maternal mortality ratio (i.e. the number of maternal deaths per 100,000 live births) declined by only 3.1 percent per year. This is far from the annual decline of 5.5 percent required to achieve MDG 5.[3] Though it is doubtful that the MDG 5 goal will now be reached, the overall progress towards it has been substantial and very encouraging; in 1990, the global figure for maternal mortality was 543,000; by 2010, the figure had fallen to 287,000 (see Fig. 2).[6] This is a really remarkable achievement, particularly in low and middle-income countries, where more than 90 percent of maternal mortality occurs. India has made significant progress in reducing its maternal mortality rate (MMR) from 254 (SRS 2004–06) to 212 (SRS 2007–09) per hundred thousand live births (LB); however, there is a long way to go on this journey to meet the millennium development goal.[7] The success in reducing maternal mortality has been achieved through tireless efforts by clinicians, policy-makers, donors, academics and private and nongovernmental organizations.

Strategies Towards Safer Motherhood: Maternal Health Ecosystem

A clear set of priority health interventions which are key to achieving the desired targets has emerged across three areas: family planning, safe abortion and appropriate maternity care.[1] They are low cost interventions and if properly implemented, they save a great many lives every year. It is also important to realize that the solution is not purely medical; the key is to create a 'maternal health ecosystem', where such interventions are not just available, but also high-quality, desirable, affordable and accessible to those in need.[1] Creating such an ecosystem needs political will and a committed government. It also depends on close collaboration between government, professionals, donors, voluntary organizations and the private sector.

There are four aspects to this ecosystem[1]:

1. *Providing quality healthcare:* Including delivery of essential interventions, task-shifting to create a sufficient workforce and investigations into each maternal death.
2. *Creating a desire for care:* By conducting campaigns on family spacing and institutional delivery, as well as by making clinical care culturally appropriate.

3. *Ensuring that care is financially affordable for all:* Free if possible for those most in need, but also drawing on microinsurance and community contributions where appropriate.
4. *Making care physically accessible:* Such as by the use of temporary accommodation near medical facilities and emergency transportation.

Interventions to Reduce Maternal Mortality

The most common causes of maternal deaths globally are hemorrhage, sepsis, obstructed labor, unsafe abortions, malaria, HIV and hypertensive disorders. There are seven specific interventions that address these causes directly. If countries make these interventions widely accessible, they can significantly reduce maternal mortality.[1]

The interventions are: Prevention of hemorrhage, treatment of hemorrhage, prevention/treatment of pre-eclampsia, prevention/treatment of infection, cesarean sections, contraception and vacuum aspiration/medical abortion.

Each of these seven health interventions can be broken down into a set of specific tools and actions and can be mapped to sites of care in the community, at primary-care level and in hospitals.

The seven interventions can also be grouped into three core areas highlighted above—family planning, safe abortion and maternal care. Of the three, family planning is probably the most effective at improving women's health, in terms of both costs and maternal outcomes. It also drastically reduces the need for abortion services. Currently, an estimated 220 million women around the world are unable to time and space their families, because of a combination of a lack of the necessary information on contraception and the inability to regularly access contraceptives.[8] However, since many users of family planning will experience accidental pregnancies, owing to method or user failure; family planning on its own will not fully prevent all unintended pregnancies. Rwanda is an example of a country which managed to reduce maternal mortality by 50 percent within three years, and one major factor in that achievement was that the country implemented an integrated family planning and maternal health programme.[1]

The second core area, safe abortion, can also play a crucial role in reducing maternal mortality, given that 14 percent of maternal deaths globally result from unsafe abortions. In Romania, the legalization of abortion caused maternal mortality rates to plummet. Thanks to the combination of safe abortions, family planning and teenage sexual education, the country's maternal mortality declined by 85 percent in the 20 years from 1990 to 2010.[1]

Tamil Nadu state in India is an example of how enhancement of maternal healthcare services leads to remarkable reduction of maternal mortality. 24/7 availability, transportation, infrastructure upgrade, training in cultural appropriateness and involvement of private services has seen the maternal mortality in the region fall by 75 percent during the 1990 to 2010 period.[1]

During the United Nations MDG summit in September 2010, UN Secretary General Ban Ki-moon launched a 'Global strategy for women's and children's health', aimed at saving the lives of more than 16 million women and children over the next four years. WHO is working with partners towards this goal.

World Health Organization Recommended Interventions for Improving Maternal and Newborn Health

The world health organization (WHO) has enlisted the key interventions to improve maternal and newborn health and survival in the form of five tables.[9] These key interventions can be delivered through health services, family and the community.

Table 1 lists interventions delivered to the mother during pregnancy, childbirth and in the postpartum period, and to the newborn soon after birth. These include important preventive, curative and health promotional activities for the present as well as the future. Routine essential care refers to the care that should be offered to all women and babies, while situational care is dependent on disease patterns in the community. Some women and babies with moderately severe diseases or complications require additional care while those with severe diseases or complications require specialized care.

Table 2 lists the places where care should be provided through health services, the type of providers required and the recommended interventions and commodities at each level.

Table 3 lists practices, activities and support needed during pregnancy and childbirth by the family, community and workplace.

Table 4 lists key interventions provided to women before conception and between pregnancies.

Table 5 addresses unwanted pregnancies.

Further information on these interventions is available in WHO's Integrated Management of Pregnancy and Childbirth (IMPAC) clinical guidelines: pregnancy, childbirth, postpartum and newborn care—a guide for essential practice (http://www.who.int/maternal_child_adolescent/documents/who_mps_0705/en/index.html).

Table 1 Care in pregnancy, childbirth and postpartum period for mother and newborn infant

	Routine care (offered to all women and babies)	*Additional care (for women and babies with moderately severe diseases and complications)*	*Specialized—obstetrical and neonatal care (for women and babies with severe diseases and complications)*
Pregnancy care—4 visits *Essential*	• Confirmation of pregnancy • Monitoring of progress of pregnancy and assessment of maternal and fetal well-being • Detection of problems complicating pregnancy (e.g. anemia, hypertensive disorders, bleeding, malpresentations, multiple pregnancy) • Respond to other reported complaints. • Tetanus immunization, anemia prevention and control (iron and folic acid supplementation) • Information and counseling on self care at home, nutrition, safer sex, breastfeeding, family planning, healthy lifestyle • Birth planning, advice on danger signs and emergency preparedness • Recording and reporting • Syphilis testing	• Treatment of mild to moderate pregnancy complications: - Mild to moderate anemia - Urinary tract infection - Vaginal infection • Post abortion care and family planning • Prereferral treatment of severe complications - Pre-eclampsia - Eclampsia - Bleeding - Infection - Complicated abortion • Support for women with special needs e.g. adolescents, women living with violence • Treatment of syphilis (woman and her partner)	• Treatment of severe pregnancy complications: - Anemia - Severe pre-eclampsia - Eclampsia - Bleeding - Infection - Other medical complications • Treatment of abortion complications

Contd...

Contd...

	Routine care (offered to all women and babies)	*Additional care (for women and babies with moderately severe diseases and complications)*	*Specialized—obstetrical and neonatal care (for women and babies with severe diseases and complications)*
Situational	• HIV testing and counseling • Antimalarial intermittent preventive treatment (IPT) and promotion of insecticide treated nets (ITN) • Deworming • Assessment of female genital mutilation (FGM)	• Prevention of mother to child transmission of HIV (PMTCT) by antiretroviral treatment (ART), infant feeding counseling, mode of delivery advice • Treatment of mild to moderate opportunistic infections • Treatment of uncomplicated malaria	• Treatment of severe HIV infection • Treatment of complicated malaria
Childbirth Care (labor, delivery, and immediate postpartum) *Essential*	• Care during labor and delivery - Diagnosis of labor - Monitoring progress of labor, maternal and fetal well-being with partograph - Providing supportive care and pain relief - Detection of problems and complications (e.g. malpresentations, prolonged and/or obstructed labor, hypertension, bleeding, and infection)	• Treatment of abnormalities and complications (e.g. prolonged labor, vacuum extraction; breech presentation, episiotomy, repair of genital tears, manual removal of placenta) • Prereferral management of serious complications (e.g. obstructed labor, fetal distress, preterm labor, severe peri- and postpartum hemorrhage) • Emergency management of complications if birth imminent	• Treatment of severe complications in childbirth and in the immediate postpartum period, including cesarean section, blood transfusion and hysterectomy): - Obstructed labor - Malpresentations - Eclampsia - Severe infection - Bleeding • Induction and augmentation of labor

Contd...

Contd...

	Routine care (offered to all women and babies)	*Additional care (for women and babies with moderately severe diseases and complications)*	*Specialized—obstetrical and neonatal care (for women and babies with severe diseases and complications)*
	- Delivery and immediate care of the newborn baby, initiation of breastfeeding - Newborn resuscitation - Active management of third stage of labor • Immediate postnatal care of mother - Monitoring and assessment of maternal well-being, prevention and detection of complications (e.g. hypertension, infections, bleeding, anemia) - Treatment of moderate post-hemorrhagic anemia - Information and counseling on home self-care, nutrition, safe sex, breast care and family planning - Postnatal care planning, advice on danger signs and emergency preparedness • Recording and reporting	• Support for the family if maternal death	

Contd...

Contd...

	Routine care (offered to all women and babies)	*Additional care (for women and babies with moderately severe diseases and complications)*	*Specialized—obstetrical and neonatal care (for women and babies with severe diseases and complications)*
Situational	• Vitamin A administration	• Prevention of mother-to-child transmission of HIV by mode of delivery, guidance and support for chosen infant feeding option	• Management of complications related to FGM
Postnatal maternal care (up to 6 weeks) *Essential*	• Assessment of maternal well-being • Prevention and detection of complications (e.g. infections, bleeding, anemia) • Anemia prevention and control (iron and folic acid supplementation) • Information and counseling on nutrition, safe sex, family planning and provision of some contraceptive methods • Postnatal care planning, advice on danger signs and emergency preparedness • Provision of contraceptive methods	• Treatment of some problems (e.g. mild to moderate anemia, mild puerperal depression) • Prereferral treatment of some problems (e.g. severe postpartum bleeding, puerperal sepsis)	• Treatment of all complications - Evere anemia - Severe postpartum bleeding - Severe postpartum infections - Severe postpartum depression • Female sterilization
Situational	• Promotion of ITN use	• Treatment of uncomplicated malaria	• Treatment of complicated malaria

Contd...

Contd...

	Routine care (offered to all women and babies)	*Additional care (for women and babies with moderately severe diseases and complications)*	*Specialized—obstetrical and neonatal care (for women and babies with severe diseases and complications)*
Newborn care (birth and immediate postnatal) *Essential*	• Promotion, protection and support for breastfeeding • Monitoring and assessment of well-being, detection of complications (breathing, infections, prematurity, low birth weight, injury, malformation) • Infection prevention and control, rooming-in • Eye care • Information and counseling on home care, breastfeeding, hygiene • Postnatal care planning, advice on danger sign and emergency preparedness • Immunization according to the national guidelines (BCG, HepB, OPV-0)	• Care if moderately preterm, low birth weight or twin: support for breastfeeding, warmth, frequent assessment of well-being and detection of complications e.g. feeding difficulty, jaundice, other perinatal problems • Kangaroo Mother Care follow-up • Treatment of mild to moderate - Local infections (cord, skin, eye, thrush) - Birth injuries • Prereferral management of infants with severe problems: - Very preterm babies and/or birth weight very low - Severe complications - Malformations • Supporting mother if perinatal death	• Management of severe newborn problems—general care for the sick newborn and management of specific problems: - Preterm birth - Breathing difficulty - Sepsis - Severe birth trauma and asphyxia - Severe jaundice - Kangaroo Mother Care (KMC) • Management of correctable malformations

Contd...

Contd...

	Routine care (offered to all women and babies)	*Additional care (for women and babies with moderately severe diseases and complications*	*Specialized—obstetrical and neonatal care (for women and babies with severe diseases and complications)*
Situational	• Promotion of sleeping under ITN	• Presumptive treatment of congenital syphilis • Prevention of mother-to-child transmission of HIV by ART • Support for infant feeding of maternal choice	• Treatment of: - Congenital syphilis - Neonatal tetanus
Postnatal newborn care (visit from/at home) *Essential*	• Assessment of infant's well-being and breastfeeding • Detection of complications and responding to maternal concerns • Information and counseling on home care • Additional follow-up visits for high risk babies (e.g. preterm, after severe problems, on replacement feeding)	• Management of: - Minor to moderate problems and - Feeding difficulties • Prereferral management of severe problems: - Convulsions - Inability to feed • Supporting the family if perinatal death	• Management of severe newborn problems: - Sepsis - Other infections - Jaundice - Failure to thrive

Table 2 Place of care, providers, interventions and commodities

Health care	*Level of health care*	*Venue/place*	*Provider*	*Interventions and commodities*
Pregnancy (antenatal) care				
Routine	Primary	• Health center in the community • Outpatient clinic of a hospital • Outreach home visit	• Health worker with midwifery skills*	• On site tests (Hb, syphilis) • Maternal health record • Vaccine • Basic oral medicines
Situational	Primary	• Health center in the community • Outpatient clinic of a hospital • Outreach home visits	• Health worker with midwifery skills*	• On site tests (HIV) • Insecticide treated nets (ITN)
Additional	Primary	• Health center in the community • Outpatient clinic of a hospital	• Health worker with midwifery and selected obstetric and neonatal skills*	• IV fluids • Parenteral drugs (antibiotics, $MgSO_4$, antimalarial) • Manual Vacuum Aspiration (MVA) • Antiretroviral therapy (ART)
Specialized	Secondary	• Hospital	• Team of doctors, midwives and nurses	All of the above plus: • Blood transfusion • Surgery • Laboratory tests • Obstetric care

Contd...

Contd...

Health care	*Level of health care*	*Venue/place*	*Provider*	*Interventions and commodities*
Childbirth (mother and baby)				
Routine	Primary	• Health center in the community • Maternity ward of a hospital • Outreach home care	• Health worker with midwifery skills*	• Delivery set • Oxytocin • Partograph
Situational	Primary	• Health center in the community • Maternity ward of a hospital • Outreach home care	• Health worker with midwifery skills*	• ART
Additional	Primary	• Health center in the community • Maternity ward of a hospital	• Health worker with midwifery and selected obstetric and neonatal skills*	• Vacuum extraction • Manual removal of placenta • Repair of genital tears • IV fluids • $MgSO_4$, parenteral uterotonics, and antibiotics • Newborn resuscitation
Specialized mother	Secondary	• Hospital	• Team of doctors, midwives and nurses with neonatal care skills	All of the above plus: • Surgery • Blood transfusion

Contd...

Contd...

Health care	*Level of health care*	*Venue/place*	*Provider*	*Interventions and commodities*
Specialized newborn	Secondary	• Hospital	• Team of doctors and nurses with obstetric and nursing skills	• Oxygen • IV fluids • Parenteral antibiotics • Blood transfusion • Laboratory—biochemical and microbiology (small blood samples)
Postpartum (mother), postnatal (newborn infant)				
Routine	Primary	• Health center in the community • Outpatient clinic of a hospital • Outreach home visit	• Health worker with midwifery skills*	• On site tests (Hb, syphilis) • Vaccines • Basic oral medicines
Situational	Primary	• Health center in the community • Outpatient clinic of a hospital	• Health worker with midwifery skills*	• On site tests (HIV) • ART
Additional	Primary	• Health center in the community • Outpatient clinic of a hospital	• Health worker with midwifery and selected obstetric and neonatal skills*	• IV fluids • Parenteral drugs (antibiotics, $MgSO_4$, antimalarial) • Manual removal of placenta

Contd...

Contd...

Health care	*Level of health care*	*Venue/place*	*Provider*	*Interventions and commodities*
Specialized mother	Secondary	• Hospital	• Team of doctors, midwives and nurses	All of the above plus: • Blood transfusion • Surgery • Laboratory tests • Obstetric care
Specialized newborn	Secondary	• Hospital	• Team of doctors, midwives and nurses with neonatal skills	• Oxygen • IV fluids • Parenteral antibiotics • Blood transfusion • Laboratory—biochemical and microbiology (small samples)

* Health worker providing maternity care only or a health worker providing other services in addition to maternity care

Table 3 Home care, family, community and workplace support for the woman during pregnancy and childbirth and for the newborn infant

	Home/family	*Community and workplace*
Pregnancy	• Safe and nutritive diet • Safe sexual practices • Support for quitting smoking • Protection from passive tobacco smoking • Support for avoiding hard work • Planning for birth, and emergencie—mother and baby • Knowledge and support for the birth and emergency plan • Recognition of labor and danger signs • Support for compliance with preventive treatments • Support/accompaniment for pregnancy care visits • Adolescent girls encouraged to continue going to school • Participation in improving quality of services • Participation in transport and financing scheme	• Maternity protection • Time off for antenatal care visits • Safe and clean workplace • Tobacco free working environment • Pregnant adolescents kept at school
Situational	• Support for taking ART and for coping with its side effects	• Support for HIV positive women
Childbirth	• Accompanying and supporting the woman in childbirth • Support and care for the rest of the family • Organize transport and financial support	• Support for the family during childbirth and immediate postpartum

Contd...

Contd...

	Home/family	*Community and workplace*
Postpartum and beyond	• Support for exclusive breastfeeding/replacement feeding • Personal hygiene • Safe disposal/washing of pads • Support for rest and less work load • Safe and nutritive diet • Safe sexual practices • Motivation for prescribed treatments • Recognition of dangers signs, including blues/ depression • Optimal pregnancy spacing • Reporting birth and death (vital registration) • Participation in improving quality of services • Participation in transport and financing scheme	• Maternity leave • Breastfeeding breaks • Time off for postpartum and baby care visits • If mother referred to hospital, support that she is accompanied with the baby
Newborn and young infant	• Exclusive breastfeeding • Hygiene (cord care, washing, clothes) • Avoiding contacts with sick family members • Clean, warm and quiet place, tobacco and fire smoke free • Extra care for small babies (preterm, low birth weight) including KMC • Support for routine and follow-up visits • Motivation for home treatment of minor problems • Recognition of danger signs • Safe disposal of baby stool • Care seeking at health facility or hospital	• Promotion, protection and support for breast feeding • Keeping mother with the baby in hospital for breastfeeding • Supporting the family during maternal absence • Support for referral care for sick newborn.
Situational	• Sleeping under ITN	

Table 4 Care for the woman before and between pregnancies

	Care by health services	*Home/family*	*Community and workplace*
Adolescence	• Immunization according to national policy (tetanus and rubella) • Family planning • HIV prevention including VCT	• Delayed childbearing • Healthy lifestyle • Balanced diet, including iodized salt	• Education • Information on prevention of HIV and STI infections
All women of reproductive age	• Family planning • Assessment and management of STIs • HIV prevention including testing and counseling	• Optimal pregnancy timing	

Table 5 Pregnant women not wanting child

	Care by health services	*Home/family*	*Community and workplace*
Pregnant woman not wanting child	• Safe abortion (where legal) • Postabortion care and family planning	• Care for unwanted pregnancy	

FIGO LOGIC Initiative in Maternal and Newborn Health: A Key Role for Professional Organizations

The International Federation of Gynecology and Obstetrics (FIGO) was founded in 1954 and is the umbrella organization for 124 national professional associations of obstetrics and gynecology around the world. One of FIGO's seven commitments is "to strengthen the capacity of its associations to enable them to play a pivotal role in the development and implementation of sustainable programs aimed at the improvement of care available to women and newborns, especially for poor and underserved populations". The FIGO LOGIC (Leadership in Obstetrics and Gynecology for Impact and Change) initiative[10] in maternal and newborn health has been working to strengthen the organizational capacity of eight national professional associations in African and Asian countries, where maternal and neonatal mortality rates are high. LOGIC's main partner in organizational capacity improvement has been the Society of Obstetricians and Gynecologists of Canada (SOGC).

The project objectives are as follows:

- Evidence informed policy strategy and action plans on maternal and newborn health influenced and supported through member associations advocating to raise and maintain awareness of, and investment in, maternal and newborn health, and engaging in dialogue with health sector stakeholders.
- Progress in delivering evidence informed policy, strategic objectives and operational/annual plans with the member associations' active role in implementation, monitoring and evaluation.
- National and subnational member association organizations strengthened to enable effective participation in national and sub-national strategic and operational fora related to maternal and newborn health.
- FIGO's facilitative role with member associations strengthened.
- Dissemination phase.

Participating Member Associations (MAs) include-Burkina Faso (SOGOB); Cameroon (SOGOC); Ethiopia (ESOG); India (FOGSI); Mozambique (AMOG); Nepal (NESOG); Nigeria (SOGON) and Uganda (AOGU).

Leadership in obstetric and gynecology for impact and change (LOGIC) has decided to organize the different tools and approaches used into an easily accessible web based toolkit.[10] Reflecting on LOGIC's and other earlier experiences and lessons learnt from organizational capacity building in health professional associations, this toolkit is intended to be a starting point and reference for other health professional associations that want to enhance their capacity. Using the toolkit will lead to better understanding of what makes an organization strong; what are the different elements of organizational capacity building?; how a change process can be initiated; and how practical activities can be conducted to support such change process?

The toolkit consists of seven chapters, which, taken as a whole, provides a comprehensive approach to enhance the impact and performance of health professional associations.

The following provides a summary of each chapter of the toolkit:

- *Capacity of building health professional associations:* This section describes what is meant by 'capacity building' and explains its importance for health professional associations who are seeking to improve their impact and performance. It presents the SOGC's organizational capacity improvement framework (OCIF), the tool used throughout this document to guide professional associations in their capacity building efforts.
- *Enriching culture:* This section focuses on culture, and more specifically, on what motivates an association to succeed, function and survive. It explores how an organization's mission, vision, values and rewards and incentives used to recruit and maintain members can contribute to enhancing an association's culture.
- *Strengthening operations:* This section addresses the complex relationship of eight capacity areas that support the ability of an association to perform, to remain relevant, to grow and to survive. It addresses issues related to governance, leadership, strategic planning, human and financial resource management, program/project management, communication and infrastructure.
- *Enhancing performance:* This section looks at the four capacity areas that enable an association to meet its goals and objectives and to move toward long term sustainability. Issues related to the association's effectiveness, efficiency, relevance and financial position are considered within this section.
- *Building external relations:* The focus of this section will be placed on addressing issues related to the environment within which the association functions and its potential impact on the association's performance and how it is perceived externally.
- *Improving functions:* This section addresses the essential functions of a health professional association as described by its goals and objectives. Capacity areas addressed include membership services; promotion of quality and standards of care; advancing the professional practice; and influencing medical practice and health policy.
- *Managing crises:* This last section, although not part of the OCIF, will focus on risk management and on how an association can be better prepared to respond if a crisis was to occur.

Guiding Principles for Improving Maternal Health (Saving Mothers' Lives: Transforming Strategy into Action—Report of the Maternal Health Working Group, 2012)

Five guiding principles that every country leader can follow to bring about change and improve healthcare for women and children were identified by the group (Table 6).[1] These are:

1. Entrench maternal health as a national priority by strengthening existing coalitions.
2. Focus on selecting and implementing a few, targeted initiatives.
3. Strengthen ownership at the grass-roots level.
4. Continually innovate to maximize available resources.
5. Reinforce accountability by consistently measuring what matters.

Of the five principles, the group suggested that two should be

Table 6 Five principles that can further improve maternal health (Saving Mothers' Lives: Transforming strategy into action—Report of the Maternal Health Working Group 2012)[1]

1. Entrench maternal health as a national priority by strengthening existing coalitions	Leverage groups of individuals who are passionate about maternal health and unite them around a shared vision of success
2. Focus on selecting and implementing a few, targeted initiatives	Several innovative solutions to reduce maternal mortality have been successfully implemented around the world. Select and focus on the ones that will work for your local context
3. Strengthen ownership at the grass-roots level	Inspire your people to continue to make a difference in maternal health and ensure they have the skills and power to drive the solution locally
4. Continually innovate to maximize available resources	Focus on using current assets creatively and efficiently, while also leveraging the power of the private sector and other contributors
5. Reinforce accountability by consistently measuring what matters	Regularly track leading indicators for maternal health and establish seamless and sustainable monitoring to ensure accountability throughout the system

the responsibility of national government—the first and last. In addition, given that MDG 5 is measured on a country level, it is national government that must take primary responsibility for the fifth guiding principle. Many donors and technical groups are well-suited to help achieve the second principle. Similarly, professional organizations, NGOs and local advocacy groups are often well-positioned to help achieve the third principle. And the private sector and other organizations can contribute to implementing the fourth principle.[1]

WHO—Global Strategy for Women's and Children's Health

World health organization (WHO) has issued a call to action emphasizing that we all have a role to play in improving the health of the world's women and children.[11]

Governments and policymakers at local, national, regional and global levels must:

- Develop prioritized national health plans, and approve and allocate more funds.
- Ensure resources are used effectively.
- Strengthen health systems, including the health workforce, monitoring and evaluation systems and local community care.
- Introduce or amend legislation and policies in line with the principles of human rights, linking women's and children's health to other areas (diseases, education, water and sanitation, poverty, nutrition, gender equity and empowerment).
- Encourage all stakeholders (including academics, healthcare organizations, the private sector, civil society, healthcare workers and donors) to participate and to harmonize their efforts.
- Work with the private sector to ensure the development and delivery of affordable, essential medicines and new technologies for health.

Donor countries and global philanthropic institutions must:

- Provide predictable long-term support (financial and programmatic) in line with national plans and harmonized with other partners.
- Advocate for focusing global health priorities on women and children.
- Support research efforts.

The United Nations and other multilateral organizations must:

- Define norms, regulations and guidelines to underpin efforts to improve women's and children's health, and encourage their adoption.

- Help countries develop and align their national health plans.
- Work together and with others to strengthen technical assistance and programmatic support, helping countries scale up their interventions and strengthen their health systems, including health-care workers and community-level care.
- Encourage links between sectors and integration with other international efforts (such as those on education and gender equality), including harmonized reporting.
- Support systems that track progress and identify funding gaps.
- Generate and synthesize research-derived evidence, and provide a platform for sharing best practices, evidence on cost-effective interventions and research findings.

Civil society must:

- Develop and test innovative approaches to delivering essential services, especially ones aimed at the most vulnerable and marginalized.
- Educate, engage and mobilize communities.
- Track progress and hold all stakeholders (including themselves) accountable for their commitments.
- Strengthen community and local capabilities to scale up implementation of the most appropriate interventions.
- Advocate increased attention to women's and children's health and increased investment in it.

The business community must:

- Scale up best practices and partner with the public sector to improve service delivery and infrastructure.
- Develop affordable new drugs, technologies and interventions.
- Invest additional resources, provide financial support and reduce prices for goods.
- Ensure community outreach and mobilization, coordinated with health-care workers.

Health care workers and their professional associations must:

- Provide the highest-quality care, grounded in evidence based medicine, share best practice, test new approaches, use the best tools possible and audit clinical practice.
- Collaborate to provide universal access to the essential package of interventions, addressing the needs of the vulnerable and marginalized.
- Identify areas where services could be improved and innovations made.
- Ensure that women and children are treated with respect and sensitivity when they receive health care.

- Advocate better training, deployment and retention of workers.
- Work with academics responsible for training and continuing education.
- Provide information to track progress and hold authorities and donors to account.

Academic and research institutions must:

- Deliver a prioritized and coordinated research agenda.
- Encourage increased budget allocation for research and innovation.
- Build capacity at research institutions, especially in low and middle-income countries.
- Strengthen the global network of academics, researchers and trainers.
- Help policy development by reporting on trends and emerging issues.
- Disseminate new research findings and best practice.

CONCLUSION

The world has recognized the need to further reduce the burden of maternal mortality. The target, specified in the fifth millennium development goal (MDG 5), is a 75 percent reduction from the 1990 level, and should be reached by 2015. While great progress has been made so far, the current pace of improvement is insufficient. If it continues unchanged, nearly 90 percent of countries will fail to meet MDG 5 on time. There is a need for more effort on the part of national as well as international governments and organizations to achieve the desired targets. It is also necessary to effectively measure performance and achieve accountability throughout the health care delivery system. Good healthcare alone is not enough to save large numbers of lives. Each country should work towards creating a maternal health ecosystem, which will ensure that women and their families have both the desire for healthcare and the ability to access that care. FIGO has launched the LOGIC initiative to improve policy and practice by strengthening FIGO member associations and using their position and knowledge to facilitate and contribute to improvements, leading to better maternal and new born health for under-served populations in low- and middle-resource countries. International organizations such as WHO and governments all over the world are working harder than ever before to take the safe motherhood initiative to the next level and realize the ultimate goal of avoiding all preventable maternal deaths across the globe.

REFERENCES

1. Arulkumaran S, Hediger V, Manzoor A, May J. Saving Mothers' Lives: Transforming Strategy into Action. Report of the Maternal Health Working Group 2012 at The Global Health Policy Summit (http://www3.imperial.ac.uk/global-health-innovation).
2. Starrs AM. Safe motherhood initiative: 20 years and counting. Lancet. 2006;30:368(9542):1130-2.
3. World Health Organisation. Maternal mortality. Fact sheet N°348, May 2012. http://www.who.int/mediacentre/factsheets/fs348/en/.
4. WHO. World Health Statistics: A snapshot of global health, WHO, 2012.
5. United Nations. United Nations Millennium Development Goals, available at http://www.un.org/millenniumgoals/maternal.shtml.
6. WHO, UNICEF, UNFPA and the World Bank. Trends in Maternal Mortality: 1990 to 2010, 2012.
7. Purandare CN. Maternal Near Miss Review: A Way Forward. The Journal of Obstetrics and Gynecology of India 2013;63(4):213–5.
8. Singh S, et al. Adding It Up: The Costs and Benefits of Investing in Family Planning and Maternal and Newborn Health, Guttmacher Institute and United Nations Population Fund, 2009.
9. World Health Organisation. WHO Recommended Interventions for Improving Maternal and Newborn Health. 2nd edn., 2009. Guidelines: Integrated management of pregnancy and childbirth (IMPAC) WHO/MPS/07.05 (http://www.who.int/maternal_child_adolescent/documents/who_mps_0705/en/index.html).
10. FIGO International Federation of Gynecology and Obstetrics. Strengthening Organisational Capacity of Health Professional Associations. FIGO LOGIC Initiative in Maternal and Newborn Health www.figo-toolkit.org.
11. World Health Organisation. The partnership for maternal, newborn and child health. Global Strategy for Women's and Children's health. A call to action – We all have a role to play (http://www.who.int/pmnch/activities/advocacy/fulldocument_globalstrategy/en/index8.html).

2

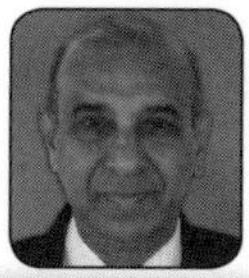

Task Shifting and Sharing in Obstetric Care for Safe Motherhood: Sri Lanka Experience and Global Perspective

Harshalal R Seneviratne

INTRODUCTION

Millennium Development Goals for Safe Motherhood

Since adoption of the millennium development goals (MDGs) by the General Assembly of the United Nations on 18th September 2000 at its 55th session (Agenda item 60 *b*) as a Resolution and Declaration 55/2, awareness of the need for safer motherhood has been accepted[1] by international health agencies, governments, national policy makers and health care providers. This has always been the expectation of the global public who have been the passive recipients of the services provided. At present however the results are far short of the goals set for 2015. With a view to making recommendations to accelerate the process of reaching the MDGs a paper was prepared by the Institute of Development Studies for the United Nations Development Group MDG Task Force in September 2010.[2] This document discusses Country priorities on Health MDGs: Health system strengthening, with the importance of 'competent and motivated human resources'.

Safe motherhood can be achieved only via a series of interactive health and nonhealth interventions where family planning is linked to and interacts with both these groups.[3] The health interventions are a range of facilities such as provision of clinical services, human resource development, health infrastructure establishment and maintenance, health information management, health service administration, etc. Amongst the nonhealth interventions general education is a leading factor while life skills development, economic enhancement, infrastructure development such as transport and communications play a major role. In fact initial reduction of maternal mortality can be shown to be due to parallel improvement of essential health and nonhealth interventions while the reduction in the total fertility rate (TFR) by family planning interventions has been associated with a corresponding reduction of the maternal mortality rate (MMR). In the context of reproductive health family planning interventions no doubt play a central role as contraception and contraceptives interact at all stages of the lifecycle of women from adolescence through the reproductive phase and beyond.

The ground realities for providing 'safe motherhood' care has been clearly demonstrated and discussed for many decades in the past. In the declaration of the global round table 'Countdown 2015' the second item in defining the world we have[4] it is stated that *"we have seen more attention to maternity care, but we have seen no decline in maternal mortality in the poorest countries"*. In this document the other items further reflect the poor facilities including deficient accessibility to reproductive health care for the economically and socially deprived populations. This chapter is meant to deal with human resources for reproductive health including safe motherhood for such populations.

HUMAN RESOURCE FOR QUALITY OBSTETRIC CARE

Human resource for safe motherhood is an essential health intervention which should be supported by adequate financial resources, training capabilities and other nonhealth interventions. Human resource development and management are the important activities which ensure staff coverage for the provision of reproductive health care as well as safe motherhood in particular. While the training of staff for safe childbirth has taken precedence in the package for the provision of health care in all countries in South Asia staff coverage is always in a negative balance. Many reasons have been responsible for this situation. The most serious barriers to adequate staffing are:

- Poor resources for training
- Brain drain
- Suboptimal commitment of Government and policy makers, etc.

Of all issues government commitment and leadership in setting the policy for reproductive health care in general and safe motherhood in particular would be the driving forces in achieving positive changes. The commitment of the Sri Lanka government over the years is described in the Womens' Report 2000 of FIGO.[3]

In the traditional manner training medical staff for safe motherhood has been by graduation from medical school. Similarly nursing training has been via nursing school. Analyzing the evolution of medical education (applicable also to nursing and paramedical). The Lancet Commission Report 2010,[5] describes the changes over the past century and the gaps in the training for adequate provision of health care (Table 1) which are also applicable to the provision of human resources for safe motherhood.

Table 1 New challenges in health needs

Global fresh health challenges	*Continuing system failures*
• Rapidly expanding new infections • Environmental risks • Behavioral risks • Epidemiological transitions • Rapid changes in demography, etc.	• Persistent professional status gender stratification • Static curricula • Narrow technical focus than broader conceptual idea of health • Sporadic patient encounters vs. continuous care • Hospital care rather than community/primary care • Mismatch of professional competencies to patient/population needs • Professions working in isolation and no integration • Lack of team work • Deficient leadership to solve management problems • Incompetency of medical professionals • Costly and complex health services • Regional inequities in provision of health care

CURRENT SCENARIO IN DEVELOPING AND POOR COUNTRIES

These challenges are very much applicable to the South Asia Region. Ensuring adequate numbers of staff to provide the services for safe motherhood appears to be an unachievable goal. This was demonstrated very clearly by Professor Tipu Sultan of Pakistan in relation to the provision of anesthesia for safe motherhood at the second consultation networking meeting between professional societies and the UN agencies organized by the South Asia Federation of Obstetrics and Gynecology on 29 March 2008 at Kathmandu, Nepal. The ground situation in Pakistan at that time was stated by him[6] as "while approximately 1400 fully and part qualified anesthetists were serving a population of 160 million people, only 46 to 60 new anesthetists were being trained annually, it would take about 220 years for Pakistan to be self-sufficient in terms of anesthesiologist (Human Resource) at the present rate of production and disappearance (Export-Loss) and with the brain drain in operation".

Similar and additional important issues on human resources have been highlighted in a study performed in Africa.[7] The study involved the assessment of availability and coverage by nurses and midwives taken as one group and doctors as the other in 12 Sub-Saharan African countries where data was available. This study, which was the first to examine whether current preservice training can improve the situation, took into account population increases and attrition due to premature death among health workers, retirement, resignation and dismissal. The results for all 12 countries combined shows that, for every 1000 physicians practicing in these countries, 59 medical graduates are produced each year. The rate is marginally higher for nursing and midwifery staff, at 66 new graduates per 1000 practicing nurses and midwives. The regional average, however, masks the diverse patterns in the study countries. Moreover, countries that have a relatively high graduation rate for one type of health worker do not necessarily have a relatively high rate for the other. As an example the study quotes the situation in Côte d'Ivoire which has the highest graduation rate for physicians (14%) but ranked only 7th in the regeneration rate for nurses and midwives (2.7%). Only 3 countries (Ethiopia, Liberia and Sierra Leone) unequivocally trained sufficient workers to replace those leaving the workforce. The study also demonstrated an important situation common to all developing countries which is generally in all countries evaluated the outflows are slightly lower for nurses and midwives than for physicians. Training capacity was inadequate in all countries analyzed. Even the 2 countries where current rates of training would increase health worker density will not be able to meet the target level of 2.28 physicians, nurses and midwives per 1000 population until well after 2015.

Governments could go further to improve human resources by implementing the existing global mechanisms to stop or minimize the brain drain. While modifying the local health structure and introducing socioeconomic developments to help in retaining the qualified professional in the country, global strategies suggested towards minimizing brain drain could also be implemented. It is now a necessity that the WHO Global Code of Practice on International Recruitment of Health Personnel[8] be implemented urgently and as suggested "recipient countries recruit doctors only via a Memorandum of Understanding (MOU) with each country". Active and targeted recruitment of doctors from countries which are experiencing shortages is discouraged by the WHO resolution (57.19).[9] The supply countries could also interact with the international agencies (International Organization for Migration (IOM)[10] to define the country specific issues and solutions. The possible effects on recipient countries of implementing the WHO Global Code of Practice on International Recruitment of Health Personnel was analyzed in an interesting paper[11] where the main conclusion was that those involved in recruitment were largely unaware of the global code.

A different aspect of human resource availability was studied using data from Zambia and Sri Lanka.[12] The justification for the study was that there was suboptimal utilization of health system indicators related to staffing in many developing countries which therefore resulted in misdistribution of maternity staff particularly those required for emergency obstetric care (EmOC). The study was intended to demonstrate their use at sub-national levels in two contrasting countries regarding human resources for health and geographical accessibility to EmOC facilities. Interesting results were obtained where both countries were shown to perform adequately on coverage of EmOC while in one the staffing situation in terms of number and distribution was very inadequate while the other was shown to be over staffed when compared to WHO bench mark for staffing.

UNFPA AND SAFOG WORKSHOP ON QUALITY ENHANCEMENT TO ACHIEVE MDG GOAL: EXPERIENCE AND CONSENSUS

In an effort to reach a consensus on staff training and coverage in general and task shifting in particular in the Asia and Pacific Regions a Workshop on Quality Enhancement to Achieve MDG 5 was held in Colombo, Sri Lanka from 27th to 29th April 2012. The workshop was organized by the South Asia Federation of Obstetrics and Gynecology (SAFOG) and United Nations Fund for Population Activities (UNFPA)—Asia Pacific Regional Office in collaboration with the Sri Lanka College of Obstetricians and Gynaecologists.[13] The presentations highlighted some very diverse situations in staffing among the countries. With an institutional delivery rate 99 percent and cesarean delivery rate of 22 percent in Mongolia it appears that only specialist obstetricians would be attending on all cesarean deliveries. It therefore appeared that with 70,538 deliveries annually of which 15,518 are cesarean deliveries covered by 568 specialist obstetricians each one would be performing an average of 28.8 operative deliveries annually. Such a staffing situation would be beyond the capabilities of most countries in the world and in particular those of the Asia and Pacific regions. The report of the workshop includes a 24 item consensus statement which focuses on future actions for the provision of emergency obstetric care including obstetric anesthesia by professional societies and governments.

The most pressing needs for staffing in many developing countries appear to be:

- Skilled birth attendance
- Provision of safe obstetric anesthesia
- Managing obstetric and medical emergencies.

At the Workshop in Colombo conducted from 27th to 29th April 2012 the efforts made by the countries represented were most revealing. The extracts from the report dealing with presentations on short-term training programs highlighted some interesting features. The grade and type of staff who received training varied in different countries. The training concentrated on nonspecialist doctors (n = 3), nurses and midwives (n = 2), both types (n = 2) and none of the above (n = 1). Two countries viz. India and Bangladesh had well defined training programs (one each for nurses and doctors), while two others (Nepal and Sri Lanka) regularly updated the knowledge and skills of nonspecialist care providers but the programs did not follow an organized academic track. The Indonesian program which trains doctors, nurses and midwives was well organized and included general practitioners as well. Cambodia also trained both doctors and nurses but their program to fast track training failed due to lack of infrastructure development especially in the rural areas.

In the provision of obstetric anesthesia only Bhutan and Papua New Guinea (PNG) had shifted tasks to nonmedical staff. Bhutan had nurse anesthetists trained overseas from the 1980s. The program in PNG is considered as being unique as it "permits a range of nonmedical professionals such as Anesthesia Technical Officers (ATO), Nursing Officers, Health Extension Officers, Health Officers, Medical Students and Community Health Workers (Year 12) to be recruited for training". Most countries did not have a process for accreditation following training except a Diploma in PNG and a voluntary MD 1A examination in Sri Lanka. Registration after training and accreditation by the Medical Council was provided only by Bhutan, PNG and Bangladesh.

What should the ideal organizational structure be for task shifting to cover the services for safe motherhood? For this purpose the presentation by Dr Mathews Mathai of the WHO at the workshop held in Colombo from 27th to 29th April 2012 gave a clear educational track which could be used by all countries (Flow chart 1). It is clear that the training should be based on the need for defined safe motherhood services such as components of skilled birth attendance, obstetric anesthesia, etc. This would also help to eventually define the tasks to be provided by the care provider after training. The entry criteria will be determined by the current professional training and expertise of the category of staff selected for the task. Each country should determine whether a basic medical qualification is required for the services to be provided. Sri Lanka recruits doctors with the basic MBBS degree for training to perform cesarean deliveries and to provide obstetric anesthesia while Bhutan covers the latter service requirement by trained nurse anesthetists.

Flow chart 1 Educational track for training to provide safe motherhood care

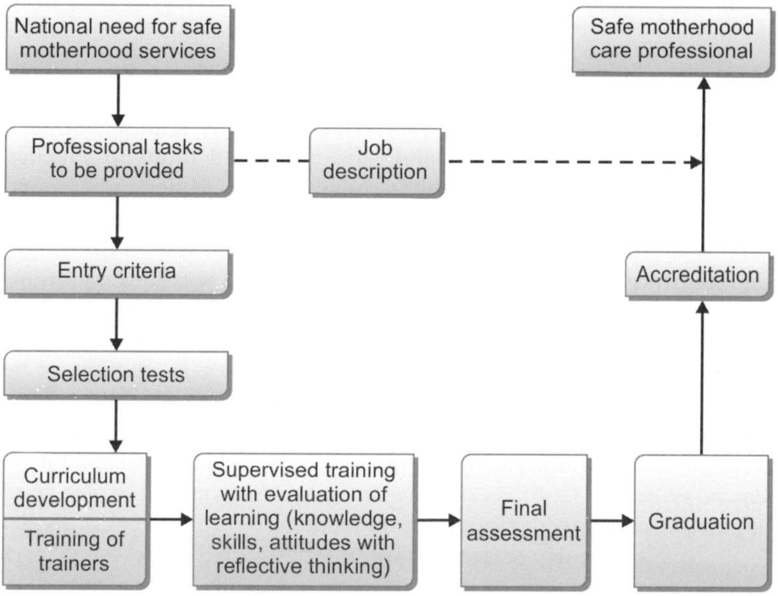

Since it would be some grades of health staff who would be selected for re-training it is very necessary that an appropriate selection test is performed to ensure that the correct person is selected to perform the task. This includes assessing their basic knowledge on the topic as well as an aptitude test(s) to determine the ability to perform key tasks and for trouble shooting.

The development of the curriculum for the training program needs meticulous planning. It is done on the basis of focused objectives of the training program. The teaching/learning sessions are designed based on these objectives. As the need is for task based provision of care hands on practical sessions are mandatory. These could be done by simulations, in mannequin based skills laboratories or as live sessions. Parallel to the development of the curriculum there should be conscious efforts to train the trainers to appreciate the correct academic content and to use the appropriate teaching methods.

Evaluation of training should be done parallel to the conduct of the course. As in the training a major portion of the assessment would involve skills. Direct observations as well as documentation of skills are evaluation methods which are mandatory. Portfolios, log books, case records are examples of such continuous evaluation. An appropriately designed final examination is necessary to ensure that the training has been successfully completed. The trainee could be then graduated from the program.

Graduation does not totally complete the process of skills transfer for practice. To permit legal and regulatory processes it would be necessary that accreditation by a proper authority is obtained. The regulatory authority should define the levels and limits of practice permitted so as to protect the public and also to avoid inter-professional conflicts. The trainee could then be authorized to provide that specific service to the public. At the workshop held in Colombo in April 2012 this was the process that was found to be most deficient in all countries. It is necessary that governments, professional societies, global health organizations and other responsible establishments ensured that the process of accreditation is implemented for task shifting to be established in a meaningful manner.

The Indian program by FOGSI presented at the Colombo 2012 workshop by Dr Prakash Bhatt, the National Technical Consultant—EmOC Project—FOGSI is extensive and could be expected to give good supervised care provider training at an academic setting (6 weeks), district level (10 weeks) and in-service distant supervision at the trainee's of work place. Assessments are in place at every level with final accreditation being after 12 months service in the work place. The professional body has planned and is responsible for the conduct of the course as well as evaluation. The program appears to be staff-intensive which has been a barrier. If resources, including staff and training venues, etc. could be arranged this program is a good model to follow.

CONCLUSION

An important issue to be considered before embarking on a program of shifting of tasks for safe motherhood is the future professional development of those care providers who receive the training and are entrusted with the new tasks. Their future in the health care structure of the country should be preplanned. This is of particular relevance if the country is subsequently able to complete its requirement for staffing.

It is clear that the technical inputs for training should come from the academic institutions and professional organizations while the government plays a pivotal role in the initiation, coordination, legislation as well as monitoring and follow-up supervision of the training process as the 'guardian' of quality services for EmOC. The drive towards teamwork at ground level and also at policy and administrative level is mandatory if the coverage of safe motherhood services is to be fulfilled.

REFERENCES

1. Millennium Development Goals Report 2013. Compiled by an Inter-agency and Expert Group on MDG Indicators led by the Department of Economic and Social Affairs of the United Nations Secretariat, Geneva.
2. Grealey Martin. "Accelerating progress on the MDGs: Country priorities for improving performance". Paper prepared for the United Nations Development Group MDG Task Force. September 2010, Institute of Development Studies.
3. Seneviratne HR, Rajapaksa LC. Safe motherhood in Sri Lanka: a 100-year march. Womens' report 2000 International Federation of Gynaecology and Obstetrics. International Journal of Gynaecology and Obstetrics. 2000;70: 113-4.
4. Countdown 2015, sexual and reproductive and rights for all. ICPD at 10 advocacy toolkit. Declaration of the global Round Table, Countdown 2015.
5. Health professionals for a new century: Transforming education to strengthen health systems in an independent world. The Lancet Commission Report. 2010.DOI:10.1016/50140-6736(10)6184-5.
6. Sultan T. Emergency Obstetric Care (EmOC) in Pakistan : Ground Realities and Anaesthesia Perspective. Consultation between Professional Societies and United Nations Health Agencies in South Asia. Organised by the South Asia Federation of Obstetrics and Gynaecology. 29 March 2008, Kathmandu, Nepal.
7. Kinfu Y, Dal Poz MR, Mercer H, Evans DB. The health worker shortage in Africa: are enough physicians and nurses being trained? Bulletin of the World Health Organization. 2009;87:225-30. doi: 10.2471/BLT.08.051599.
8. WHO Global Code of Practice on International Recruitment of Health Personnel. 63rd World Health Assembly 2010, Geneva.
9. Fifty-Seventh World Health Assembly 2004. International Migration of Health personnel : A challenge for health systems in developing countries. WHO Resolution 57.19.
10. International Organization for Migration (IOM)17, Route des Morillons, CH-1211 Geneva 9, Switzerland.
11. Edge JS, Hoffman SJ. Empirical Impact Evaluation of the WHO global code of practice on the international recruitment of health personnel in Australia, Canada, UK and USA. Globalization and Health. 2013;9:60-80. doi 10.1186/1744-8603-9-60.
12. Gabrysch S, Zanger P, Seneviratne HR, Mbewe R, Campbell OMR. Tracking progress towards safe motherhood: meeting the bench mark yet missing the goal? An appeal for better use of health-system output indicators with evidence from Zambia and Sri Lanka. Tropical Medicine and International Health. 2011;16:83-83. doi: 10.1111/j.1365-3156.2011.02741.x.
13. Report of the Workshop on Quality Enhancement to Achieve MDG 5. United Nations Fund for Population Activities – Asia Pacific Regional Office. 2012. South Asia Federation of Obstetrics and Gynaecology and United Nations Fund for Population Activities – Asia Pacific Regional Office in collaboration with the Sri Lanka College of Obstetricians and Gynaecologists April 27 to April 29, 2012.

3

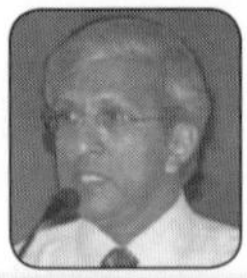

Safe Motherhood Initiative in Sri Lanka: A Success Story to Share

Hemantha Parera

INTRODUCTION

Every day almost 800 women die in pregnancy or child birth. Every loss of a mother shatters a family and threatens the well-being of surviving children. All women deserve the care they need to be safe and healthy throughout the pregnancy and child birth which is termed Safe Motherhood. It could be regarded as a right of every mother. However in the backdrop of social and cultural factor, including political governance, health system and health policy, there is huge inequality of care received by mother across the globe.

In a last decade there has been a lot of progress towards a better understanding of problem of maternal mortality. However only a few South Asian countries could make significant strides towards a safe motherhood. Sri Lanka is in the forefront of these countries. This chapter gives glimpse to their road map towards success.

Historical Perspective of Sri Lankan's Maternity Care

Sri Lanka has a long history with objective evidence to it running into over 2550 years. There have been following facts noted in history of Sri Lanka notifying sensitivity and measures for safe motherhood in Sri Lanka from the beginning:

1. *Pre-Europe era:* A long chain of kingdom encouraged Buddhist way of living, which preaches mother to be the most sacred of all. Sri Lanka had established system of health care including hospital as far back as 9th century AD. Traditional nature medical care, later supplemented by Ayurveda from India was cornerstone of health delivery system.

2. *European era*: Sri Lanka, than Ceylon was under Portugal, Dutch and then since 1815 to 1947 till independence was under British rule. Followings are few landmarks at his period.
   - Western system of medicine was introduced by Portugese in 1506
   - The foundation of present health system was rooted by British in 1858 with creation of civil medical department
   - Registration of birth and death under Registrar general began in 1887 and made compulsory in 1897
   - Maternal mortality was included in the annual report in special section as way back as 1921
   - Universal health coverage of all including women was introduced as way back as 1931 in Sri Lanka, only 3 years after UK well ahead of its neighbor like India (1950), Nepal (1951), Pakistan (1956), Bhutan (1953), Bangladesh (1972).

Registration of midwives and training of nurses and midwives was made compulsory from 1897, A separate maternal and child health department was started in 1906, and trained midwives were made available in Colombo city municipality. Figures 1 and 2, show data of MMR in Sri Lanka from 1930 to 1996.

It shows marked reduction of MMR from 2200 death/100,000 live birth in 1920 to 34 death/100,000 live births, in present time one of lowest in developing factor despite general poverty still prevalent in country.

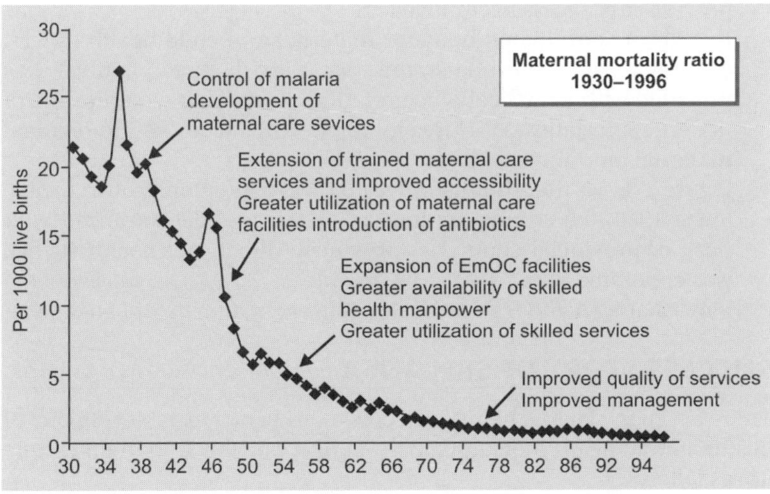

Fig. 1 Maternal mortality ratio in Sri Lanka from 1930–1996

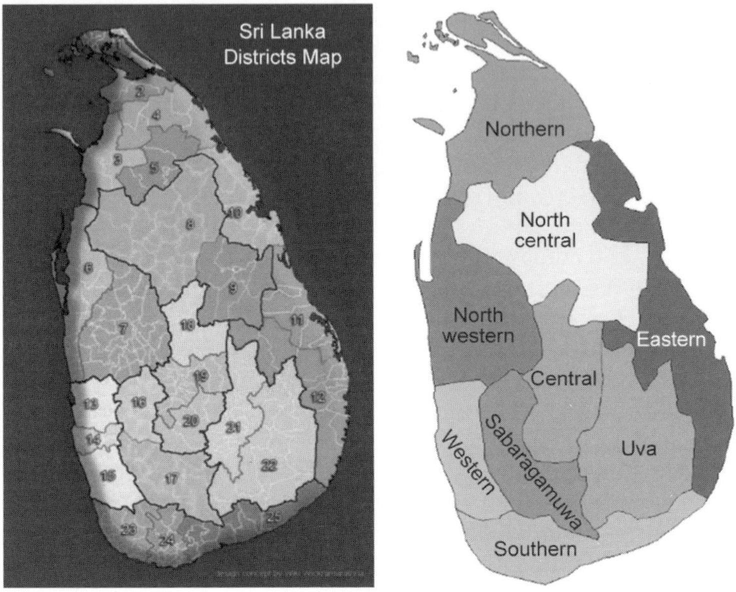

Fig. 2 Political demography of Sri Lanka *(for color version see Plate 1)*

Postindependence Period

- In 1948, village hospitals (Peripheral units) were introduced to provide easy access to curative care
- In 1968, a coordinated body for maternal and child health (MCH) services were established. Same year every district of country was provided with a medical officer of MCH. Central line monitoring of maternal mortality (MM) was initiated with a team sent to regional maternal mortality meetings.

  Figure 2 shows the administrative political demography of Sri Lanka.
- Since 1989, the administration of country was decentralized with birth of provincial council. A provincial director of health service was appointed to each of the 09 provinces.

  Flow charts 1A and B show health delivery system in Sri Lanka.

SUCCESS STORY OF SRI LANKA

There are many factors behind success of Sri Lanka in achieving one of best maternal heath indicators in Sri Lanka. The few important factors are as follows:

- Government's historical emphases on meeting the basic needs of its population in area of infrastructure—health and education, with the

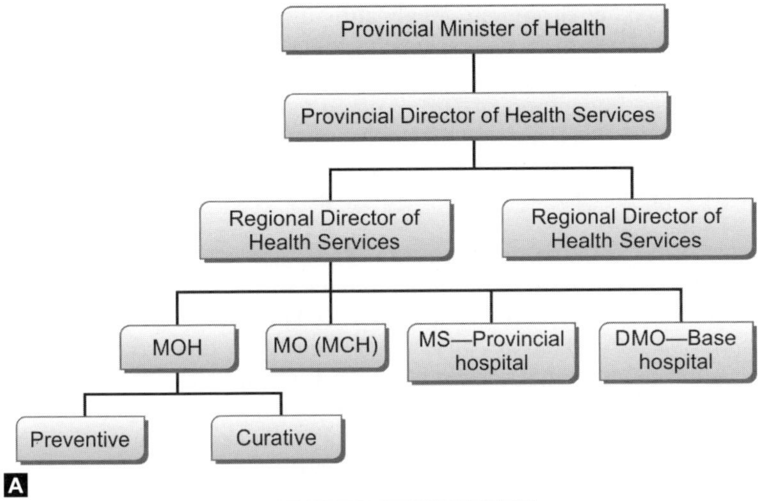

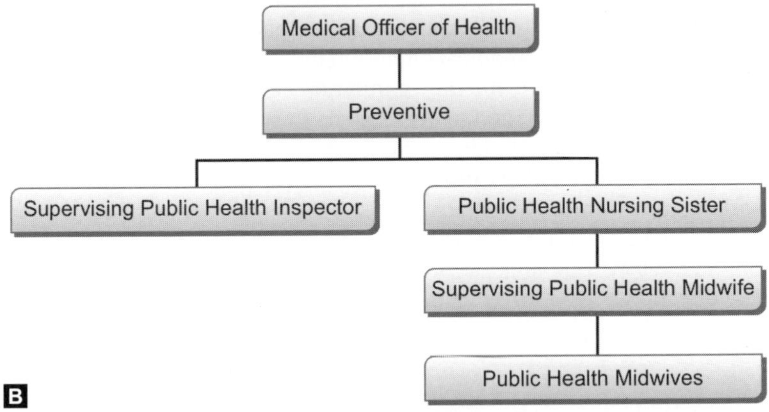

Flow charts 1A and B Health delivery system in Sri Lanka

Abbreviations: MS, Medical Super in tendent; DMO, District Medical Officer; MOH, Medical Officer of Health; MCH, Maternal and Child Health

relatively high status of women in society. High female literacy, free education and opportunity for girls and increased age at marriage for girls (25.1 year in 1993) has substantiated the improvement in women health

- A comprehensive and high quality family planning program which offer contraception through wide range of channel. As a result contraceptive prevalence rate is 66 percent, fertility rate is 2.3 birth/women

- Focussed environment in health intervention generally and maternal health services specially
- A good road network, community local maternal child health free services, integration of family planning with maternal and child health services, institutional delivery up to 90 percent, and use of appropriate technology like home-based mother's record and partograph are few implemented focussed interventions in Sri Lanka.
- *Literacy in Sri Lanka:* Education in Sri Lanka has history of 2300 years. Today there is free education for all and literacy rate for with male and female has reached nearly 100 percent.

Health master plan, November 2003: The clear demarcation of the preventive and curative section of the health system from the beginning was instrumental in service delivery and recognition of priorities for health expenditure. Having trained birth attendant in form of government midwives, posted to every village was the first major step in bringing down MMR. Midwives were divided into the preventive and curative sections with interchange for regular exposure to all aspect of maternity care.

On preventive side medical officers of health (MOH) were appointed to every district, based on the population ratio and apex preventive health officer was provided to every MOH to supervise and oversee the midwifery team appointed to the field service.

There are MOH officer per district and 5725 public health midwives working in community level.

Midwives role has been broadened to encompass a major preventive role like early booking of pregnant mother, contraceptive service delivery and vaccination (Figs 3A and B)

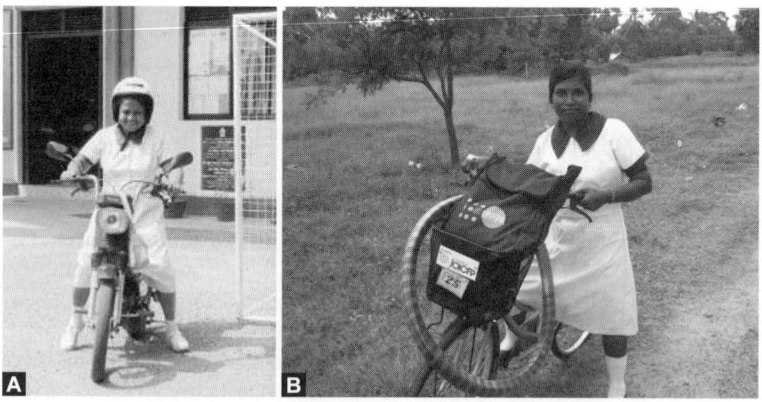

Figs 3A and B Midwife role in MCH care is broadened

Box 1 Decrease in domiciliary delivery from 2007 to 2012 in Sri Lanka

Percentage of home deliveries	2007	0.5
	2008	0.4
	2009	0.3
	2010	0.2
	2011	0.1
	2012	0.1

On curative side, maternity homes were built in every village and with trained midwives, there was a rapid transition from home delivery to institutional deliveries, creating an immediate impact on MMR.

Box 1 shows marked reduction in home deliveries from 2007 to 2012 in Sri Lanka.

There were smaller hospitals in the periphery called peripheral units with a medical officer-in-charge and a labor room with midwives as a mandatory component.

The referral system: It was planned with expenses of specialist care centers as well as planning of the obstetrician was and gynecologist to cater to ever increasing need based on demographics.

SOCIOCULTURAL AND DEMOGRAPHIC IMPROVEMENT

This improvement added to improvement in maternal child health. The good registration system and statistics gives very clear objectivity to the planning, implementation and analysis of health services.

Figures 4 to 6 mark the distribution of specialist care center, peripheral units in district and health institutions in Sri Lanka respectively.

PROFESSIONAL BODIES IN SRI LANKA

The first association of obstetric and gynecologist was founded in 1953, called Ceylon Obstetrical and Gynecologist Association (COGA).

The editorial of the first journal (1954) is testimony of its aim and high principles.

'The association of obstetric and gynecologist is not a trade union, nor does it exist for main purpose of fighting for the right and privilege of its members. The only fight that figures in our aim is that against maternal and infant mortality.'

In May 1970, the association was elevated to status of college and became known as Ceylon College of Obstetric and Gynecologist (CCOG), which was renamed Sri Lanka College of Obstetrician and Gynecologist as it stands today with 1972 constitutional reforms of Sri Lanka. Today the college with 245 members stands out among rest as a beacon in

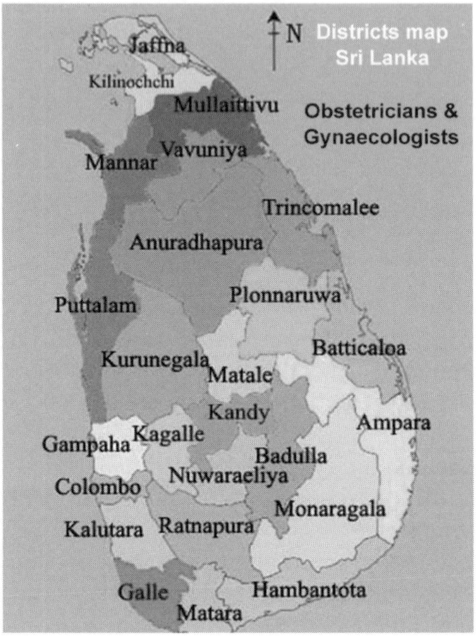

Fig. 4 Specialist care centers in Sri Lanka *(for color version see Plate 1)*

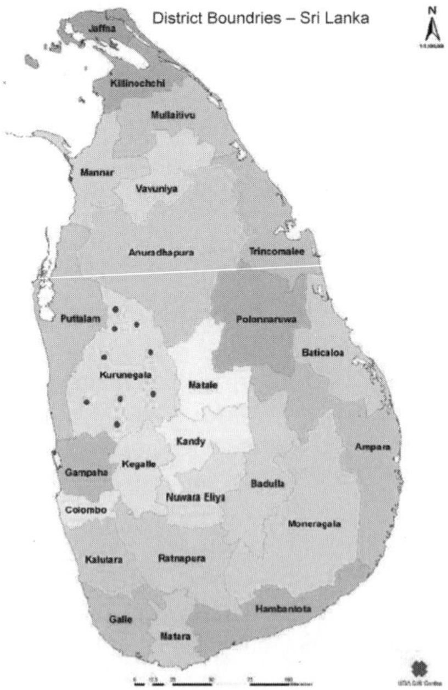

Fig. 5 District-wise peripheral units in Sri Lanka *(for color version see Plate 2)*

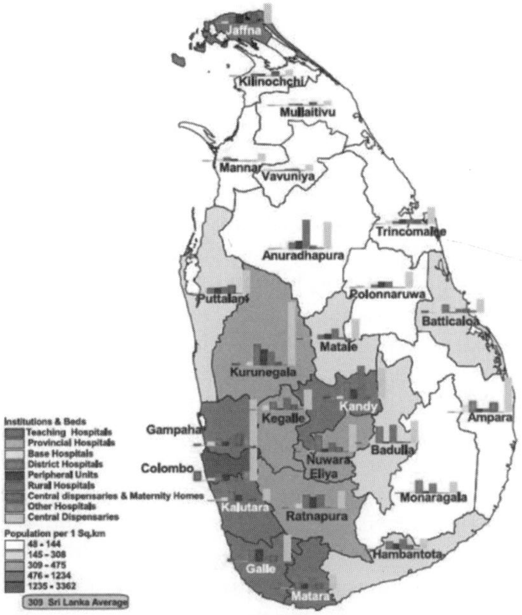

Fig. 6 Health institutions in Sri Lanka *(for color version see Plate 2)*

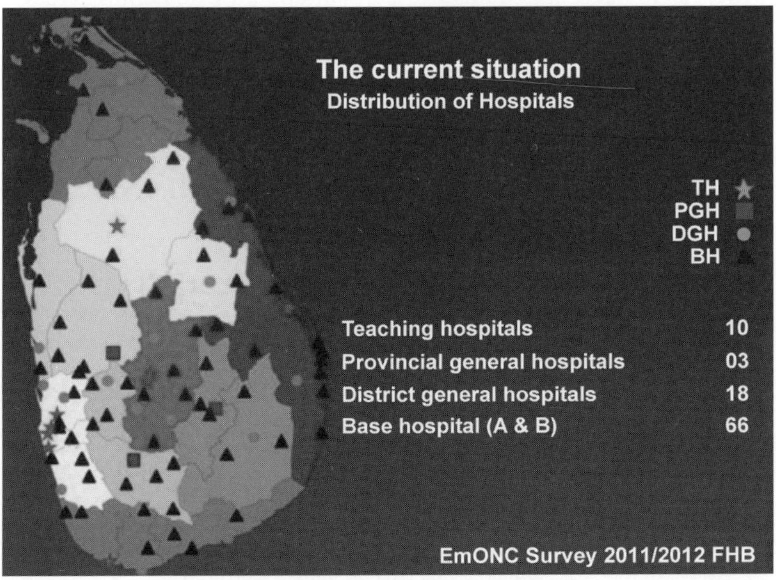

Fig. 7 Current distribution of hospitals in Sri Lanka *(for color version see Plate 3)*

directing the maternal and child health services in country. Its members work in 68 hospitals, along with a fully fledged private sectors, providing the women care of a caliber with the country could be proud of (Fig. 7)

SCOG was geared to action by the very first international initiative at Nairobi, Kenya in 1987. In 1985 both AOFOG conference held in Colombo with major lead by doctor Shiva, Chimathamby and Professor S Ratnam. AOFOG supported Island wide workshops on maternal and perinatal health with tag quality of care in safe motherhood. First was held in Colombo 1989 and second at Ratnapura 1993. Over the years this single aspect of action of SCOG has remained constant with workshops held in various parts of Island prioritize on regional MMR.

The objectives were broadened with changing causes as well as reduction of MMR. With very high institutional delivery, the focus has shifted to EMOC as well as reduction of maternal morbidity, perinatal morbidity and mortality. Hands on training on essential emergency obstetric procedure have been incorporated into the workshop. As a step of galvanizing the next generation of obstetrician to need of quality of care in obstetrics as well to expose the different facilities and the need of different regions of the country, all the postgraduates are expected to take part in these intense workshops. Figure 8 shows author and members of SCOG providing skills and training to health care providers.

SCOG has come to an understanding with Ministry of Health (MOH) as to need to update any health attendant who comes across a laboring mother on the management of obstetric emergencies. Further development of program is expected with the assistance of RCOG, with whom the SCOG signed a historic MOU in 2012. Box 2 summarizes the purpose of this partnership.

Box 2 SCOG and RCOG partnership

The purpose of this partnership is to:

- Strengthen knowledge and clinical skill development by:
  - Facilitating placement of trainees from Sri Lanka to participate in the RCOG sponsorship scheme.
  - Facilitating short-term placement of Board certificated specialists serving in Sri Lanka on their own funding in pre-arranged centers in the UK with the objective of updating knowledge and skills.
  - Exchanging of trainees to gain knowledge and skills including medical elective placements.
  - Establishing active and genuine collaboration inclusive of other professional and professional bodies involved in health issues of women, newborns and reproduction, such as the organization of joint conferences, development of guidelines and exchange of opportunities.

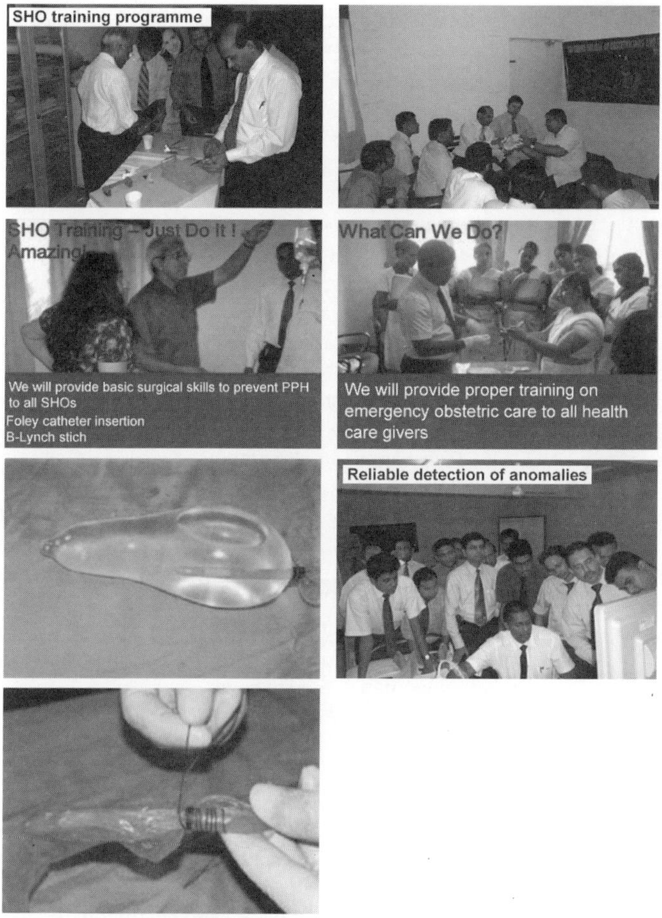

Fig. 8 SCOG training workshop

SCOG plan for 2012 to 2016: In 2012, a strong effort was made by SCOG to make the MOH to initiate confidential enquiry into maternal death as well as to maternal morbidity, SCOG plans to develop mechanism for it, coordinate legal authorities, to obtain indemnity of participants, provide assessors and scrutinize the final report and ensure it's publication within a year. Beside SCOG and MOH wishes to have many more health initiatives like universal sexual and reproductive health education, independent adolescent and youth friendly clinics, universal contraceptive availability, comprehensive abortion services

Box 3 Strategic goal of SCOG

Strategic goal 4	By 2015 we want all children, adolescents and youth to have mandatory sexual and reproductive health education
Strategic goal 5	By 2017 we want independent adolescent and youth-friendly reproductive health services
Strategic goal 6	By 2014 we want contraceptive services to be available, accessible and be utilized by all sexually capable people irrespective of age, parity and marital status
Strategic goal 9	By 2014 we want all eligible for parenthood to receive satisfactory preconception care
Strategic goal 10	By 2014 we want all pregnant mothers to receive antenatal, intrapartum, postnatal care and emergency obstetric care at an appropriate standard set by the SLCOG
Strategic goal 11	By 2014 we want postabortion care to be delivered at an appropriate standard set by the SLCOG
Strategic goal 12	By 2014 we want all single mothers to receive equal care and assistance
Strategic goal 15	SLCOG stands for eradication of Gender Based Violence (GBV) from Sri Lanka. By 2015 we want women victims of GBV to be managed in an appropriate manner safeguarding the principles of human rights.
Strategic goal 16	To mobilize necessary resources to assist women undergoing psychological repercussions of obstetrical and gynecological and other women ralated life events
Strategic goal 17	By 2013 we want all maternal death inquiries to be carried out in the internationally accepted standard confidential reporting format
Strategic goal 18	By 2015 we want severe acute maternal morbidity inquiries to be carried out in the internationally accepted standard confidential reporting format
Strategic goal 19	We want to incorporate and promote evidence-based practice into the undergraduate and postgraduate curriculum and the clinical practice of obstetrics and gynecology

and eradication of gender based violence. Box 3 summarizes strategic goal of SCG in coming years.

CONCLUSION

Sri Lanka has shown a remarkable improvement of quality of maternal health care over the years from the colonial era to present time. Sri Lanka is a country which achieved remarkable reduction in level of maternity during second half of 20th century, despite total expenditure on maternal health care (recurrent and capital expenditure) average 0.23 percent of GDP or around 12 percent of total government expenditure on health. Cost were higher at the beginning of the program during 1950 and gradually decreased at a result of combination of increased efficiency and growth of private sector.

The universal and free of cost health care, women-friendly sociocultural, demographic and political influences introduced to country have given benefits to multitude of women in the country. A mother in Sri Lanka is safer than most of her counterpart in the region and in many part of the world. She could be safer further and continual address of the objective of safe motherhood initiative will be way forward.

BIBLIOGRAPHY

1. Historical overview of education in Sri Lanka - Ancient period (543 BC–1500 AD) Ministry of Education.
2. http:www.unfpa.org/public/cache/offomce/home/mother/pid/4381.
3. Launch of World Health Report 2013: Research for universal health coverage; Dr Margaret Chan, Director General of WHO; Remarks at the launch of the world health report; 2013, Beijing, China 15th August 2013.
4. Maternal Survival, Maternal Mortality: Who, When, Where, and Why; Carine Ronsmains, Wendy J. Graham, on behalf of the Lancet Maternal Survival series stering group, Lanup 2006;368:1189-2000.
5. Safe Motherhood: A Review the safe motherhood initiative 1987-2005.
6. Safe Motherhood; A brief history of global movement 1947-2002; Carla AbouZahr WHO, Geneva, Switzerland, British Medical Bulletin 2002;67:13-25.
7. Safe Motherhood Initiative: 20 year and counting, Ann.M. Starrs, Family Care International, NewYork NY 10012, USA, astarrs@familycareintl.org; www.thelancet.com; Vol. 368, Sept 30, 2006.
8. Safe Motherhood Program: Options and Issues, Deborah Main Program direction, Prevention of maternal mortality, centre for people, PHC 1991,99.

4

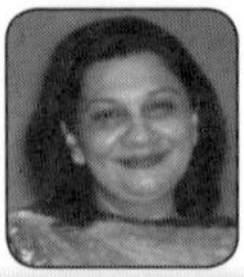

Safe Motherhood Initiative in Pakistan: A Long Journey to Go

Lubna Hassan, Lauren Woodbury-Jamal, Syed Ghazi Ghazan Jamal

"No power can save a country where education and health become a highly profitable business."

—Nelson Mandela

INTRODUCTION

Investing in women's and children's health is not only the right thing to do; it also builds stable, peaceful and productive societies. The status of women in society is the best indicator for assessing overall health outcomes of that country. Evidence from many countries confirms that increasing investments in the health of women and children has many benefits, i.e. it reduces poverty, stimulates economic productivity and growth, is cost-effective, and helps women and children realize their fundamental human rights.[1] Investing in health is also about holding ourselves accountable.

Despite limited progress, the overall health situation for the majority of the women of Pakistan is bleak. The Government of Pakistan appears to regard both health and population planning as core elements of its development agenda; both are reflected in broader frameworks of planning,[2] respective sectoral policies,[3] and international commitments.[4] However, despite stated commitments, successive governments have been unable to unable to cascade policies and plans into concrete action, as a result reproductive health including safe motherhood has eluded the women of Pakistan.

Pakistan spans an area of more than 796,000 square kilometers. There are four provinces—Punjab, Sindh, Khyber Pakhtunkhwa (KPK) and Balochistan, federal units which include district Islamabad, Federally Administered Tribal Area (FATA), and two regions Gilgit—Baltistan and Azad Jammu and Kashmir (AJK) Pakistan is classified as a lower middle income country.[5] Now in its 66th year of independence, the country's political landscape remains plagued by instability. Pakistan's geopolitical position and ongoing tensions with two of its neighbors have a direct bearing on the low status accorded to health and other social sectors. The fact that the first national health policy was not created until 43 years after independence, speaks volumes. Currently, Pakistan spends 67 percent of its GDP on defense and debt servicing, and under 2 percent on education and less than 1 percent on health clearly demonstrating the priority for successive governments has not been social development, and women and children have suffered the most severely from this neglect. Pakistan has the worst maternal health indices in South Asia, and the repercussions go well beyond conventional health determinants. The average Pakistani woman is illiterate, under nourished, over worked, and discriminated against, with high fertility and little access to quality health care. She carries the double burden of productive and reproductive work. Economic returns from her productive work are often usurped by the male members of her family further degrading her autonomy. Yet, when lawmakers have no sense of people's rights, then the first challenge is to capture these deeply entrenched realities as determinants of the inequalities that prevail. Only then can these inequalities begin to be addressed.

LAWS, HEALTH POLICIES AND INTERNATIONAL COMMITMENTS

The pledge of the government of Pakistan to safeguard the health of women is enshrined in the Constitution which guarantees that all citizens are equal before the law and empowers the state to make special provisions for the protection of women and children and the vulnerable sections of the society (Articles 25, 27, 34, 35 and 37).[6]

In 1990, the first national health policy focused on primary health care, with emphasis on universal immunization of children; drugs for 22 common diseases, training for health personnel, especially for maternal health. The 1997 policy speaks of universal immunization; an increase in trained personnel, but interestingly does not target improvement in the doctor-nurse ratio. The 2001 policy is more comprehensive, as it strives for preventive and promotive measures in health, rather than relying entirely on curative care. It also proposes to overcome the urban bias in health care. The 2001 policy identified ten areas for attention, and they include: reducing communicable diseases, promoting preventive care, improving the quality of primary health care, and regulating the private sector. A major shift to address inequities was also taken by setting a goal of removing three areas of inequities, namely: urban-rural, gender, and income differences. How this would be done, and what changes in the health management information system would be possible to capture and monitor inequities is yet to be seen.

In 2002, the National Policy for Development and Empowerment of Women was adopted. The goal of the policy is—"Empowerment of Pakistani women, irrespective of caste, creed, religion, or other consideration for the realization of their full potential in all spheres of life, especially social, economic, personal and political and in keeping with our Islamic way of life." The section on health (4.2) focuses on the provision of primary as well as emergency obstetric care in order to reduce maternal mortality rates. It also calls for ensuring quality health coverage for women and promotes family planning and a small family norm within a rights based approach.[7] Additionally, the Protection of Women Act (Criminal Laws Amendment) of 2006 further compels the government to protect women. In short, on paper at least the women of Pakistan enjoy a high level of protection and an equal status as men.

Pakistan has also ratified a number of international conventions and agreements which emphasize the health of women and obligate the government to take necessary steps to improve the access to and the quality of reproductive health care. These agreements include: the convention on the elimination of all forms of discrimination against women (CEDAW), the Program of Action established at the International Conference on Population and Development (ICPD), the Beijing Declaration and Platform for Action agreed at the Fourth World Conference on Women, the ECOSOC Ministerial Review on Global Health, the Millennium Development Goals (MDG) established at the United Nations Millennium Summit.[8] MDGs three and five set explicit targets for improvements in women's rights and health to be achieved by 2015.

Pakistan's Development Indicators and Health Financing Landscape

According to the human development index (HDI) 2013, Pakistan's ranking has dropped to 146 in the world and it holds the lowest rank in its region. The Government of Pakistan spent only 0.8 percent of GDP on health and 1.8 percent on education. In comparison, Bangladesh and India both spent 1.2 percent on health and 2.2 percent and 3.1 percent on education respectively.[9] The low spending on education and health by Pakistan is not the only cause for alarm; of concern is also the fact that a major chunk of this meager amount is squandered because of corruption and inefficiency.

Taking into account public and private sector health services the total expenditure ranges roughly between 2.4 percent and 3.7 percent of GDP. As a percentage of the government's total budget health has received between 2.6 and 4 percent of total government expenditures. Health currently receives 3.2 percent.[10] In 2005 to 06 the government's expenditure on maternal and child healthcare facilities was 0.55 percent of the total public health budget[11] (Tables 1 and 2 for the breakdown of the expenditure on health). If Pakistan is to comply with the recommendations by the WHO Commission on Macroeconomics and Health it must increase spending on health by 2 percent of GDP by 2015. This amounts to a 285 percent increase in Pakistan's health budget.[12]

Table 1 Health expenditure breakdown in Pakistan

Ministry of Health and the Department of Health	0.67%
Public expenditure	33.32%
Out-of-pocket payments (Private)	57.33%
External support	4–16%
Philanthropy	0.92%
Commercial profits (health insurance)	1.64%
Employers contribution (social security)	5.07%

Table 2 Systems and financing in Pakistan

Costed national implementation plan(s) for maternal, newborn and child health available		Yes
Density of doctors, nurses and midwives (per 10,000 populations)	13.7	(2009)
National available of emergency obstetric care services (percentage of recommended minimum)	–	–
Per capita total expenditure on health (Int$)	88	(2010)
General government expenditure on health as percentage of total government expenditure (%)	4	(2010)
Out-of-pocket expenditure as percentage of total expenditure on health (%)	50	(2010)
Official development assistance to child health per child (US$)	8	(2009)
Official development assistance to maternal and neonatal health per live birth (US$)	12	(2009)

An estimated 73.38 percent of the population does not have healthcare costs fully covered. The other modes of financing health within the country include out-of-pocket payments, social security contributions from private sector sources, and donor contributions. Private sector expenditure on health as a percentage of the total expenditure on health has averaged above 67 percent over the last several years; 98 percent of this is out-of-pocket expenditure. This is clearly a significant burden for a sizable portion of the Pakistani population, which lives below the poverty line.[13]

Health and Family Planning Infrastructure

Each district of Pakistan has a four tiered health services delivery system. The first level is the basic health unit (BHU); the next level is the rural health center (RHU); the third level is a secondary level hospital, and the fourth level is the district/teaching hospital. A district, however, could also take its own initiative, and many established dispensaries where BHUs had not been established. These dispensaries were financed by the respective district. This rather elaborate web of facilities is for the most part unconnected through a formal referral system. This results in a lack of a complete continuum of care throughout the pregnancy, delivery and the post-partum period including PAC and family planning (FP) greatly contributing to the high maternal mortality. This not withstanding the system is a public/private mix with 70 percent of services provided by a largely unregulated private sector and 43 percent of poor women access middle order professionals. The Population Welfare Ministry, on the other hand, provides FP services via family welfare centers (FWC) at the district level and Reproductive Health Units Type A centers at the tertiary level.

Formidable geographical constraints pose a major challenge for health service provision since many families live in remote communities that are inaccessible for parts of the year. There is duplication and wastage with some areas slipping through the cracks while some (usually urban) areas are over served and the difficult to access rural, poor areas under served or not served at all. For example, at least one district, Kohistan, of Khyber Pakhtunkhwa Province has no hospital. The first institutional delivery was conducted by us at RHC Dobair during the floods of 2010 (Fig. 1).

Family planning, in the context in which it is understood today, was not a core consideration at the time of Pakistan's inception. In 1990 the Ministry of Population Welfare was established and made responsible for FP service delivery; whereas maternal and child health were the domain of the health ministry. Effective June 28, 2011 the 18th Amendment to

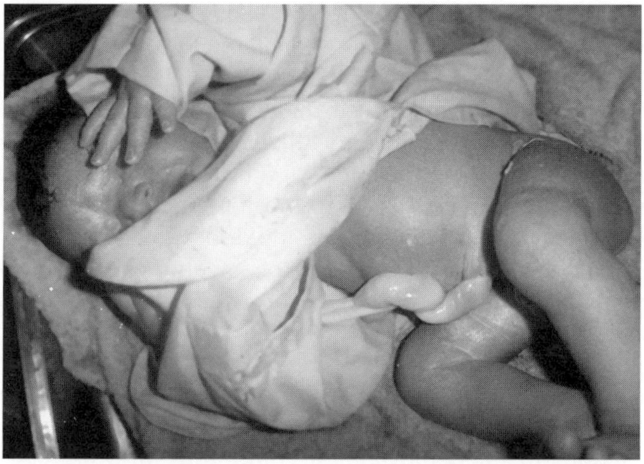

Fig. 1 The first institutional delivery done at Rural Health Center at Dobair during the flood of 2010 *(for color version see Plate 3)*

the Constitution devolved the services related public sectors including the health sector. The Federal Ministry of Health was dissolved and the overall responsibility for health services policy direction and planning lies with the provincial governments.

Maternal Health Program

Over the two last decades the government efforts around maternal, newborn and child health have centered on expanding the program for Family Planning and Primary Health Care. The program has recruited about 110,000 lady health workers (LHWs) to date. More than 60 percent of total population and 76 percent of the target population is covered by LHWs. About 16 million children out of the 30 million target are immunized by LHWs during National Immunization Days (NIDs). Similarly, in high risk districts 4.5 million out of the 5 million target women are vaccinated by LHWs. Thus, their role in improving mother and child health is by now well recognized.

The LHW programs have been lauded internationally but have failed to achieve several objectives. A recent survey revealed that the LHWs did not have the intended impact on hygiene, sanitation behaviors, breast-feeding, growth monitoring or skilled attendance at birth.[14] One of the reasons behind the failure of the LHW program to provide free neonatal and antenatal care is that the LHWs tend to engage in polio and other campaigns shifting resources from their central purpose.[15]

To meet the target of skilled attendance at birth the government launched the National Maternal, Neonatal, and Child Health Program (MNCH) in all four provinces to ensure the training and recruitment of a new cadre of community-based midwives. The government aims to institutionalize quality ambulatory midwifery care at the community level by providing one local resident midwife/lady health visitor per a population of 3500. In order to improve maternal and neonatal health services particularly for the poor and the disadvantaged it aims to train 10,000 community midwives, and to offer comprehensive emergency obstetric and neonatal care (EmONC) services in 275 hospitals/health facilities, basic EmONC services in 550 health facilities, and family planning services in all health outlets.[15] It was envisioned that the program would ensure progress toward achieving the millennium development goals by:

- Comprehensive and integrated MNCH services at the district level
- Development and deployment of community midwife
- Comprehensive family planning services at health facilities
- Advocacy and demand creation
- Strengthening of management.

Maternal Health Human Resource Crisis

Having the sixth highest number of maternal deaths in the world, Pakistan is far from achieving the fifth MDG. The main reason for which is a chronic shortage of skilled personnel at the service centers. Adequate health human resources (HHR) are a vital ingredient in the strengthening of health systems.

Numerical Deficiency

Pakistan has a deficit of health workers on all cadres: doctors, nurses, paramedics including Lady Health Visitors (LHV), LHWs, Community Midwives (CMWs,) (midwifery as a discipline does not exist). In all these fields Pakistan falls short of the universal standard of 2.5 per 1000 population. The shortage, although prevalent throughout the country, is most acutely felt in rural areas, particularly in the provinces of Balochistan and Khyber Pakhtunkhwa. Pakistan is listed among the 57 countries with critical HHR deficiencies.[16]

Skill Imbalance

Pakistan has the classic inverted pyramid structure of health work force by skills. Specialist obstetricians are not available in many of the 134 districts and yet the specialty of Obstetrics/Gynecology is the fastest growing specialty in the country. The very expensive to train doctors far outnumber the other cadres. There remains an acute shortage of the middle order professionals such as nurses, midwives, LHVs and LHWs which should be the backbone of maternity/RH services in a low resource country like Pakistan.

Questionable Quality of Care

The number, range and quality of training programs for health workforce development are very limited. The basic training including the curricula and training methodology in maternal health, across the board from postgraduates to the newest cadre of CMWs, is outdated and inappropriate. For instance CMWs/LHVs, a cadre for home deliveries, are quite often trained in teaching hospitals.

The often unsympathetic and hostile attitude of health care providers to the poor in the public sector hospitals combined with the lack of privacy and trained female health staff discourages women from accessing the facilities that are available. In most public sector hospitals the obstetrics and gynecology (Obs/Gyn) departments account for about a quarter of the workload but are invariably allotted inadequate premises/facilities with an acute shortage of beds causing two and at times three patients to occupy the same bed. This compromises not only the quality of health care provided but also the training environment of the postgraduate trainees and other skilled birth attendants (SBAs).

The Current State of Women's Health

Findings from the largest household survey ever conducted in Pakistan show some improvement where antenatal care is concerned, increasing the antenatal care from 50 percent in 2004–2005 to 58 percent in 2008–2009; almost 61 percent women have had at least one visit and 44 percent have at least 4 or more visits. Another sign of progress is the decrease in the total fertility rate (TFR) from 4.1 percent (2006–2007) to 3.75 percent (2008–2009); however, this is still unacceptably high compared to other developing countries and Pakistan remains unlikely to meet the MDG target of 2.1 percent by 2015.[17] Figure 2 for the overall trends in antenatal care from 1996 to 2013 and Figure 3 for access to care along the continuum from prepregnancy to postpregnancy. Figure 4 shows the number of births attended by the skilled birth attendants from 1990 to 2013.

An evaluation of the progress Pakistan has made thus far indicates there is a widening gap between performance and the targets set by the MDG. This is due in part to various disruptions that have confronted the country since 2006.[18] The 2010 report by the Government of Pakistan on the MDG sheds light on various events since 2006 including

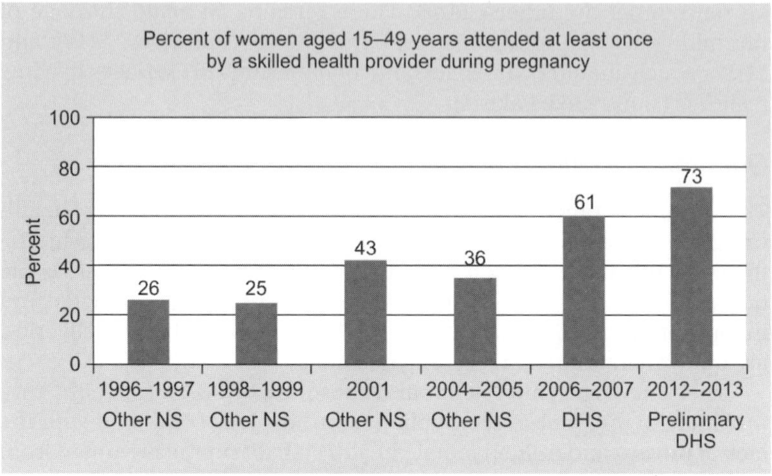

Fig. 2 Antenatal care; DHS and other NS in Pakistan

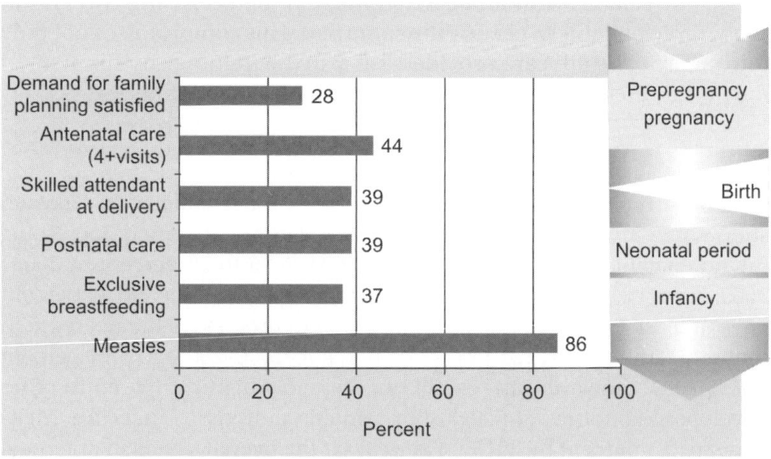

Fig. 3 Coverage along the continuum of care in Pakistan (*Source*: DHS, MICS, Other MS)

worsening political instability, economic recession, a deteriorating security situation nationwide, major military operations in the FATA, and large scale natural disasters including earthquakes and the 2010 flood which devastated one-fifth of the country. The combined impact of such factors has been a stagnation of Pakistan's progress in meeting

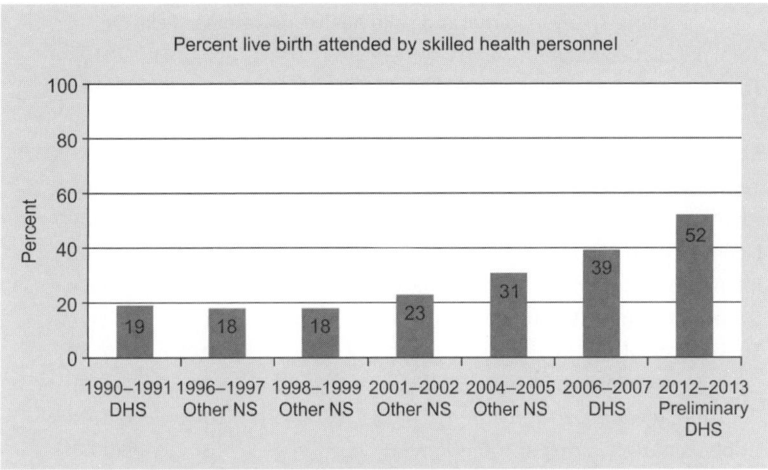

Fig. 4 Skilled attendant at delivery in Pakistan

the MDG. Table 3 in the appendix includes key statistics on maternal and newborn health in Pakistan.

Maternal and newborn health care statistics in Pakistan are some of the poorest in South Asia with a MMR of 276 per 100,000 women in 2007.[19] Figure 5 shows the trends for the MMR in Pakistan since 1990. Nationally the numbers remain staggering: each year there are at least 46 stillborn babies per 1000 LB, 42 neonatal deaths per 1000 LB and more than thirty thousand maternal deaths.[20] Postpartum hemorrhage accounts for most of the maternal deaths which is compounded by high incidence of anemia in women. The time spent in labor and giving birth, the critical moments when a joyful event can suddenly turn into an unforeseen crisis, needs more attention, as does the often-neglected postpartum period. These periods account not only for the high burden of postpartum maternal deaths, but also for the associated large number of stillbirths and early newborn deaths. According to UNICEF one in every 110 Pakistani women will die of childbirth related causes compared to one in 8000 in the developed world.[21] This disparity demonstrates that majority of the maternal deaths in Pakistan are avoidable with proper care. Figure 6 in the annexure shows a pie chart that gives the breakdown of the reasons for maternal deaths in Pakistan.

Population Control and Family Planning

In terms of reproductive health outcomes, the fact that Pakistan has a separate ministry for population welfare can be viewed positively as it

Table 3 Key maternal and child health indicators in Pakistan

Total population (000)	173,593	(2010)
Total under-five population (000)	21,418	(2010)
Births (000)	4,741	(2010)
Birth registration (%)	27	(2006–2007)
Total under-five deaths (000)	423	(2010)
Neonatal deaths: Percent of all under-5 deaths	46	(2010)
Neonatal mortality rate (per 1000 live births)	41	(2010)
Infant mortality rate (per 1000 live births)	70	(2010)
Stillbirth rate (per 1000 total births)	47	(2009)
Total maternal deaths	12,000	(2010)
Lifetime risk of maternal death (1 in N)	110	(2010)
Total fertility rate (per woman)	3.4	(2010)
Adolescent birth rate (per 1000 women)	16	(2007)
Malaria during pregnancy – intermittent preventive treatment (%)	NA	–
C-section (total, urban, rural; %) (Minimum target is 5% and maximum target is 15%)	7, 13, 5	(2006–2007)
Neonatal tetanus vaccine (%)	84	(2010)
Postnatal visit for baby (within 2 days for all births, %)	–	–
Postnatal visit for mother (within 2 days for all births, %)	39	(2006–2007)

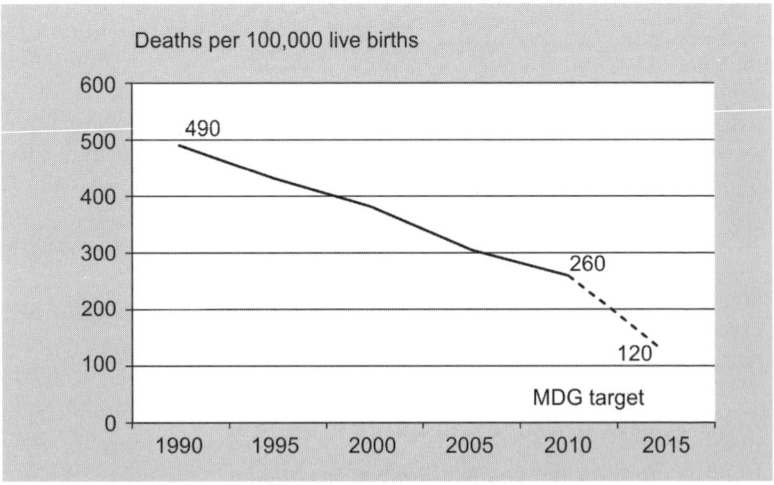

Fig. 5 Maternal mortality ratio and MDG goal for Pakistan

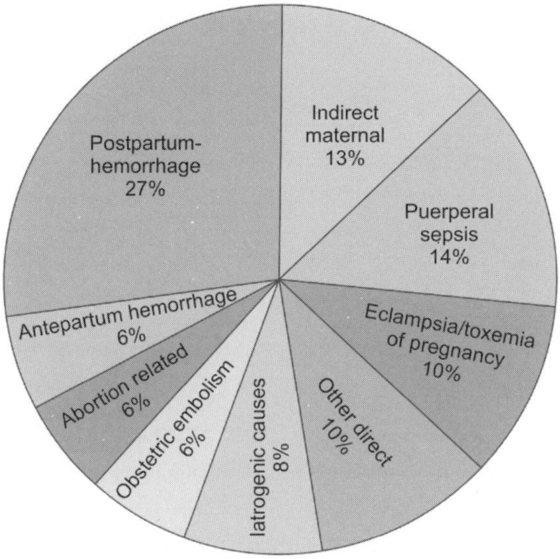

Fig. 6 Causes of maternal deaths in Pakistan
(*Source*: 2006–2007 PDHS, NIPS and Macro International)

gives population planning an additional concerted institutional focus. Nevertheless, it has proved to be counterproductive due to the lack of availability of both the RHMNCH and Family planning services at the same locations. As a result family planning has been marginalized. Moreover family planning has been culturally and socially stigmatized in many underprivileged rural and urban areas where it is not viewed as a health intervention.[22] Therefore, public health experts believe that if family planning and reproductive health services are provided through a recognized health service delivery network rather than institutions created for population control, better health and population outcomes can be achieved. Removing FP from the purview of respected health care providers has only served to strengthen the negative connotations associated with family planning. On the other hand, the provision of health is socially esteemed. Thus, globally the necessity to integrate vertical programs is being emphasized by stressing that better health and population outcomes can be achieved if family planning and reproductive health services are provided through a functional health system (Fig. 7).

Family planning efforts have failed in Pakistan when compared to other countries in South Asia including Bangladesh and Sri Lanka. In 1950 Pakistan had a population of 37 million and was the world's 13th largest country. The current population is estimated at 191 million,

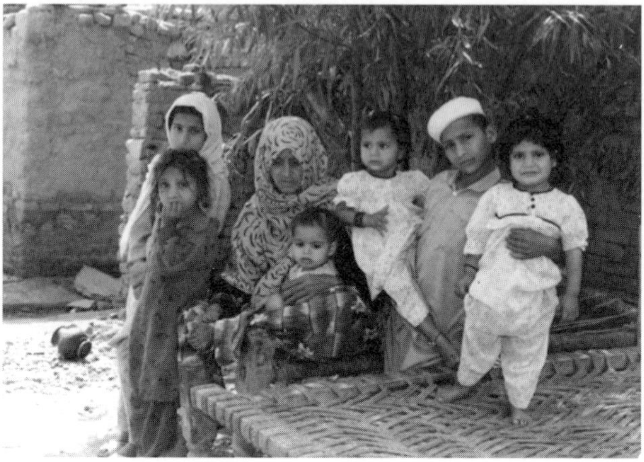

Fig. 7 Family planning and health services difficult to reach in rural areas

and the Population Reference Bureau projects that by 2050 Pakistan will have a population of 363 million people and be the sixth most populous country in the world after India, China, Nigeria, the USA, and Indonesia.[23] This inadequate progress is due at least in part to the low contraceptive prevalence rate.

The provision of comprehensive, voluntary family planning and reproductive health services is a fundamental human right, and yet today these services still remain out of reach for millions of Pakistanis. In fact, one-quarter of married women want to either wait before having another child or end childbearing altogether, but are not using a method of contraception. In 1990 to 1991 twelve percent of couples used contraceptives. This increased to 28 percent in 2000 to 2001 and has remained at around 30 percent ever since. The low usage rate is in spite of a high level of awareness about contraception. Among currently married women 96 percent are aware of at least one modern method of contraception yet only half of Pakistani women had ever used contraception; only 22 percent of married women said they were currently using a modern contraceptive method, and 8 percent were using less effective traditional methods.[24] This suggests that knowledge alone does not always translate into contraceptive use.

In the socio-structural context of Pakistan there are many factors potentially affecting fertility regulation. The extent of communication between husbands and wives, early marriage, early pregnancy, son preference, religious beliefs, female autonomy, family planning service and supply variables can all serve to limit women's access and even their willingness to use contraceptives. Instead, induced abortions appear to be a common and accepted choice for Pakistani women when they have an unwanted pregnancy. It is often the case that induced abortion increases simultaneously with increases in contraception, both satisfying increasing demand for fertility control.

Social Determinants of Health: The Challenge of Inequities

Gender disparities in the form of delayed access to health services, restrictions on women's mobility, domestic violence, and women's workload are central to poor maternal health outcomes. Although very important gender disparities, represent only one facet of disparities that plague Pakistani society. Given the state of health of the poor in Pakistan, there is a need to understand why Pakistan has not built on the foundation it received (unlike the development of the health sector by Sri Lanka which too was under the British rule). Identifying and monitoring inequities in Pakistan has yet to become rigorous or to become part of the formal discourse. Living in a rural area is itself associated with a greater risk for mortality than living in an urban area; being a woman places one at a higher risk than being a man, and being poor makes you more vulnerable than middle and high income individuals. It is thus not sufficient to focus on improving national averages. Instead the underlying disparities have to be targeted.

Poverty is the most reliable predictor of poor health, premature death and disability. The more equally wealth is distributed, the better the health of that society. Unfortunately, the disparity between rich and poor in Pakistan is growing which will only contribute to disparate health outcomes. According to the Human Development Index 2013, income inequality in Pakistan increased from 0.27 to 0.29 (Gini-coefficient) from 2000 to 2010. This indicates that Pakistan is trending in the wrong direction in terms of income disparity.

Thus far, national level programs have failed to address inequalities in access to maternal care between rural and urban women. In rural areas the maternal mortality ratio (MMR) is 319 per 100,000 of live births (LB), almost twice as high as that of urban areas which is 175 per 100,000 LB. An estimated 22.9 percent of deaths in rural women of reproductive age are due to pregnancy and child birth as compared to 14 percent among those in urban areas. Most of the deliveries take place at home usually without any assistance of a skilled birth attendant.

The Way Forward

Globally the gender perspective in health is now recognized: women have distinct health needs, and causes and outcomes differ by gender. Health inequities affect them the most. Pakistan needs to ensure equal treatment, overcome biases that impede well-being and desist from blunt, across-board solutions which often miss the mark and waste money. Instead Pakistan should undertake to enhance the sensitivity of its health systems to women's health issues along with ensuring appropriate gender sensitive medical care. The essential core of the Pakistan Safe Motherhood initiative should be an inter-sectoral multilevel programmatic framework that links the common women and men in the community, the obstetricians, midwives, nurses and educators and, is supported by a strong political commitment at the national level.[25]

The World Health Organization's "Global Strategy for Women's and Children's Health" recommends an integrated package of essential interventions and services for women and children delivered through functioning health systems.[26]

The WHOs Commission on Information and Accountability for Women's and Children's Health gave clear recommendations about what still needs to be done as we approach the 2015 deadline for achieving the MDG.[27] One such recommendation was that countries accomplish civil registration and keep records of all births, deaths, and marriages. It is the most basic of human rights to exist officially, but according to UNICEF only 27 percent of births were officially registered in Pakistan between 2000 and 2009. Moreover, Pakistan does not currently have a national policy requiring specific notification of maternal deaths. Without such records we are left dealing with data gaps and guess estimates of the magnitude of the maternal health crisis. Accurate data is essential to tracking trends in maternal health and evaluating the success of programs. Early marriage is a major concern in Pakistan, and a key strategy to saving women's lives, to delay their first pregnancy until they have reached adulthood, is dependent upon accurate birth data. It is, after all, harder to marry off a child if her age is known through proper documentation.[28]

Pakistan must also highlight the links between women's health and their social and economic circumstances. If as a society Pakistan is serious about making Pakistani women the healthiest people in the world, then we have to be serious about closing the gap between rich and poor via sustainable development programs that emphasize education and job training to help build a middle class.

The solution to the crisis in health human resources is not straightforward. Addressing the shortages in each district will involve a chain of cooperation and shared intent between the various stakeholders: the government of Pakistan, which is ultimately responsible for health service staffing, the private sector, and UN agencies and other donors. It is essential donors make financial and technical commitments to enhance the sustainability of health services to ensure successful projects are not simply closed down when the finances run out. Furthermore, there is a need for a comprehensive human resource strategy for emergency obstetric care (EmOC) particularly in rural areas. Task shifting of EmOC services has been effective in expanding access to care in South Asia. Doctors competent in providing EmOC are required to establish first referral units at district/tehsil level. Very few public sector obstetricians work in rural areas, but the infrastructure does exist. This gap can be filled by women medical officers. The Society of Obstetricians and Gynaecologists of Pakistan (SOGP) is prepared to take up the challenge and has proposed a program for training nonspecialist medical officers to provide EmOC in rural Pakistan where skilled obstetricians are not available.

To solve the problem of inadequate training a strong component of MNCH/Family planning in the curricula of all health professionals must be introduced and used uniformly across the country. Training of non-specialists including medical officers, nurses, LHVs, LHWs, FMTs, CMWs must all be improved and standardized. Investments in counseling skills must be made and trained specialists utilized appropriately.

The solution to the structural constraints between the ministry of health and population welfare will require a paradigm shift in family planning from a demographic objective to a reproductive health goal. Health and population policies have shared agendas, with maternal, child and reproductive health being core themes of both as well as common intervention paradigms. Therefore, the effective merger of the ministries of health and population welfare is imperative to reduce waste and duplication of effort as well as to align family planning and reproductive health into the more culturally acceptable paradigm, namely public health as opposed to population control. An FP package should be offered as part of a total MNCH package of services. A substantial amount of the funds of the population welfare department should be invested in female education. Programs must also emphasize greater involvement of the male partner in his wife's health.

It is important to note that both the Population Welfare Ministry's FWCs and the Health Ministry's BHUs have critical management issues, which are more critical in the short-term than attempts aimed at merging them. Institutional reorganization and reform of BHUs and FWCs should, therefore, be actively pursued. Rather than a merger of BHUs and FWCs, the integration of vertical programs which, at least in one province is underway, will ensure minimum service delivery including RH MNCH, immunization through the health system and other outlets. Any restructuring arrangement should group health and family planning into a set of services to be delivered by the agency mandated with service delivery responsibilities at the primary health care level.

A long-term commitment to reform is needed to realize the above mentioned changes. Over the short to medium-term, a number of measures should be undertaken to build capacity for the needed long-term changes—these centers on enunciation of a joint health, population and well being policy, broadening the remit of the NCPW, revitalizing the Joint Committee for Health and Population Welfare and exploring, where feasible, joint proposals for funding. Additional measures in the right direction include addressing governance issues at the level of requisitioning, procurements and supplies, where a significant collaboration is already underway and incorporating family planning into the mandate of the health sector; this can be done by further reinforcing family planning as a LHW mandate, augmenting the field force through appropriate linkages with male mobilizers and mobile service units, mandating synchronous communication campaigns and by fostering ownership of RHS-A centers in the health sector. The potential to develop bridges through training should also be capitalized. However, sustained political and institutional resolve will be needed to implement these recommendations.[29]

CONCLUSION

This chapter provides an overview of the status of maternal health in the entirety of Pakistan. However, to gain a more complete understanding of the situation one must be aware of the vast differences that exist between provinces, urban and rural areas, and income levels. One key difficulty in the endeavor is that there is often a lack of data specific to the populations most in need of maternal health intervention, such as those with an ongoing insurgency and IDP crisis. For example, data from FATA, some parts of KP province, and areas of Balochistan was not even included in the latest Demographic Health Survey. Thus, when Pakistan has been able to demonstrate significant progress on maternal health it is often based on very incomplete data gathered in areas that already have access to the best infrastructure in Pakistan.

Unlike the situation for disease-specific programs, for maternal and child health very little attention has been paid to monitoring progress and evaluating programs, even for the analysis and use of existing data. Policy decisions and program planning are therefore often carried out without evidence-based information and program evaluation.

A key constraint limiting progress is the gap between what is needed and what exists in terms of skills and geographical availability of human resources at provincial and district levels. Other challenges are how to address deteriorating infrastructures; how to maintain stocks of drugs, supplies and equipment in the face of increased demand; lack of transport; ineffective referral to and inadequate availability of 24-hour quality services—particularly emergency obstetric care services—and weak management systems. We need to challenge our policy-makers and program managers to refocus program content and to shift focus from development of new technologies towards development of viable organizational strategies that ensure a continuum of care and account for every birth and death.

The challenges Pakistan faces do not require new technologies or new knowledge about effective interventions; we mostly know what needs to be done to save the lives of mothers and newborns (Fig. 8).

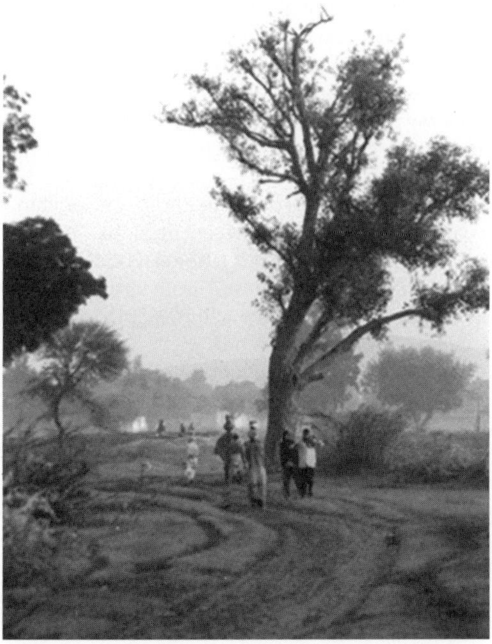

Fig. 8 A long journey ahead in Pakistan for safe motherhood

Effective health interventions exist for mothers and babies such use of misoprostol, magsulf, PPIUCD and several proven means of distribution can be used to put these in place. The crux of the challenge is how to deliver services and scale up interventions, particularly to access those who are vulnerable, hard to reach, marginalized or excluded. However, none will work if political will is absent where it matters most: at national and district levels.

REFERENCES

1. The Partnership for Maternal Newborn and Child Health. (2013). Knowledge Summary #24 The economic benefits of investing in women's and children's health. Retrieved from http://www.who.int/pmnch/knowledge/publications/summaries/knowledge_summaries_24_economic_case/en/index.html.
2. See for example Ministry of Finance, Government of Pakistan. (2003). Accelerating Economic Growth and Reducing Poverty: The Road Ahead. Islamabad, Pakistan; Government of Pakistan. (2005). Medium Term Development Framework. Islamabad, Pakistan; Government of Pakistan. (2007). Vision 2030. Islamabad, Pakistan.
3. Ministry of Population Welfare, Government of Pakistan. (2002). Population Policy. Islamabad, Pakistan; Ministry of Health, Government of Pakistan. (2001). National Health Policy 2001, The Way Forward. Islamabad, Pakistan.
4. United Nations Population Fund. (1994). Report of the International Conference on Population and Development United Nations. Re.trieved from http://www.un.org/popin/icpd/conference/offeng/poa.html
5. World Bank. (2013). Pakistan Data. Retrieved from: http://data.worldbank.org/country/pakistan.
6. Government of Pakistan. (2012). Constitution of Pakistan. Retrieved from http://www.pakistani.org/pakistan/constitution/.
7. Government of Pakistan. (2002). National Policy for Development and Empowerment of Women. Retrieved from http://sgdatabase.unwomen.org/uploads/National%20Policy%20for%20Development%20and%20Empowerment%20of%20Women.pdf.
8. United Nations. Millennium Development Goals Overview. Retrieved from http://www.un.org/millenniumgoals/; UNFPA. International Conference on Population and Development Overview. Retrieved from http://www.unfpa.org/public/icpd; United Nations. Fourth World Conference on Women Overview. Retrieved from http://www.un.org/womenwatch/daw/beijing/platform/; ECOSOC. (2009). Annual Ministerial Review Overview Retrieved from http://www.un.org/en/ecosoc/newfunct/amr2009.shtml/.
9. UNDP. (2013). Human Development Report-2013 The Rise of the South: Human Progress in a Diverse World. Retrieved from http://hdr.undp.org/en/content/human-development-report-2013.

10. Nishtar, Sania. (2010). Choked Pipes: Reforming Pakistan's Health System, Oxford University Press.
11. Akram, Muhammad and Faheem Jehangir Khan. (2007). Health Care Services and Government Spending in Pakistan. Pakistan Institute of Development Economics, Islamabad, Pakistan. Retrieved from http://www.pide.org.pk/pdr/index.php/wp/article/viewFile/2447/2420.
12. WHO. (2003). Investing in Health: A Summary of the Findings of the Commission on Macroeconomics and Health. Retrieved from: www.who.int/macrohealth/infocentre/advocacy/en/investinginhealth02052003.pdf.
13. Ibid Nishtar, Sania (2010).
14. Government of Pakistan. (2010). Development Amidst Crisis: Pakistan Millennium Development Goals Report 2010. Retrieved from http://www.undp.org/content/dam/pakistan/docs/MDGs/UNDP-PK-MDG-Pakistan-2010.pdf.
15. Government of Pakistan. (2013). Health, Nutrition and Population Annual Plan 2012-13. Islamabad, Pakistan.
16. UNICEF. (2011). Universal Children's Day - Children in Pakistan have the right to be counted. Retrieved from www.unicef.org/pakistan/media_7393.htm.
17. National Institute of Population Studies (NIPS) Pakistan and Macro International Inc. (2008). Pakistan Demographic and Health Survey 2006-07. Islamabad, Pakistan.
18. Government of Pakistan. (2010). Development Amidst Crisis: Pakistan Millennium Development Goals Report 2010. Retrieved from http://www.undp.org/content/dam/pakistan/docs/MDGs/UNDP-PK-MDG-Pakistan-2010.pdf.
19. UNICEF. (2012). Annual Report 2012 for Pakistan. Retrieved from http://www.unicef.org/about/annualreport/files/Pakistan_COAR_2012.pdf.
20. UNFPA. (2011). State of the World's Midwifery Pakistan Country Profile. Retrieved from www.unfpa.org/sowmy/resources/docs/country_info/profile/en_Pakistan_SoWMy_Profile.pdf.
21. UNICEF. (2009). The State of the World's Children. Retrieved from http://www.unicef.org/sowc09/docs/SOWC09-FullReport-EN.pdf.
22. Ministry of Population Welfare, Government of Pakistan. (2002). National Population Welfare Programme—Handing over note for Punjab. Islamabad, Pakistan.
23. Population Reference Bureau. (2013). World Population Data Sheet. Retrieved from http://www.prb.org/pdf13/2013-population-data-sheet_eng.pdf.
24. National Institute of Population Studies (NIPS) Pakistan and Macro International Inc. (2008). Pakistan Demographic and Health Survey 2006-07. Islamabad, Pakistan.
25. Fikree FF (2002). Safe Motherhood in Pakistan: Past Failures and Future Challenges. Journal of Pakistan Medical Association. Retrieved from ile:///Users/LubnaHassan/Desktop/safemotherhood%20in%20Pakistan%20/

Safe%20Motherhood%20in%20Pakistan:%20Past%20Failures,%20Future%20Challenges.webarchive.

26. United Nations Secretary General. (2010). Global Strategy for Women's and Children's Health. Retrieved from http://www.who.int/pmnch/topics/maternal/201009_globalstrategy_wch/en/index.html
27. World Health Organization. (2011). Commission on Information and Accountability for Women's and Children's Health. Keeping promises, measuring results. Geneva.
28. Stenberg, Karen, et al. (2013). Advancing social and economic development by investing in women's and children's health: a new Global Investment Framework. The Lancet. Retrieved from http://www.thelancet.com/journals/lancet/article/PIIS0140-6736(13)62231-X/fulltext.
29. Nishtar, Sania, et al. Synergizing health and population in Pakistan. 2009;59(9)Suppl.3:S-2.

5

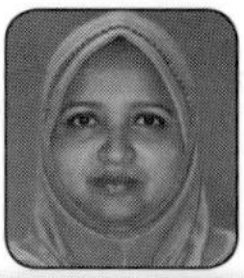

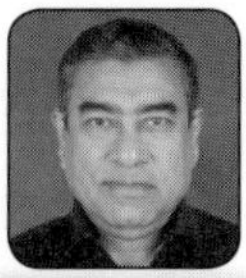

Achievements and Challenges for Safe Motherhood in Bangladesh

Fatema Shabnam, Abu Jamil Faisel

INTRODUCTION

Every 2 minutes a woman dies of causes related to pregnancy or childbirth. She is most likely to be young, already a mother, and living in a developing country. Women who survive is afflicted by disease, disability, or physical damage caused by pregnancy-related complications. Bangladesh is not far away from this situation, 194 mothers still dying per 100,000 births each year. Bangladesh has made progress in achieving certain family planning and maternal health indicators in the last three decades. Total fertility fell from 5.1 to 2.3 during the period 1989 to 2011, seven out of ten pregnant women have had at least one antenatal care (ANC) visit, 32 percent delivered with a medically trained provider, and one in three women received post-natal care (PNC) within two days of delivery. Though maternal mortality declined from 322 in 2001 to 194 in 2010, a 40 percent decline in nine years but this figure still has unexpectedly high.

Bangladesh has been taking different steps to draw attention to the dimensions and consequences of poor maternal health and to mobilize action to address high rates of death and disability caused by the complications of pregnancy and childbirth that was the objectives of the global Safe Motherhood Initiative launched in 1987.

SAFE MOTHERHOOD INITIATIVES

Bangladesh has a long history of maternal and child health (MCH) activities dating back to 1946 and the first MCH unit was established in the Directorate of Health in 1952 to 1953 (NIPORT et al. 2003). Throughout the time, various changes have been introduced in the provision of maternal health services like integration of MCH services in the health arena, the use of a community-based approach to providing maternal health services by training traditional birth attendants (TBAs), and a facility-based approach to safe motherhood with a primary focus on emergency obstetric care (EmOC) services.

The Bangladesh National Strategy for Maternal Health formulated in 2001 focused explicitly on EmOC based on three key considerations: all pregnant women are at risk of developing life-threatening complications, most complications can neither be predicted accurately nor prevented, and once a woman develops complications, she needs prompt access to EmOC services if death or disability is to be prevented.

During 2001 to 2011, following four special initiatives were introduced which have had a significant impact on the provision of maternal health services in the country.

Emergency Obstetric Care Programs/Interventions

In line with global goals for the provision of safe motherhood, the Government of Bangladesh (GOB) initiated an EmOC program during the 4th Population and Health Project (1992–1997, then extended to 1998). In 1994, the Ministry of Health and Family Welfare (MOHFW) began upgrading existing government facilities in a phased-in manner under two development projects: a UNICEF-funded EmOC project to strengthen district hospitals and selected upazila health complexes (UHCs) to provide comprehensive EmOC services, and a UNFPA-funded project to strengthen maternal and child welfare centers (MCWCs) to provide comprehensive EmOC services. In 2000, a national target was set for one comprehensive EmOC and four basic EmOC facilities per 500,000 population, per World Health Organization (WHO) global targets. Currently, all the Government of Bangladesh facilities provide comprehensive EmOC services at the district level and one-third sub-districts facilitates have been upgraded to provide comprehensive EmOC.

MOHFW—UN Joint Project on Maternal and Child Health Initiative

In 2006, the MOHFW of the GOB started the Joint GOB-UN-MNH initiative for "Accelerating Progress Towards Maternal and Neonatal Mortality and Morbidity Reduction". The overall goal of Maternal and Child Health Initiative (MNHI) is to reduce maternal and neonatal mortality and morbidity in Bangladesh with an emphasis on equity issues in order to achieve MDGs 4 and 5. In phase I (2006–2011), the program was implemented in four districts. In phase II (2011–2016), programs were implemented in seven districts and plan to expand the program into 13 other districts.

Demand Side Financing Maternal Health Voucher Scheme

The demand side financing (DSF) maternal health voucher scheme was initiated by the MOHFW with technical assistance from the WHO in 2006. The main objective of the program was to accelerate progress towards MDG 5 by stimulating increased utilization of maternal health services by the poor and other vulnerable groups in the community.

The vouchers cover the cost of three ANC visits, safe delivery at a facility or at home by skilled birth attendants, management of complications including the cost for cesarean sections from designated providers, and one postnatal check-up within six weeks of delivery. Users also receive reimbursement for transportation, referral and cash incentives for the mother's nutrition and a gift box for the newborn. In addition, the service providers receive benefits for providing services to the voucher beneficiaries. The DSF program has been expanded with financial support from the World Bank, DFID, and pool funding from HNPSP 2003 to 2010 and now covers 73 upazilas across different districts including Joint GOB–UN collaborative MNHI districts. Under the current Health Population Nutrition Sector Development Program (HPNSDP) 2011 to 2016, the DSF program will be scaled up in phases in other rural upazilas in Bangladesh.

Community Skilled Birth Attendant Program

A program called the "Skilled Birth Attendant Training Program" was initiated by the Directorate General of Health Services (DGHS) and the Obstetrical and Gynecological Society of Bangladesh (OGSB) during 2001 to 2002 with technical and financial assistance from WHO and UNFPA. The purpose of this program was to increase access to skilled attendance at birth and provision of ANC and PNC at home. Under the program, existing family welfare assistants (FWAs) and female health assistants (FeHAs) were trained in basic midwifery skills in order to provide home-based maternal health services in addition to their regular assignments. The program was initiated as pilot in 2003 provided training for 90 workers from six districts, which had a positive evaluation (Bhuiyan, 2005), the program was expanded gradually throughout the country. More than 8000 Community Skilled Birth Attendant (CSBA) Program have been trained so far. In the HPNSDP 2011 to 2016, although the emphasis is upon facility delivery, the CSBA training program will be expanded further, particularly for the geographically hard-to-reach areas and that will include private and NGO candidates along with public sector candidates.

OBSERVANCE OF NATIONAL SAFE MOTHERHOOD DAY

In 1997, Prime Minister Sheikh Hasina announced observance of the Safe Motherhood Day on May 28 every year with a view to enhancing awareness on mothers' health and prevent mothers' mortality. The main objective is to reduce maternal mortality rates of mothers and newborn babies establishing safe motherhood as a right for a woman. Since then the day is being observed with extensive program every year throughout the country. The day is started with a colorful procession at early morning with participation of the government and non-government organizations representatives. Important places and street intersections are decorated with colorful banners, placards and festoons to mark the day. Prime Minister distributes award among individuals and institutions of different districts, upazilas and community level health care bodies for providing special maternity services. Special services are provided to the expecting mothers at district hospitals, UHCs and MCWCs. Every year a theme is declared considering the Safe Motherhood initiatives."Take care expecting mother, prevent mother mortality" is the theme for this year 2013.

SAFE MOTHERHOOD CAMPAIGN

Safe Motherhood Campaign is a package of simple evidence based maternal and neonatal mortality reduction interventions that could be implemented throughout the country. A planning workshop was organized on 17th June, 2009, where 104 participants from government, development partners, national and international NGOs attended and developed the nucleus of the draft action plan.

The working group members divided themselves into several teams and developed action plan by interventions keeping in mind the five prioritize technical interventions areas and five domains. The plan was for all level starting from national level the community level (Figs 1A and B).

SUCCESS IN MATERNAL MORTALITY: REASONS FOR DECLINING

The risk of a maternal death is now down to 1 in 500 births. Programmatic effort goes to encourage all pregnant women to minimize risk by delivering with a skilled birth attendant, preferably in a facility, and under certain circumstances to have a C-section.

According to Bangladesh Maternal Mortality Survey (BMMS) 2001 the two major causes, accounting for over half of maternal deaths, were hemorrhage (29%) and eclampsia (24%). Both of these normally require management at facility by a medically trained provider. In BMMS 2010 it

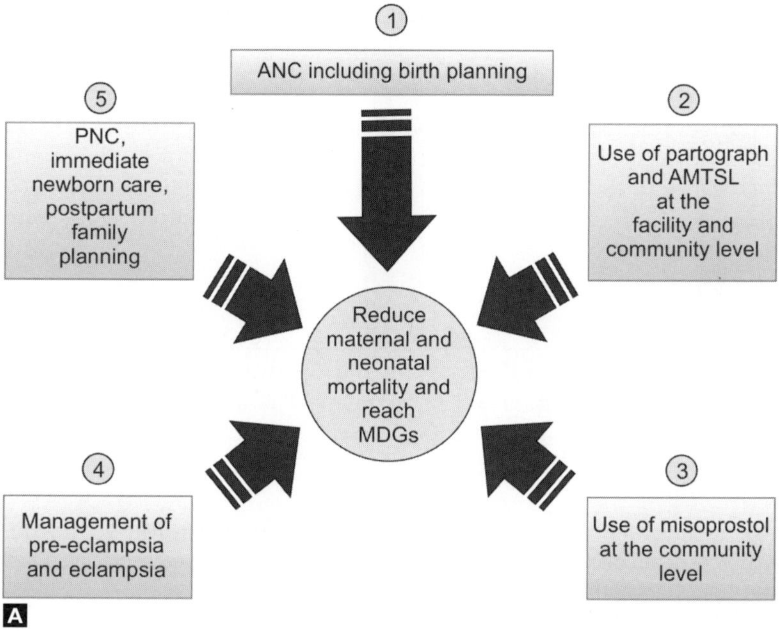

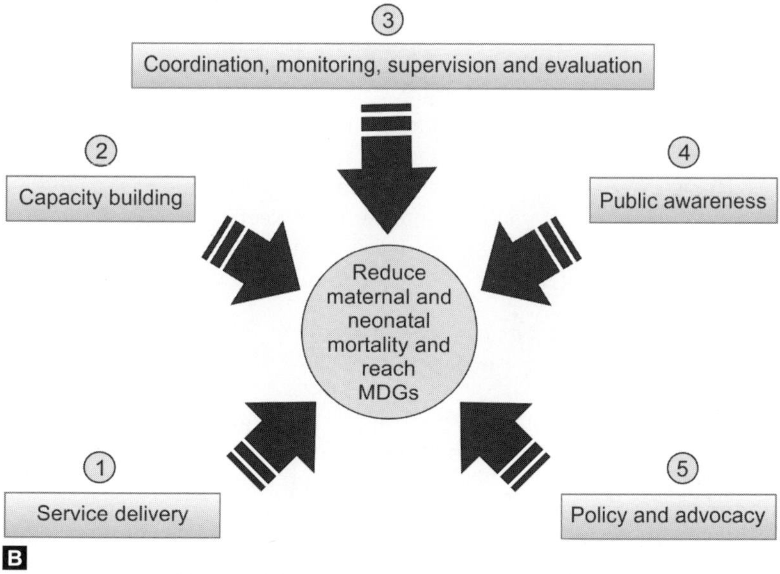

Figs 1A and B (A) Five prioritized technical interventions areas; (B) Five thematic domains. Action plan drafted on June 2009 to reduce maternal mortality

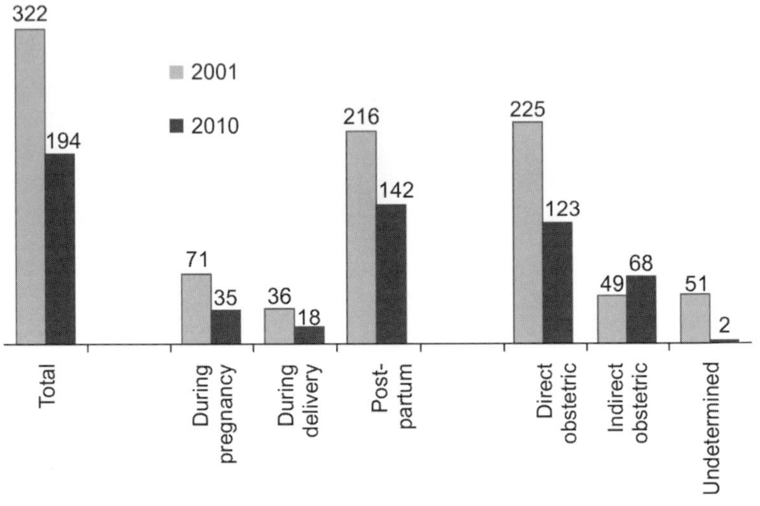

Fig. 2 Survey on maternal mortality in Bangladesh in between 2001–2010. Maternal death declined in all three periods. Direct obstetric deaths declined but not indirect obstetric deaths

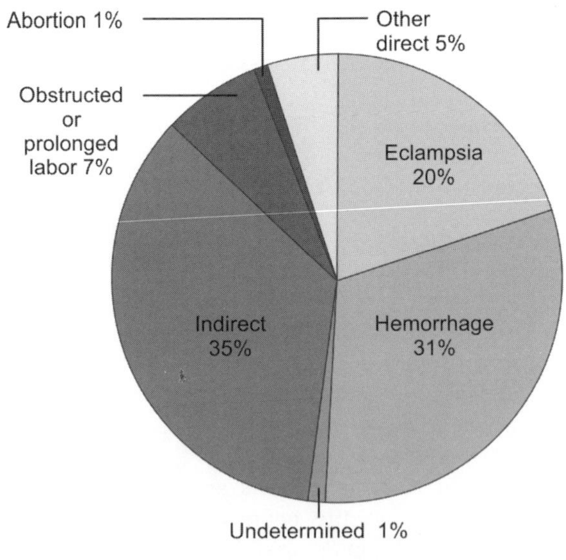

Fig. 3 Causes of maternal deaths in Bangladesh, (Bangladesh Maternal Mortality Survey)

is seen that very substantial declines have occurred in both these causes, a 35 percent reduction in hemorrhage and a 50 percent reduction in eclampsia. This implies greater use of facilities for delivery, and for management of obstetric complications. The entire decline in MMR has been due to reductions in direct obstetric deaths (Figs 2 and 3).

Reasons for Declining Maternal Mortality 40 percent by Nine Years

Behavior Change in Seeking Health Care

Facility Delivery

After persisting at historically low levels, the proportion of women delivering in a facility has finally begun to rise in the past decade, more than doubling from 9 percent in 2001 to 23 percent in 2010. Much of that increase has come through the private sector (2.7–11.3%).

Skilled Birth Attendant at Delivery (SBA)

As facility delivery has increased, it would be expected that births with SBA would increase, and it has doubled (12.2–26.5%). Only a small proportion of women use a medically trained provider to attend deliveries at home (4.4%) which has changed little since 2001 (3.5%). Almost the entire increase in skilled attendance at delivery has been through facility deliveries—which suggest that strategic investments in improving services at health facilities may provide the greatest and quickest returns in terms of skilled attendance at delivery.

While the rise in facility delivery is welcome, it still leaves some 2.4 million births at home annually. But the decline in maternal deaths suggests that many pregnancies with complications may now be selectively going to facilities, as is intended.

Treatment Seeking for Complications

There has been a substantial increase in women experiencing obstetric complications seeking treatment (53–68%). This includes home-based treatment, purchasing medicines from pharmacies, and treatment seeking outside the home. Seeking treatment from a facility has greatly increased (16–29%), indicating that both awareness and referral systems are improving. This positive trend is consistent across the economic scale. However, not all treatment seeking is effective; as the qualitative study showed that many of the maternal death cases sought treatment at a non-CEmOC facility which could not manage their problem (e.g. hemorrhage).

What Accounts for these Behavioral Changes?

Improved Access to Health Programs

It has been mentioned that a huge number of facilities are now providing comprehensive EmOC services. This definitely improved availability of maternal health care services within the district headquarters as well as the sub-district level (upazilas).

There is evidence from the qualitative study that better communications, particularly the widespread availability of mobile phones, has contributed to more rapid contact with service providers—though not always the desired medically qualified providers, as sometimes contact was made with village doctors who were unable to resolve obstetric complications. Overall, improvements in road communications seem to have increased the use of facilities, though further spatial analysis of travel times, etc. will be needed to confirm this. Health behaviors are not simply determined by the availability of facilities and services, but are also influenced by socioeconomic factors.

Higher Education Levels

Globally, higher female education is associated with behaviors which reduce the risk of maternal (and child) mortality. The investments made by the Government (and some NGOs) over the past several decades in female primary and secondary education are starting to show positive impacts on risk behaviors.The levels of education of recent mothers have risen dramatically in the past decade as well educated young women enter their childbearing years. The proportion of mothers with no education has halved since 2001, and the proportion with secondary schooling has nearly doubled. It is estimated that this trend alone has contributed to the impressive increases in facility delivery (25% of the increase), in the use of medically trained attendants at delivery (33%), and intreatment seeking for obstetric complications.

Increased Awareness

Not only are there fewer uneducated women giving birth, but among the uneducated, their awareness and behavior is changing positively. For example, seeking care for complications at a facility has doubled (8.6–16.9%) among uneducated women, while remaining unchanged among women with secondary plus education (56.1–52.2%). This differential improvement is reducing inequities by education.

Better Economic Conditions

Bangladesh has undergone an improvement in overall economic well-being since 2001 [gross national income (GNI) per capita up from $350 in 2000 to $550 in 2008], which is reflected in better housing, greater access to electricity, and presumably greater ability to mobilize funds for medical emergencies. This will be reflected in increases in many of the indicators among the poorest. Virtually all indicators of use of health services by the poorest quintile show considerable improvement and reductions in inequity between rich and poor, from a tripling of facility delivery (2.5% in 2001 to 7.5% in 2010), to use of medically trained assistance at delivery (3.6–9.2%), to seeking care for complications (7–15%).

Demographic Factors

Between BMMS 2001 and BMMS 2010 the total fertility rate fell from 3.2 to 2.5 that is a 22 percent decline in 9 years. The fall in fertility has some implications on reductions of risks of maternal deaths. The risk of maternal mortality increases as maternal age and order of the pregnancy rise. As fertility has fallen, the proportion of births to women of higher parities has fallen, e.g. birth order 4+ down from 30 to 19 percent. This shift away from high parity births, which are at high mortality risk, reduces the overall risk of maternal deaths.

Steps for the Next

Not a single death is desirable due to pregnancy but it has been happening as it is closely linked with pregnancy risks other socioeconomic conditions of the country. Bangladesh has made some progress and on the way to further progress in maternal health. Following are the areas government has undertaken and/or planning for actions considering the barriers and existing situations.

- As fertility reduction has been as important as MMR reduction to this point, future gains in maternal mortality may be achieved by ensuring effective family planning to lower fertility to replacement level and below, which will shift births away from high parity higher risk births.
- The trend of rising education levels among young women can be expected to bring behavior changes which favor more use of skilled birth attendants, more facility deliveries, and more and quicker treatment seeking for complications.
- The decline in direct obstetric deaths is most likely the consequence of better care-seeking practices and improved access to higher level referral care. The higher proportion of maternal deaths now contributed by postpartum deaths (73%, up from 67% in 2001)

suggest the need to prioritize the strengthening of access to treatment and improving referral systems and referral level care.

- On health interventions, the leading cause of maternal death in both surveys was hemorrhage and eclampsia. Several interventions have been tested and are being made available to reduce this problem, like use of misoprostol tablets to all pregnant women shortly after delivery of bady to minimize the risk of hemorrhage; use of delivery mats have proved to be effective at aiding attendants in determining if blood loss is excessive around delivery; use of magnesium sulfate for management of (pre-) eclampsia.
- It is necessary to understand the benefits of improved access to upgraded facilities at upazila and union levels. Plans are in place to expand such access, but staffing issues will need to be addressed, as well as essential logistics, including blood transfusion, being ensured. Finally, access for the poor is essential, and as relatively expensive interventions become more widely available, some kind of health insurance (possibly like DSF or another model) may be needed to overcome the fear of heavy costs of life saving obstetric procedures.

SPECIAL INITIATIVES FOR SAFE MOTHERHOOD

Distribution of Misoprostol at the Community

It has already mentioned that about 31 percent of maternal deaths are due to hemorrhage, mostly postpartum hemorrhage (PPH), which mainly occurs during the third stage of labor. The most common cause of PPH is uterine atony (70%), which can be managed effectively by practicing active management of the third stage of labor (AMTSL). One of the components of AMTSL is injection oxytocin. It is not possible to use this in a home setting, however, where deliveries are often assisted by unskilled birth attendants. In Bangladesh, 77 percent of pregnant women deliver at home (Streatfield et al. 2011). Alternatively, taking misoprostol orally immediately following the birth of a baby also reduces the occurrence of PPH. In 2006, the National PPH Prevention Task Force was formed under the guidance of the DGHS to coordinate efforts by the government, nongovernmental organizations (NGOs) and the public sector to prevent PPH and help facilitate the introduction of international best practices, in particular AMTSL and misoprostol use.

In May 2008, the Directorate of Drug Administration approved misoprostol as a means for PPH prevention and included it in the updated Essential Drug List. National PPH Prevention Task Force and Engender Health Bangladesh in collaboration with the Directorate

General of Family Planning (DGFP) and DGHS piloted Misoprostol at the community level in two districts in the period of 2008 to 2010. Upon successful completion of the pilots, MOH and FW developed a national scale-up plan, in collaboration with the National PPH Prevention Task Force and other partners. Misoprostol for the prevention of PPH was included in the operational plans of both DGHS and DGFP in the new health sector program, with implementation budget and distribution of misoprostol distributing has been incorporated in the government's management information system. The scale-up plan will be implemented in a phased way and began with six districts in July 2011.

Introducing and Scaling-up AMTSL at the Facilities

Before 2006 little was known about the actual practice of AMTSL in Bangladesh and it was decided that before introducing this evidence-based practice, it would be important to assess current practice. In 2008, a National Assessment was conducted in nine randomly selected sample districts by the National PPH Prevention Task Force and Engender Health (Al-Sabir et al, 2008). Based on the findings and recommendations of the national assessment following steps were taken in collaboration DGHS, DGFP and PPH Task force to correctly practice all steps of *AMTSL at every vaginal delivery* including proper storage of oxytocin:

- Training of the all maternity providers throughout the country
- Orientation for the community skilled birth attendants (CSBAs)
- Followed-up the trained providers to ensure that they apply their AMTSL skills
- Issuance a government circular to ensure a system of on-the-job training for the newly recruited and untrained maternity service providers by the skilled and trained service providers who already received AMTSL training
- Issuance of circular for proper storage of injection oxytocin.

Box 1 summarize improvement in adherence to *protocol* of active management of 3rd stage of labor.

Box 1: Comparison AMTSL Situation: 2008–2013

AMTSL element assessed	*2008 national survey findings*	*2013 service delivery audit findings*
• Number of deliveries observed	• 478 deliveries in 78 facilities	• 91 deliveries in 35 facilities
• Injection oxytocin used in third stage of labor	• 83%, but use not consistent at correct time and by intramuscular route	• 100%, and consistent in time and intramuscular route

Contd...

Contd...

AMTSL element assessed	2008 national survey findings	2013 service delivery audit findings
• Use of all three components of AMTSL	• 16%	• 89%
• Availability of oxytocin	• 76%	• 100% (either in facility or nearby shop)
• Correct oxytocin storage in refrigerator	• 4%	• 100% for those facilities that have a refrigerator (50% of facilities were not found to have a refrigerator and/ or not have oxytocin stored there)

Strengthening Partograph

Prolonged labor and obstructed labor contributes 7 percent of maternal mortality; they can lead to ruptured uterus, postpartum hemorrhage, infection, obstetric fistula, and fetal injury or death.

The incidence of obstetric fistula in Bangladesh is not known. A study conducted by GOB, UNFPA and EngenderHealth Bangladesh in 2003 showed a prevalence of 1.69 per 1000 ever married women and a total of about 71000 patient with such condition. With a MMR of 194/100000 life birth and about 7300 women dying annually gives a projection of about 2000 new cases of obstetric fistula. One of the tools used to monitor labor and prevent prolonged and obstructed labor is the partograph. However, this useful tool is underutilized in many low-resource settings including Bangladesh.

In Bangladesh with the funding of USAID, an advisory committee led by Professor Dr Latifa Shamsuddin, current president of Obstetrical and Gynecological Society, Bangladesh (OGSB) formulated few action plans to strengthening partograph. Committee has undertaken a baseline situation analysis at the five different health facilities where EmOC training had taken. Based on field visit findings advisory committee drafted a simplified version of modified WHO partograph. Now the next planning is to disseminate simplified partograph at all levels of health facilities through Govt. There is a plan to involve OGSB to take the lead to training of the providers. Supportive supervision, data collation and chart review, monthly perinatal mortality meeting/verbal autopsy are also taking into account to strengthen partograph use.

FERTILITY AND FAMILY PLANNING

Maternal and Child Health (MCH) Based Family Planning Program

The Government of Bangladesh merged Maternal and Child Health (MCH) services program with family planning in 1975 with a view to organize MCH based family planning program. The merger was based on the philosophy that provision of effective MCH services would improve the health of the mothers and children leading to a reduction in the prevalence of maternal and infant morbidity and mortality. If a pregnant woman is followed through her prenatal and postnatal period, it is likely that the women would enjoy good health and deliver a healthy baby. Such a mother would have effective lactation and would be able to give better attention to her newly born baby and thus would increase the probability of survival of her baby. This, in turn, is expected to encourage the woman to limit her fertility.

Family planning is one of the pillars of safe motherhood. It has been shown that 25 percent reduction of maternal mortality has attained due decline of fertility. Use of contraception is not only important to prevent unwanted but also for minimize the risk of pregnancy, spacing and delaying pregnancy that is needed to improve overall situation of the maternal health.

Figures 4A and B show the achievement in contraceptive use and birth order of a woman.

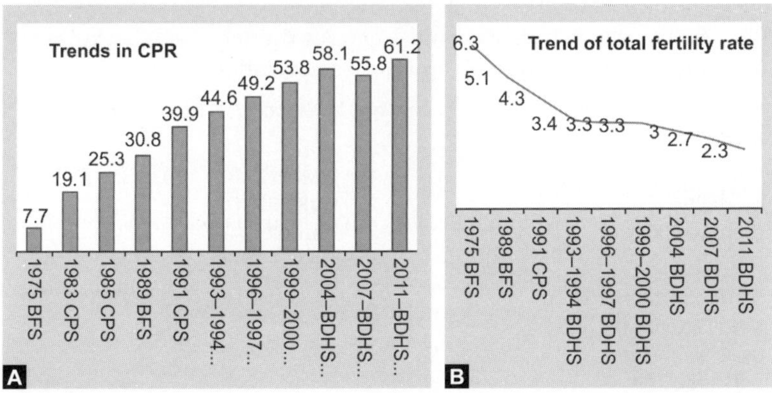

Figs 4A and B (A) Increasing contraceptive prevalence rate in Bangladesh from 1995–2011; (B) Declining trends in total fertility rate in Bangladesh from 1975–2011

Adolescent Fertility and Motherhood

Adolescent fertility in Bangladesh occupies a prime place in the design and implementation of reproductive health strategies, policies, and programs. The issue of adolescent fertility is important for both health and social reasons. First, children born to very young mothers are normally prone to higher risks of illness and death. Second, adolescent mothers are more likely to experience complications during pregnancy and are less likely to be prepared to deal with them, which can lead to maternal death. Third, early entry into reproduction denies young women the opportunity to pursue basic and further academic goals which is detrimental to career prospects. In Bangladesh 21 percent of adolescent women (age 15–19) in Bangladesh are already mothers with at least one child and 6 percent are currently pregnant, for a total of 27 percent who have started childbearing (BMMS 210).

MDG 5 AND BANGLADESH SITUATION

MDG 5 at a Glance

Box 2 summarizes the achievement of maternal health indicators from 1991 to 2011. Bangladesh despite its political instability, nature adversity like flood and poverty has been successful in reducing maternal morbidity and mortality as well total fertility rate.

Box 2 Base year 1990/91, current status and target by 2015

Goal, targets and indicators (as revised)	*Base year 1990/1991*	*Current status*	*Target by 2015*
MDG 5: Improve maternal health			
Target 5.A: Reduce by three quarters, between 1990 and 2015, the maternal mortality ratio			
5.1: Maternal mortality ratio (per 100,000 live births)	574	194 (BMMS 2010) 209 (SVRS 2011) 218 (Sample census, 2011 BBS)	143
5.2: Proportion of births attended by skilled health personnel (%)	5.0	31.7 (BDHS 2011)	50

Contd...

Contd...

Goal, targets and indicators (as revised)	*Base year 1990/1991*	*Current status*	*Target by 2015*
Target 5.B: Achieved by 2015, universal access to reproductive health			
5.3: Contraceptive prevalence rate (%)	39.7	61.2 (BDHS 2011) 58.4 (SVRS 2010)	72
5.4: Adolescent birth rate (per 1,000 women)	77	118 (BDHS 2011) 59 (SVRS 2010)	–
5.5: Antenatal care coverage (at least one visit and at least four visit) (%)			
5.5a: Antenatal care coverage (at least one visit) (%)	27.5	67.7 (BDHS 2011)	100
5.5b: Antenatal care coverage (at least one visit) (%)	5.5 (1993–94)	25.5 (BDHS 2011)	50
5.5b: Unmet need for family planning (%)	21.6 (1993–94)	13.5 (BDHS 2011)	7.6

Maternal Mortality

Maternal mortality declined from 322 in 2001 to 194 in 2010, a 40 percent decline in 9 years. The rate of decline was at an average of about 5.5 percent per year, compared to the average annual rate of reduction of 5.4 percent required for achieving MDG 5. Bangladesh appears to be on track to achieving the primary target of MDG 5 (Fig. 5).

Challenges to Achieving the Targets

- Inadequate coordination between health, family planning and nutrition services prevent the effective use of limited resources and frequently result in inefficiencies and missed opportunities.
- Human resource capacities remain a major obstacle to quality health service delivery. Key challenges include acute shortage of manpower of all categories, insufficient skills-mix and insufficient numbers of health workers especially in the rural areas.
- Further progress with CPR will require consistent and reliable access to contraceptives to reduce unmet need and dropout rates.

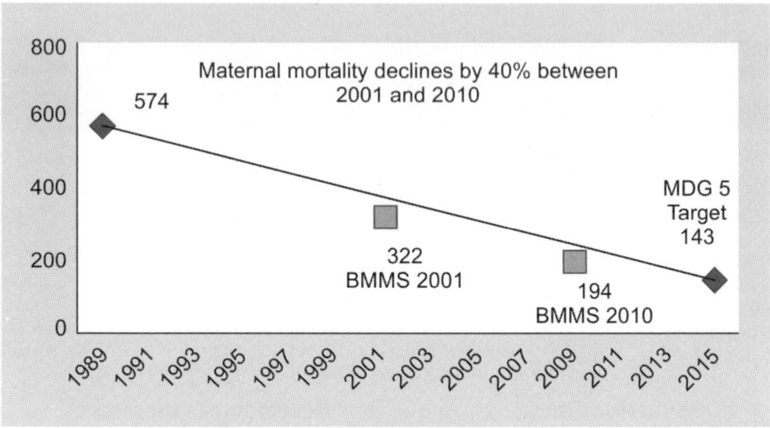

Fig. 5 Declining maternal mortality in Bangladesh from 1989–2011

- Overall, public spending on health has remained relatively low due, in part, to conditionality in project aid and government procedures. Allocation of public resources continue to be based on historical norms for facilities and staffing, rather than on accurate indicators of individual and household health needs, incidence of poverty, disease prevalence and population.
- Despite expansion of physical facilities, use of public health facilities by the poor remains low due to supply-side barriers such as lack of human resource capacities, inadequate drug supplies and logistics, and management inadequacies.
- Underlying socio-cultural factors contribute to the lack of knowledge about maternal health complications among women and families. Social marginalization, low socioeconomic status of women and lack of control over their personal lives make it difficult for many women to seek reproductive health care. Other contributing factors include early marriage and child bearing, poor male involvement in reproductive health issues and poor community participation in issues relating to maternal health.
- For all indicators, with the exception of CPR, significant disparities is observed in terms of the services women receive according to rural/urban residence, mother's education level, household wealth status and geographic location. It remains a big challenge to reduce the regional disparities.
- The legal age of marriage in Bangladesh is 18 years for women, but a large proportion of marriages still take place before the legal age.

Hence enforcement of *The Child Marriage Restraint Act 1984* remains a big challenge for Bangladesh.

Way Forward

To achieve the MDG5 goal and targets, Bangladesh must effectively address the three pillars within the health care system for reducing maternal deaths. These include: family planning, skilled birth attendants and emergency obstetric care.

- The life cycle approach should be used to address the general and reproductive health needs of women and to ensure reproductive health and rights in all phases of life. Essential health services should be provided in an integrated manner.
- Strong government commitment through national policies and program implementation needs to be continued for reduction in maternal mortality in Bangladesh.
- A holistic population planning program that addresses the challenges of the future and taking lessons from the past should be contemplated to attain replacement fertility by 2015 for population stabilization. The promotion of contraceptives along with FP services should continue and be expanded to poor and marginalized population in both rural and urban areas to respond to unmet needs. Procurement and supply management should be strengthened to avoid contraceptive shortages. Long-acting and permanent reproduction control methods should be promoted to increase the CPR and ensure further decline in the total fertility rate.
- The vast network of state facilities should be strengthened for appropriate women, adolescents and reproductive health service delivery for better utilization of MH/RH services. A mainstreamed nutrition program should target adolescents, particularly girls. Adolescents should be provided with required life-skills education and access to accurate information about health issues.
- Comprehensive EmOC facilities should be expanded by establishing such facilities in more upazila health complexes. More community skilled birth attendants (SBA) should be trained.
- The demand of ANC, institutional delivery or delivery by trained personnel, PNC should be created through strengthened health promotion involving community and different stakeholders.
- Communities should be mobilized to stimulate demand, improve care seeking behaviors and overcoming barriers to access health care. Door to door service providing may also be encouraged for greater participation.

- DSF schemes have also contributed to positive results. A recent evaluation reveals that DSF programmers have had an unprecedented positive effect on utilization of safe maternal health services by poor pregnant women, including ANC, delivery by qualified providers, emergency obstetric and postnatal care. The DSF can be expanded to all areas of Bangladesh with some modifications.
- In support of the Human Resource Development Master Plan for 2010 to 2040 to close large human resource gaps over the next 10 years, the government will need to focus on the following areas:
  - Reviewing the skills mix and deployment model for midwifery/ MH/RH services.
  - Improving the quality of education and training of health workers especially midwifes.
  - Ensure necessary regulations to protect the public from unsafe and incompetent care.
  - Addressing recruitment, career development, performance management, and retention issues to reduce staff shortages, particularly in rural areas.

CONCLUSION

The safe motherhood initiative is a worldwide effort that aims to increase attention to and reduce the devastating numbers of women that suffer death or serious illness every year. Women have the right not only to survive childbirth, but for it to be an enjoyable, rewarding and affordable experience. Making motherhood safe for the women, Bangladesh governments, funding agencies, and non-governmental organizations need to make maternal health an urgent health priority and to ensure that the necessary political and financial support is dedicated to this effort.

BIBLIOGRAPHY

1. Bangladesh Demographic and Health Survey 2007 (BDHS 2007).
2. Bangladesh Demographic and Health Survey 2011 (BDHS 2011).
3. Bangladesh Maternal Mortality Survey 2001 (BMMS 2001).
4. Bangladesh Maternal Mortality Survey 2010 (BMMS 2010).
5. Community-Based Misoprostol Distribution to prevent Postpartum Hemorrhage in Bangladesh: From Pilot to Scale, Program Brief # 03, January 2012, the Respond project under USAID.
6. Consultancy Report (draft), Strengthening Use of Partograph and Standardizing C-Section Indications, Fistula Care, EngenderHealth Bangladesh.

7. Factors Affecting Utilization of MCH Services in Bangladesh. Begum Zainab, Sayma Sharmin, M. Nurul Islam.
8. Family Planning Program Review, Eleanor Randall, January 2012.
9. Maternal, Neonatal and Child Health Program in Bangladesh. Review of good practices and lesson learned, July 2007, Hashima-e-Nasreen, Sayed Masud Ahmed, Hosne Ara Begum, Kaosar Afsana.
10. Millennium Development Goals, Bangladesh Progress Report, General Economics Division (GED), Bangladesh Planning Commission, Government of the People's Republic of Bangladesh, June 2013.
11. Presentation of National Workshop on Safe Motherhood Campaign, Bangladesh, 17 June 2009.
12. Project documents, Mayer Hashi, EngenderHealth Bangladesh.
13. Safe Motherhood, Evaluation Report, Number 15, UNFPA.
14. Special Issue: Safe Motherhood, OUT LOOK, July 1998.
15. The Safe Motherhood Action Agenda: Priorities for the Next Decade, Report on the Safe Motherhood Technical Consultation, 18–23 October 1997, Colombo, Sri Lanka.

6

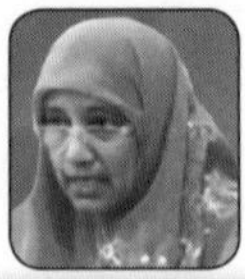

Changing Trends and Track in Bangladesh for Safe Motherhood

Ferdousi Begum

INTRODUCTION

The lives of women who get pregnant are unanchored in the sea of uncertainly, whose sorrows never sad enough, whose lives never important enough, are from all socioeconomic back grounds and are of all ages. But those who are encompassed by the vicious circle of poverty are suffering the most. During pregnancy there may be many complication which results in disability and even death if early signs are not noticed or more tragically not heeded.

Maternal mortality represents the tragic, untimely and often unnecessary end to a women's life. For us maternal mortality is not merely an abstract statistics which represents 1.94 women per thousand live births. Maternal mortality all too often is an extremely painful memory of a personal loss. It is the reminder of a face, a person lost in their prime of life. It is real risk that all women are subjected to during each pregnancy.

Maternal mortality rate (MMR) is a key indicator of progress and development of a society. On one side MMR represents the end point of a life time experience of gender discrimination. On the other hand the existence of high MMR represents the failure of the health system to effectively provide services and care for people, woman in particular. In the twenty first century maternal mortality is not a mystery. We have the tools and technology to save them.

Bangladesh is one of the new independent countries which suffered a lot of political instability and natural disaster. Despite that government, bureaucracy and health delivery system have made many policies and program which is showing in gradually reduction in maternal morbidity and mortality. Figure 1 shows the geographical and demographic characteristics of Bangladesh.

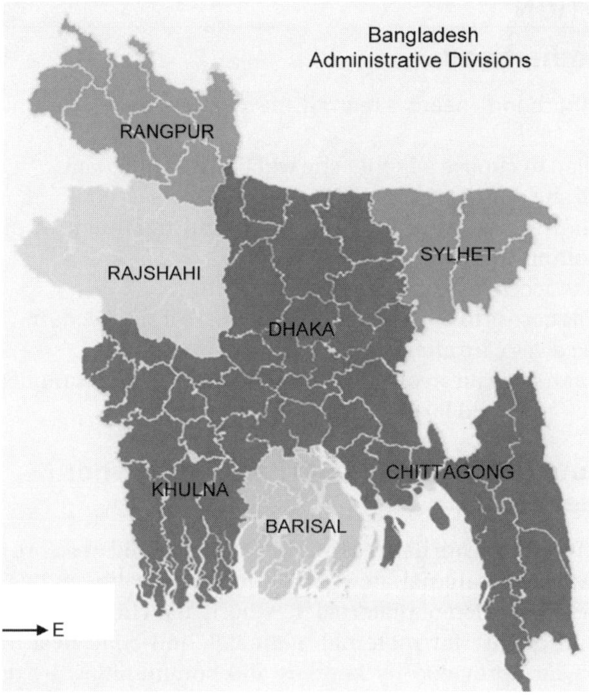

Demographics

- Area: 147,570 sq km
- Population: 150 million
- Population density: 1000/sq km
- Overall literacy rate: 50 percent
- Per capita income: US$ 600
- Life expectancy: 66.7 years
- Maternal morality ratio: 194/100000 LB
- Contraceptive prevalence rate: 62 percent
- Total fertility rate: 2.3
- Unmet need for family planning: 12 percent
- Antenatal care coverage (At least 1 visit): 67.7 percent
- Antenatal care coverage (At least 4 visit): 25.5 percent
- Delivery in health facility: 28.8 percent
- Delivery by medically trained person: 31.7 percent
- Postnatal care coverage (Within 2 days): 27 percent
- Met need (%) of Obst care in EmOC facilities: 70 percent
- Caesarean section (%) in the EmOC facilities: 12 percent
- Case fatality rate: 0.7 percent

Census 2011, BMMS 2010, BDHS 2011, DGHS 2012.

Fig. 1 Demographic characteristic of Bangladesh *(for color version see Plate 4)*

DEFINITION

Safe Motherhood

Safe motherhood means creating the circumstances within which a woman is:

- Enabled to choose whether she will become pregnant,
- And if she does, ensuring that:
  - she receives care for prevention and treatment of pregnancy complications,
  - has access to trained birth assistance,
  - has access to emergency obstetric care if she needs it,
  - receives care after birth,

So, that she can avoid death or disability from complications of pregnancy and child birth.

Continuum of Care for Maternal, and Newborn, Child Health

The continuum of care has recently been highlighted as a core principle of programs for maternal, newborn, and child health, and as a means to reduce the burden of maternal, newborn and children's deaths. The continuum of care for maternal, neonatal, and child health requires access to care provided by families and communities, by outpatient and outreach services, and by clinical services throughout the lifecycle, including adolescence, pregnancy, childbirth, the postnatal period, and childhood. Saving lives depends on high coverage and quality of integrated service-delivery packages throughout the continuum, with functional linkages between levels of care in the health system and between service-delivery packages, so that the care provided at each time and place contributes to the effectiveness of all the linked. The concept of continuum of core and its situation in Bangladesh are shown in Figure 2 (Kerber KJ, 2007).

ACHIEVEMENTS AND LACUNA

Bangladesh has made remarkable progress in the health sector over the last twenty years through effective implementation of health population sector program (HPSP) and health nutrition population sector program (HNPSP). All these improvements are evidenced by the findings of successive *Bangladesh Demographic and Health Surveys 2011* (BDHS) and *Bangladesh Maternal Mortality Survey 2010* (BMMS). But still there is long way to go. The brighter side of achievement is often shadowed by the yet high maternal and neonatal mortality and morbidity, prevailing

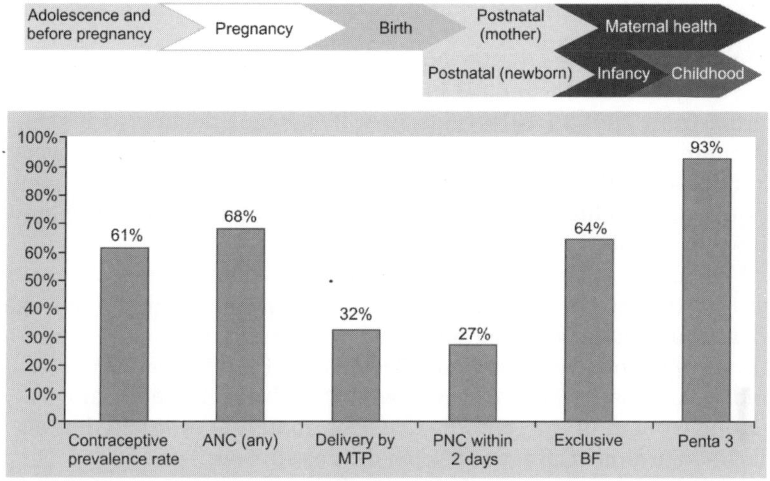

Fig. 2 Status of continuum of care for maternal, and newborn, child health in Bangladesh

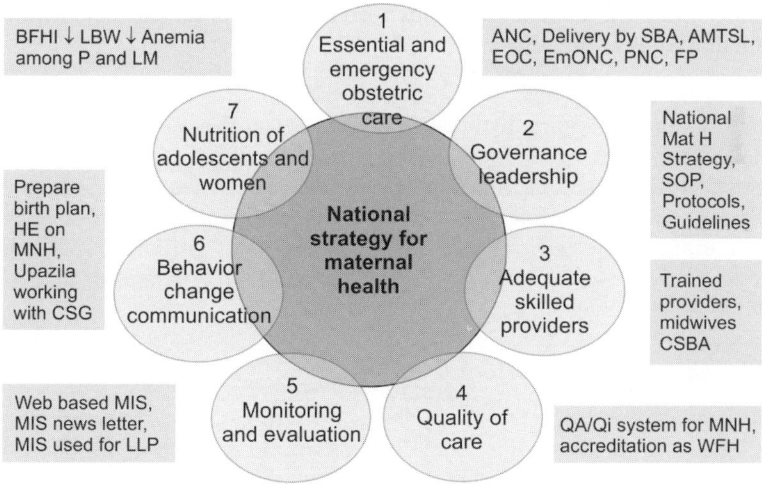

Fig. 3 Maternal health strategy in Bangladesh

malnutrition and its consequences on mother, child and society as a whole. Figure 3 shows the comprehensive maternal health strategy in Bangladesh.

Maternal Mortality

Bangladesh appears to be on track to achieve MDG5. Maternal mortality declined from 322 in 2001 to 194 in 2010 per 100,000 live births from 2001 to 2010 (Fig. 4) A 40 percent decline in 9 years. The rate of decline was at an average of about 5.5 percent per year, compared to the average annual rate of reduction of 5.4 percent required for achieving MDG5. The risk of a maternal death is now down to 1 in 500 births.

The major causes of maternal deaths are hemorrhage, eclampsia, and obstructed or prolonged labor (BMMS 2010). While hemorrage and eclampsia accounting for over half of maternal deaths (Fig. 5). This proportion was same in the BMMS 2001 (hemorrhage 29 percent and eclampsia 24%). Consistent with the trend in overall mortality among women in the reproductive ages, maternal mortality has also declined in almost all ages between the two surveys. The entire decline in MMR has been due to reductions in direct obstetric deaths. However mortality due to indirect obstetric causes has increased somewhat (Fig. 6).

The high MMR directly relates to the high perinatal (newborn) mortality rate in the country. The tragic consequence of these deaths is that about 75 percent of the babies born to these women, also die within the first week of their lives.

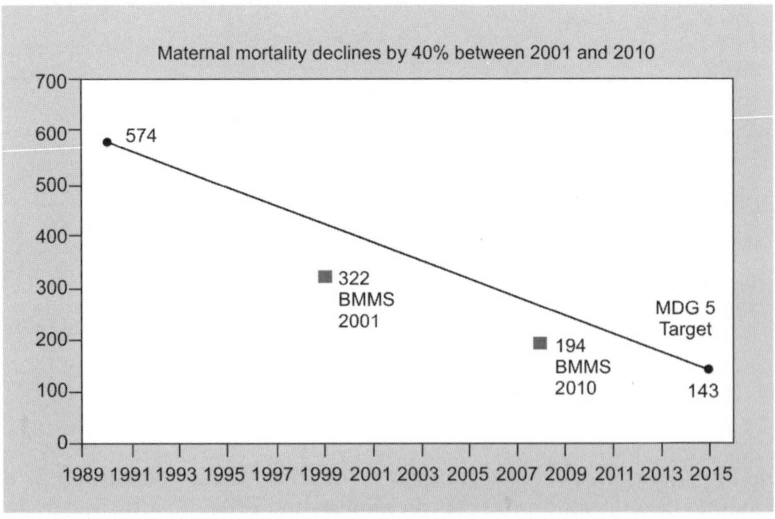

Fig. 4 Trend in maternal mortality rate (MMR) in Bangladesh

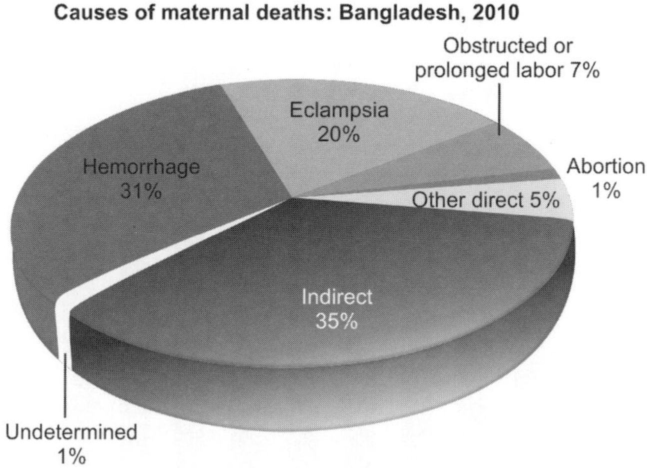

Fig. 5 Causes of maternal mortality in Bangladesh

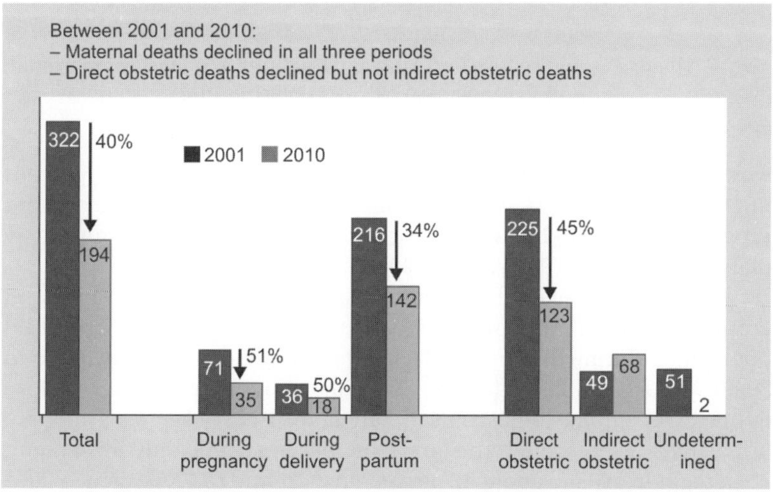

Fig. 6 Reduction of maternal mortality by cause in Bangladesh

Fertility and Fertility Regulation

Use of contraception among married women in Bangladesh has increased gradually, from 8 percent in 1975 to 61 percent in 2011, a greater than sevenfold increase in fewer than four decades (Fig. 7, Table 1). Unmet need increased from 15 percent of currently married

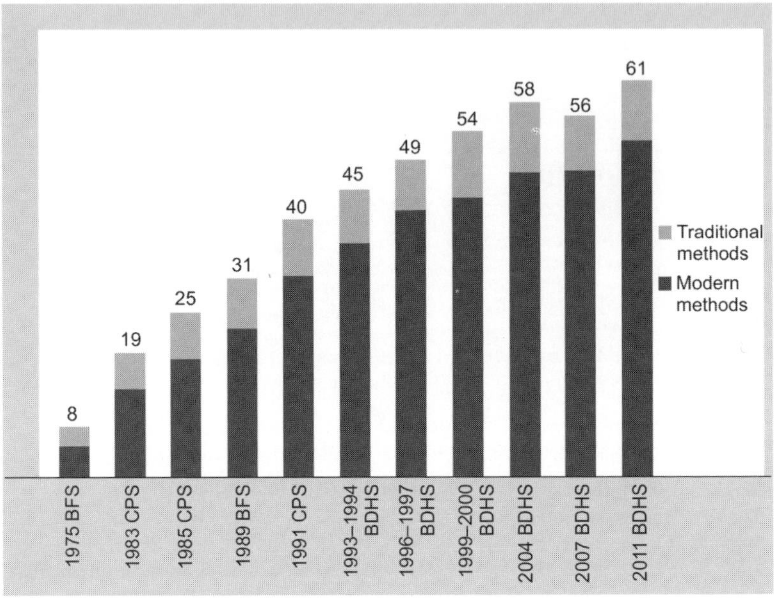

Fig. 7 Trends in contraceptive (in %) use among currently married women age 10–49, in Bangladesh 1975–2011 (BDHS 2011)

women in 2004 to 17 percent in 2007 and then decreased to 14 percent in 2011 (Fig. 8). The Health Population Nutrition Sector Development Program (HPNSDP) has set as a target reducing unmet need for family planning services to 9 percent by 2016.

Following a decade-long plateau in fertility during the 1990s, at around 3.3 births per woman, the TFR declined further by one child per woman during the current decade to reach 2.3 births per woman in 2009-2011 (BDHS 2011) (Fig. 9). Knowledge of contraceptives is close to universal among adolescents in Bangladesh. However, user rates are not as high, even though they have increased significantly from about 25 percent in 1993 to about 42 percent in 2007 and to 47 percent in 2011 among 15-19 year olds. Bangladesh's current health sector program, the Health, Population and Nutrition Sector Development Program (HPNSDP) 2011-2016 aims to reduce fertility to 2 births per woman by 2016. Khulna (1.9 births per woman) has reached that level already, and Rajshahi and Rangpur are very close (2.1 births per woman) (Fig. 10). The long history of family planning activities in Bangladesh is shown in Table 2.

Table 1 Millennium development goal 5: Goal, target and indicator

Goal 5: Improvement of maternal health	*Base year 1990/1991*	*Mid-term report 2007*	*Current status*	*Target by 2015*
Target 5.A: Reduce by three quarters, between 1990 and 2015, the maternal mortality ratio.				
5.1 Maternal mortality ratio, per 100,000 live births	574 (1990)	290 (2006)	194 (2010)	143
5.2 Proportion of births attended by skilled health personnel, percent	5.0	20 (2006)	32 (2011)	50
Target 5.B: Achieve, by 2015, universal access to reproductive health.				
5.3 Contraceptive prevalence rate, percent	39.7	58.1 (2004)	61.2 (2011)	–
5.4 Adolescent birth rate, per 1000 women		77	59 (2007)	–
5.5a Antenatal care coverage (at least one visit), percent		27.5 (1993)	67.7 (2011)	100
5.5b: Antenatal care coverage (at least four visits), percent	5.5 (1993)		25.5 (2011)	100
5.6 Unmet need for family planning, percent	19.4 (1993)		12 (2011)	9 (2016)

Indicator 5.1 (BMMS, 2001 and 2010) Indicator 5.4, (SVRS, 2007); Indicator 5.2, Indicator 5.3, Indicator 5.5, Indicator 5.6 (BDHS)

About two-thirds of couples in six of the seven divisions are protected from pregnancy either by FP or by husbands' absences. However Sylhet and Chittagong divisions are behind and need attention (Fig. 11).

Maternal Health

Sixty-eight percent of women with a birth in the three years preceding the Bangladesh Demographic and Health survey 2011, received antenatal care at least once from a provider. However, only 26 percent of those mothers make at four plus visits. The majority of women (55%) received care from a medically-trained provider, that is, a qualified doctor, nurse, midwife, paramedic, family welfare visitor (FWV), community skilled birth attendant (CSBA), medical assistant (MA), or sub-assistant community medical officer (SACMO) (Figs 12 and 13, Table 1).

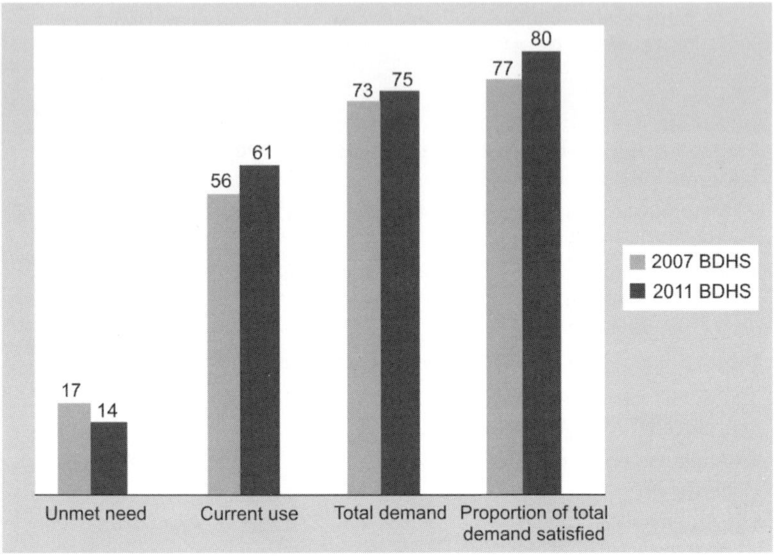

Fig. 8 Trends in unmet need for family planning (in %) among currently married women age 15–49, 2007 and 2011 BDHS in Bangladesh

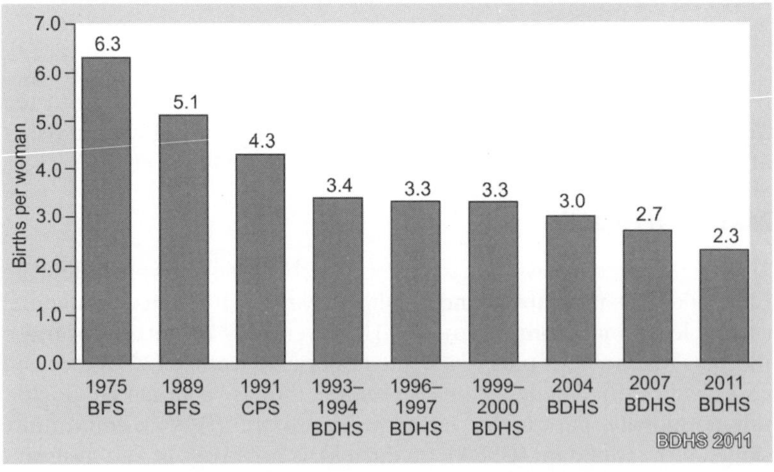

Fig. 9 Trend in total fertility rate in Bangladesh

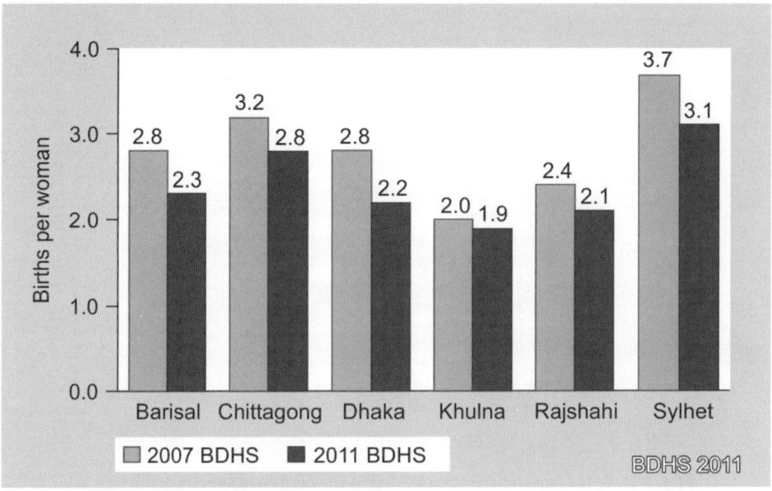

Note: Rangpur division TFR2.1 (BDHS 2011)

Fig. 10 Total fertility rate by division in different regions of Bangladesh

Table 2 History of family planning in Bangladesh

Period	*Activity /Program*
1953–59	Voluntary activities
1960–64	Clinic based Family Planning Program under GoB initiative
1965–70	Government Family Planning Program at field level
1972–74	Integrated Health and Family Planning
1975–78	MCH program Multipurpose Family Planning Program
1978–80	Development of the structure of Integrated Health and Family Planning Program from Thana and downwards
1980–85	Unified program at field level
1985–90	Family planning by community participation
1990–95	Intense FP care program
1995–98	Preparatory phase for 5th Health and Family Planning Program
1998–2003	Health and Population Sector Program (HPSP)
2003–2011	Health, Nutrition and Population Sector Program (HNPSP)
2011–2016	Health, population, Nutrition Sector Development Program (HPNSDP)

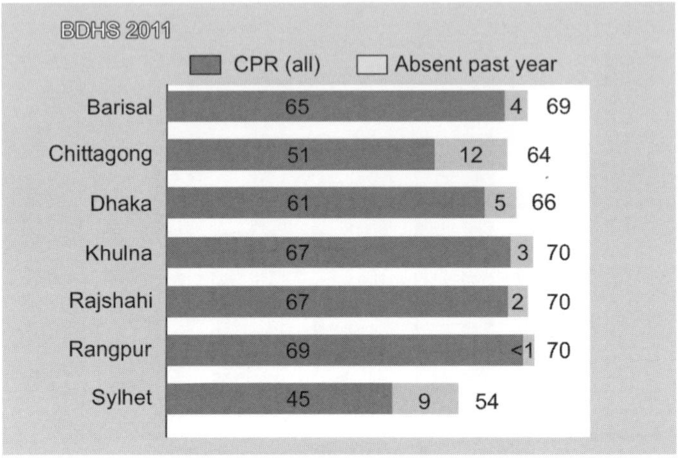

Fig. 11 Total protection (%) FP from FP and husband's absence in past year by division in Bangladesh

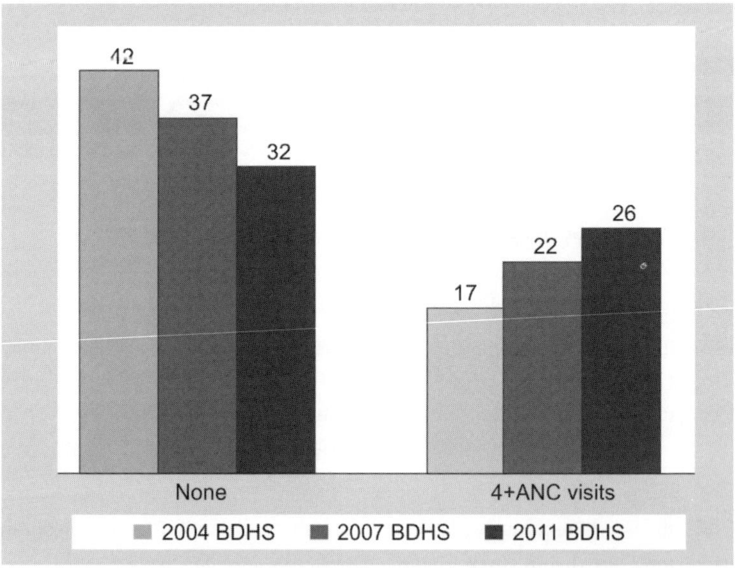

Fig. 12 Trend in antenatal care visits (in %), 2004–2011 in Bangladesh

Place of Delivery

Twenty-nine percent of births in Bangladesh are delivered at a health facility: 15 percent in a private facility, 12 percent in a public facility,

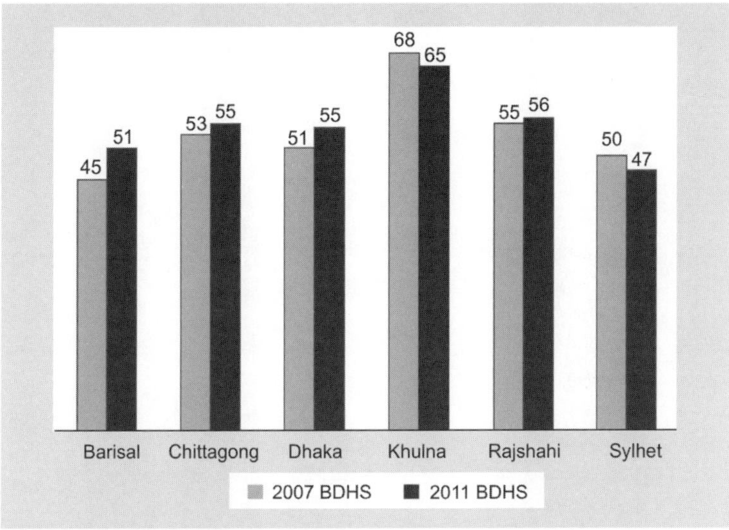

Fig. 13 Trend in utilization of antenatal care (in %) from a medically-trained provider by division, 2007–2011 in Bangladesh

and 2 percent in an NGO facility. Seventy-one percent of births are delivered at home (Table 3). The institutional deliveries have increased from 14 percent in 2007 to 29 percent in 2011. However, only 22 percent of 15–19 year old mothers received postnatal care from a medically trained provider within 42 days after delivery.

Assistance During Delivery

Obstetric care from a trained provider during delivery is critical for the reduction of maternal and neonatal mortality. Thirty-two percent of births in Bangladesh were attended by medically-trained personnel, that is, a qualified doctor, nurse, midwife, family welfare visitor (FWV), or community skilled birth attendant (CSBA). Additionally, trained traditional birth attendants assisted in 11 percent of deliveries. However, more than half of births in Bangladesh were assisted by dais or untrained traditional birth attendants (53%), and 4 percent of deliveries were assisted by relatives and friends (Table 4).

The HPNSDP 2011–2016 target for delivery by a medically-trained provider is set at 50 percent of deliveries, to be achieved by 2016 (MOHFW, 2011). Over the past seven years, the proportion of deliveries by medically-trained providers has doubled, from 16 percent in 2004 to 21 percent in 2007, and to 32 percent in 2011 (Fig. 14). This is

Table 3 Place of delivery—Bangladesh

Percent distribution of live births in the three years preceding the survey by place of delivery, percentage delivered in a health facility, and percentage delivered by C-section, according to background characteristics, Bangladesh 2011

	Health facility			*Home*	*Other/ missing*	*Total*	*Percentage delivered in a health facility*	*Percentage delivered by C-section*	*Number of births*
	Public sector	*Private sector*	*NGO*						
Total	11.8	15.1	1.9	71.0	0.2	100.0	28.8	17.1	4,956

Table 4 Assistance during delivery —Bangladesh

Percent distribution of live births in the three years preceding the survey by person providing assistance during delivery (skilled and unskilled) and percentage

	Qualified doctor	*Nurse/ midwife/ paramedic*	*FWV*	*CSBA*	*HA/ FWA*	*Trained traditional birth attendant*	*Untrained traditional birth attendant*	*Unqualified doctor*	*Relatives and friends*	*NGO worker*	*No one*	*Percent delivered by a medically trained provider*
Total	22.2	8.9	0.3	0.3	0.4	10.9	52.5	0.2	3.8	0.0	0.4	31.7

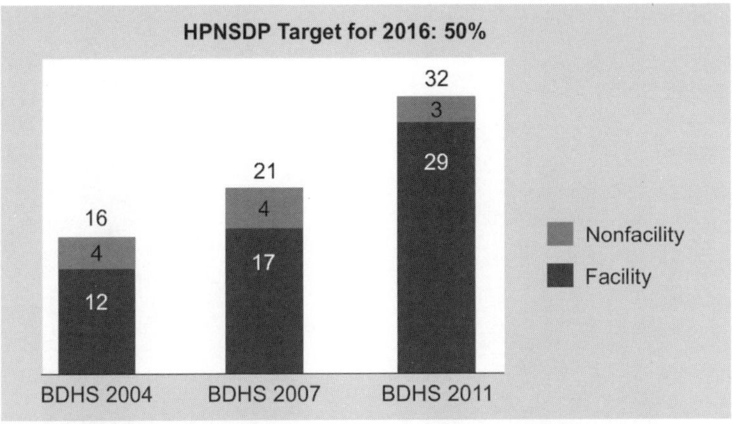

Fig. 14 Trend in skilled attendant at delivery in Bangladesh

almost solely due to an increase in institutional delivery, given that the majority of births delivered at home are mostly performed by unskilled individuals (95% in 2011) (Fig. 14).

The percentage of mothers receiving postnatal checkup from medically-trained providers within 2 days of delivery has increased from 16 percent in 2004 to 20 percent in 2007, and 27 percent. However, it is still much lower than the HPNSDP 2011–2016 target of 50 percent that needs to be achieved by 2016. Similarly, the percentage of children receiving postnatal care from a medically-trained provider within two days of delivery has increased from 13 percent in 2004, to 20 percent in 2007, and to 30 percent in 2011 (Fig. 15).

Emergency Obstetric Care

Emergency obstetric care (EmOC) comprises of life saving interventions for obstetric complications. The Obstetrical and Gynaecological Society of Bangladesh (OGSB) in collaboration with the DGHS and with UNICEF sponsorship implemented a project entitled "Strengthening of EOC services in 11 districts of Bangladesh" during July 1994–Dec. 1996. While implementing the EOC project it was realised that the maternal mortality is not a separate issue and all other issues related to women should also be addressed in order to get better and prompt result. The EmOC Project was followed by a second project "Improvement of Women and Maternal Health" by DGHS and OGSB from January 1997 covering 54 districts in Bangladesh with support from UNICEF. A two pronged approach was applied. In one hand facilities for dealing

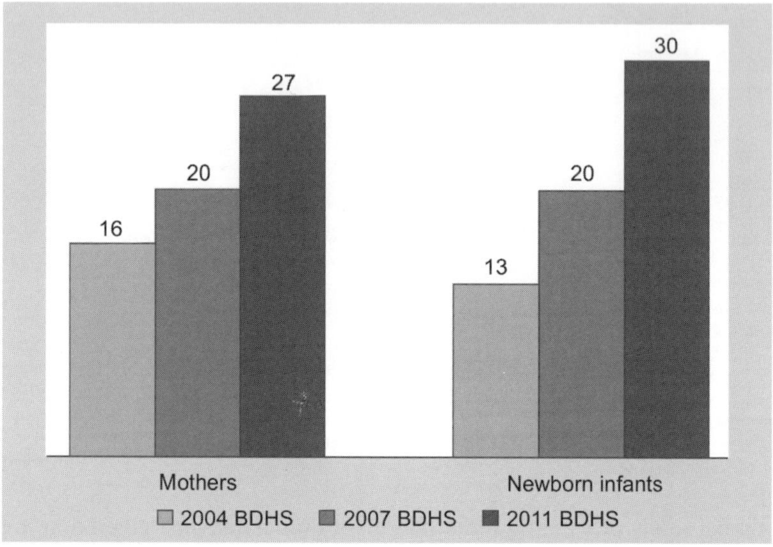

Fig. 15 Trend in utilization of postnatal care (in %) for women and children from a medically trained provider within two days of delivery, 2004–2011 in Bangladesh

with obstetric emergencies was strengthened and on the other hand measures was taken to mobilise the community to utilise the available services. Number of health facilities designated for CEmOC 59 District Headquarters and 132 upgraded health centers (105 functioning) Total-164 centers (UNICEF); MCWC-70 (UNFPA) (2006).

Nutrition

In one field Bangladesh is lagging behind is in nutrition. Maternal nutrition and child nutrition both are important. Because the growth occurs mostly in early years in life and it is often unreasonable in later life.

Comparisons of data from the three surveys BHDS, 2004, 2007 and 2011, indicate a slight improvement in the proportion of women whose height is less than 145 cm, from 16 percent in 2004 to 13 percent in 2011 (Fig. 16). At the same time, the mean BMI has increased from 20.2 in 2004 to 21.4 in 2011 (NIPORT et al. 2009). Consequently, the proportion of women with a BMI below 18.5 has decreased from 34 percent in 2004 to 24 percent in 2011. Moreover, the proportion of women who are overweight or obese has almost doubled, increasing from 9 percent in 2004 to 17 percent in 2011.

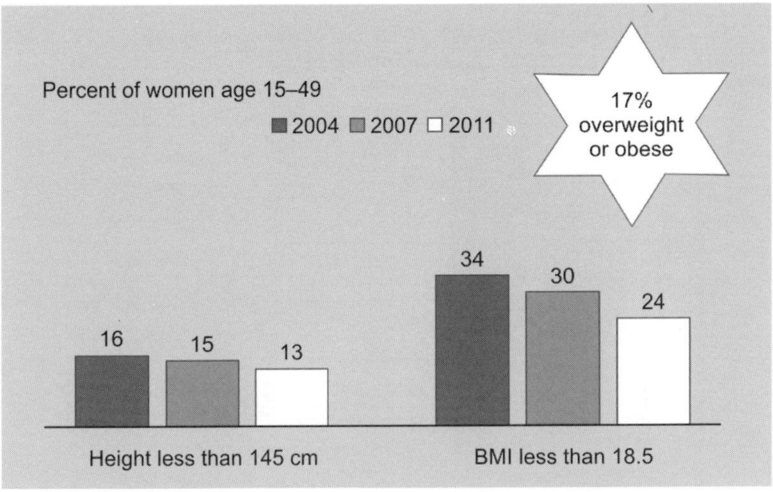

Fig. 16 Trends in nutritional status of women in Bangladesh

Prevalence of Anemia in Women

In Bangladesh, a number of interventions have been put in place to address anemia in women.

These include supplementation of iron with folic acid tablets for pregnant women from the second trimester to 45 days following delivery and deworming of pregnant women after completion of the first trimester. Figure 17 shows that 42 percent of women age 15–49 are anemic (36%: mild, 7%: moderate and < 1%: severe) (BDHS 2011).

Adolescent Reproductive Health

More than one-fifth of the population of Bangladesh is adolescents, with 13.7 million girls and 14 million boys; the adolescent population of Bangladesh constitutes over 23 percent of the population, a total of at least 32 million people (2011 Census data). From 1993 to 2011 age of marriage increased from 15.3 to 16.6 years. (+15 month). But time from marriage to first birth shortened from 3 to 2.3 years (–8 months). Net delay in age at first birth only from 18.3 to 18.9 years (+7 months) in 18 years. In past 15 years fertility declined most among older women (30); little decline in fertility among women under 25; this pattern is result of persistent early marriage and quick first birth. The percentage of women age 15–19 years who have begun child bearing has been decreased from 32.7 percent in 2007 to 30.2 percent in 2011. Adolescent

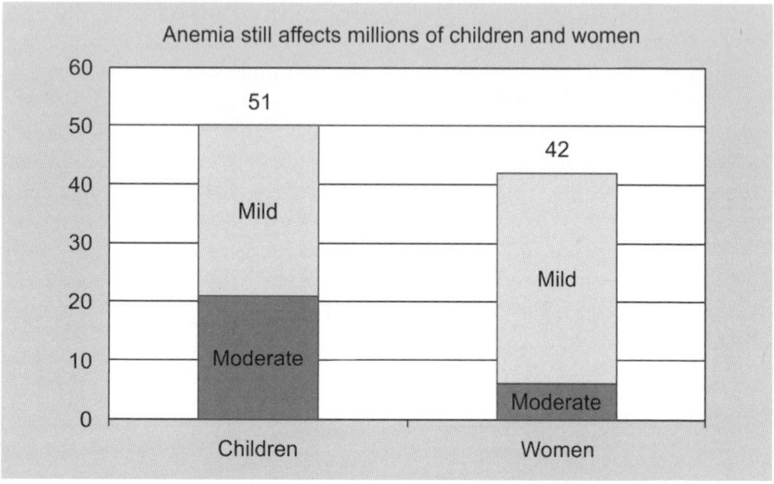

Fig. 17 Prevalence of anemia in Bangladesh

girls are vulnerable to health hazards as they suffer from malnutrition, early marriage and quicker childbearing, stillbirth, premature delivery, low birth weight baby reproductive tract infection (RTI). A large number of adolescent girls suffer from malnutrition. One fourth of ever married girls of late adolescent period (15–19 years) are underweight (BMI <18.5) and 13 percent are short statured (height <145 cm). Anemia is most common during periods of life when iron requirements are high due to rapid growth, menstruation and reproduction. About one-third (30%) of adolescent suffer from anemia.

To ensure quality of care, maternal health strategy, standard operating procedure, different protocols and guidelines are developed. Directorate General of Family Planning (DHFP) conduct regular supportive supervision through FPCST/QAT teams and Directorate General of Health Services performs accreditation of Women Friendly Hospital. National maternal health strategy serves as a guideline to provide quality maternal health services.

A number of programs/innovative activities are being conducted in Bangladesh to provide the service and meet the identified challenges. A few are mentioned below.

Demand Side Financing Maternal Health Voucher Scheme (DSF Scheme)

The Ministry of Health and Family Welfare (MOHFW) piloted the DSF scheme in 21 districts in 2007/8 which was scaled-up in 53 sub-districts in 2010. The aim was to increase utilization of maternal health care services by the poor. A voucher entitles its holder to receive free maternal health care services including ante-and postnatal care, safe delivery and treatment of complications (including cesarean sections and assisted vaginal delivery from designated facilities (public or private) or skilled providers in the community. Service recipients receive cash incentives, transport subsidies, and a gift box. Service providers also receive incentives to distribute vouchers and to provide services covered by the voucher scheme. The scheme is implemented by the Directorate General of Health Services (DGHS) with technical assistance from WHO. Comprehensive evaluation undertaken during April–July, 2013 shows the following:

Impact on use and inequity: There has clearly been a positive effect DSF scheme on utilization of maternity care services. At present, DSF facilities are performing much better than non-DSF facilities while their performances were comparable during 2007/2008. During the first half of 2013, on average, 60 deliveries were conducted in intervention UHCs while the same number was 36 per month in non-DSF UHCs. MIS data also depicts that more ANCs were provided from DSF upazilas than non-DSF upazilas and the difference was significant in 2013. But the (mean) number of PNC (post natal care) visit was similar between DSF and non-DSF upazilas. Moreover, the national level data clearly shows that the use-inequity has reduced over time which implies that the DSF scheme might have some impact in reducing access-inequity for maternal health care services.

Impact on quality of care: The quality is poor in both DSF and non-DSF facilities and there is no difference in QOC when measured in standardized summary scores. The human resource situation is poor as well in all rural health facilities irrespective of their DSF status. Vacancies and absenteeism is enormous in both DSF and non-DSF facilities (Anwar I, 2007).

Poor women defined by specific criteria (roughly 50 percent of the pregnant women) and validated by local government representatives are eligible for the voucher. Both public and nonpublic healthcare providers (NGO and private facilities) participate in the DSF scheme. There is a target to scale the program up to 100 upazilas, with a 20 percent increase each year. Strikingly, the maternal mortality rate among the voucher holder women is 12 per 100,000 live births, in sharp contrast to the national rate of 194 per 100,000 live births.

In Bangladesh skilled delivery of women are usually conducted by obstetricians. Doctors trained in obstetrics, Nurses, Family welfare visitors (FWV), and NGO paramedics. Since in 2000–2003 community based skilled birth attendants were developed. Since 2008 a cadre of midwives is also developed (Table 5).

Table 5 Milestones for development of skilled birth attendants in Bangladesh

Period	Events
1992	SMI conference at Dhaka, following1987 Nairobi conference on SM: Professional encouraged to take the charge of the situation
1994	Strengthening of EmOC in 11 districts project—OGSB, GOB, UNICEF
1994	EmOC training in MCWC
1996	EmOC was taken up in Government program as Reproductive Health Program (Following ICPD conference), Cairo ICPD, (RH redefined)
1999	Needs assessment and curriculum development for SBA by OGSB, GOB, WHO (Following 1997: Combo Conference Technical Review of Progress of SMI)
2007	OGSB proposes to develop a cadre of midwife in Bangladesh following Tunisia Conference on Midwives
2008	Midwifery training started under BNC Registered Nurse midwife (Six month training of nurses) Midwife: Three years formal course

Midwifery Training

Globally, midwifery personnel have long been recognized as a cornerstone for safe motherhood. They provide the necessary supervision, care and advice for women during pregnancy, labor and the postpartum period. They also conduct deliveries and provide care for the newborn. To improve maternal and newborn health services in Bangladesh, a strategic direction paper on midwifery was developed and approved by the Ministry of Health and Family Welfare, OGSB, BNC and BMS in September 2008. A two-pronged strategy has been suggested in the document: (i) Increase the number of midwives for midwifery services (through a 3-year direct entry midwifery education course); and (ii) Improve the skills and utilization of existing registered nurse midwives (RNMS) for midwifery services (through a 6 months advanced post basic midwifery course of the qualified nurse). Presently both type of training are going on in government and private sector which is regulated by Bangladesh Nursing Council. The proportion of deliveries with skilled birth attendants (SBA) is an indicator for progress monitoring in the achievements of MDG. Bangladesh public health sector (and recently non government sector in a limited way) struggling for many years to ensure Skilled Birth Attendants (SBA) at delivery who can conduct safe delivery and have the capacity to refer complicated cases to hospital for life saving obstetric emergencies.

The government's target established in 2006 at 50 percent delivery by SBA by 2010 has not been achieved as only 18 percent and 26.5 percent births were assisted by a medically trained person in 2008 and 2010. Achieving the increased coverage by SBAs requires a greater reservoir of educated girls and implementation of home birth with updated SBA strategy and increase in quality antenatal care.

One of ways of ensuring care to rural people is to have peripheral level health posts as near to the community as possible with skilled manpower and required materials. Community clinic is an innovative activity to ensure this.

Quality of Care

To ensure quality of care maternal health strategy, standard operating practice, different protocol and guideline are developed. Regular monitoring and supervision are done by FPCST/QOT team by DG. Family planning and accreditation as women friendly hospitals are done by Director General of Health Services (DGHS).

Gender Issues

As the recommendation made by the ICPD, Cairo'94 the important issues where attention should be needed for ensuring reproductive health is elimination of discrimination on gender. As women constitute almost half of the Bangladesh population, have little opportunity to enjoy equality. Less participation in the economic activities carry a disproportion burden of poverty, illiteracy, malnutrition and ill health. So, to accelerate the total socioeconomic development and promote the reproductive health of women Bangladesh have already given importance on gender issue aspect. Gender differentials in present program considered a major challenge. To face the challenge the present program has given importance on gender issues. Gender equity strategy has been developed and already incorporated in the main stream of the program. MOHFW has established a gender issue cell in the Ministry and nominated focal point in each program unit for effective functioning of gender related activities. Box 1 summarizes the health care implementations at community choice in Bangladesh.

Key Policy Relevant Questions

- Why the existing public sector facilities are not being able to attract the families? Whether these are adequate in numbers? Are they located at right places? Do they have a need based distribution? Are they functioning with adequate, available skilled human resources, supplies and equipments? And finally how is the quality of care?

Box 1 Community clinic (CC): Most peripheral level health facility in Bangladesh

Services of CC:

- Maternal and neonatal health care services (ANC, PNC)
- Integrated management of childhood illness (IMCI)
- Reproductive health and FP services
- EPI
- Screening of chronic noncommunicable diseases—diabetes, Hypertension, Arsenicosis, Cancer, Heart disease, etc.
- Nutritional education and micronutrient supplements
- Health, nutrition and FP education and counseling
- Treatment of minor ailments, common diseases and first aid
- Establishing referral linkage with higher facilities

No. of functional CC at present: 12460 (92.29%): Target 13500

CC catchments area has more or less 1200–1500 HH and population 6000–10000

Service period: 9 AM–3 PM

Service Providers–CHCP, HA and FWA (paramedics)

CHCP: (52% female, 48% male), minimum qualification-12 class schooling but most of them are Graduate and some are Masters

Public-Private partnership (*Community Group is the key player)*

- Land for CC construction: Community
- Construction, medicine and other inputs, service providers: GOB
- Management: Community Group + GOB

- How to ensure auality of care?
- Who will deliver the vast majority of our mother still delivering at home? CSBAs? FWVS? Midwives?
- Are the CSBAs, midwives, FWVs, surgeon-anesthetist pair deployed properly?
- Are we adhering to the standard indications of C-Sections? Are we enforcing the quality control regulations?
- Why serviced coverage is more in urban than in rural area?
- Why we are not reaching the poor adequately?
- Why Sylhet and Chittagong divisions remain consistently low performing?
- Revisit job descriptions of SBA's CSBA Program?
- Strengthen supervision and streamline CSBA related performance indicators?
- Need more task shifting, e.g. CSBAs to work in UH and FWCs? How to address adolescents with information and childbearing? How to reduce early marriage and early childbearing?

- How to ensure birth registration?
- How to improve the nutritional status? How to implement the life cycle approach to break the vicious cycle of under nutrition including IYCF (Breastfeeding and complementary feeding), nutrition of children, adolescent girls and women?
- How to take nutrition specific intervention among adolescent girls and women like food, hygiene?
- How to improve maternal nutritional status? How to ensure counseling on increased food and intake, hygiene, iron folic acid supplementation and awareness about ideal weight gain and hemoglobin level in pregnancy?
- How to improve nutrition sensitive (or indirect) interventions? Like improvement of female literacy, woman's empowerment, creating livelihoods, nutrition sensitive agriculture.
- What strategies to be taken to further reduce MMR to an acceptable level?
- How to increase the use of long acting and permanent methods including male sterilization (NSV)?
- How to improve CPR? How to address East West disparity of TFR?
- How to achieve fertility reduction by ensuring effective family planning to lower TFR to replacement level and below?
- How to expand and ensure use of evidence based practices to prevent maternal death from hemorrhage and eclampsia? How to implement interventions like active management of third stage of labor (AMTSL), distribution of misoprostol tablet to all pregnant women shortly before delivery (600 mg to be taken immediately after delivery) to minimize risk of hemorrhage, use of magnesium sulfate for preeclampsia both in hospitals and field level (before referral)?

Options to Achieve a Further 25 percent Reduction in MMR to Achieve MDG 5 (ref BDHS 2011)

As fertility reduction has been as important as MMR reduction to this point, future gains in maternal mortality be achieved by ensuring effective family planning to lower fertility to replacement level and below.

The trend of rising education level among young women can be expected to bring behavior changes which favor more use of skilled attendance at birth, more facility deliveries, and more and quicker treatment seeking for complications.

Introduction and strengthening of interventions for prevention of PPH and eclampsia related deaths.

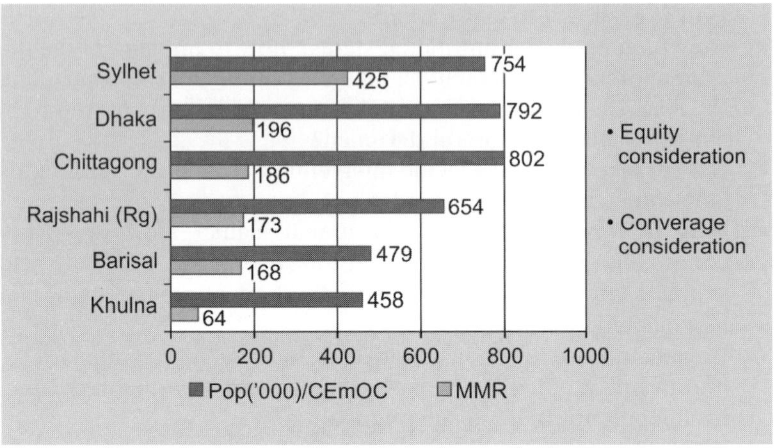

Fig. 18 MDG goal 5 for different regions of Bangladesh

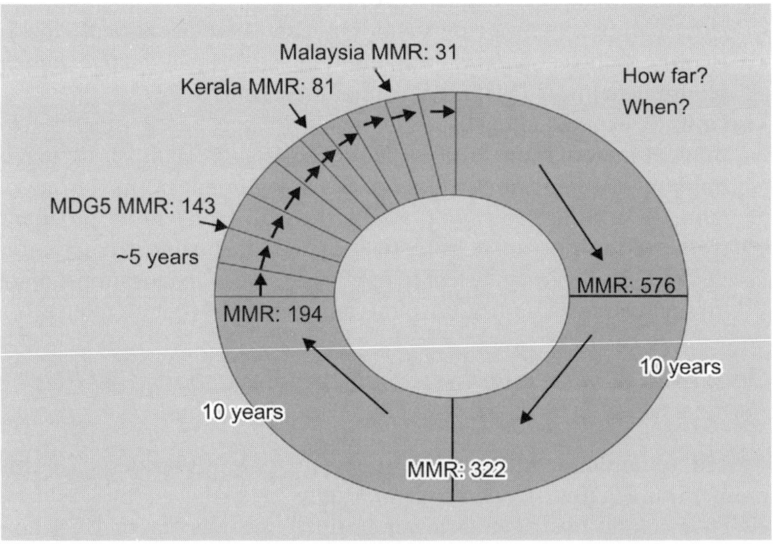

Fig. 19 MDG goal; Bangladesh may be a little behind, but on right track

Improve access to upgrade facilities with focus on quality, human resource and possibly some kind of health insurance to overcome fear of heavy costs of life saving obstetric procedures.

CONCLUSION

The final hundred meters in a marathon is really important; we must boost the input to reach the target in time, keeping in mind the differential needs (Figs 18 and 19). It is said that "The best way to predict the future is to create it". So let's create our future!

ABBREVIATIONS

ANC–Antenatal Care, BDHS–Bangladesh Demographic and Health Survey, BF–Breastfeeding, BMI–Body Mass Index, BMS–Bangladesh Midwifery Society, BNC–Bangladesh Nursing Council, CPR–Contraceptive Prevalence Rate, FP–Family Planning, FPCST/QAT–Family Planning Clinical Supervisory Team/Quality Assurance Team, FWC–Family Welfare Centre, HPSP–Health Population Sector Program (HPSP). HNPSP–Health Nutrition Population Sector Program, HPNSDP–Health Population Nutrition Sector Development Program, MNH–Maternal and Newborn Health, MCH–Maternal and Child Health, MDG–Millennium Development Goal, MMR–Maternal Mortality Rate, MOHFW–Ministry of Health and Family Welfare, MTP–Medically Trained Person, NGO–Non Governmental Organization, OGSB–Obstetrical and Gynaecological Society of Bangladesh, Penta 3–Three doses of pentavalent Vaccine taken, PNC–Postnatal Care, SMI–Safe Motherhood Initiative, SOP–Standard Operating Procedure, SVRS–Sample Vital Registration Survey, TFR–Total Fertility Rate, QOC–Quality of Care.

BIBLIOGRAPHY

1. Bangladesh Bureau of Statistics (BBS). Sample Vital Registration Survey. (SVRS 2007).
2. DGFP. 2011. Maternal and Child Health Services Unit. National Adolescent Reproductive Health. Plan of Action.
3. DGHS, UNICEF. Voice of MIS. Newsletter, MIS Health, DGHS. Emergency Obstetric Care (EmOC) Performance Report, 2012.
4. Kerber KJ, de Graft-Johnson JE, Bhutta ZA, Okong P, Starrs A, Lawn JE. Continuum of care for maternal, newborn, and child health: from slogan to service delivery. www.thelancet.com 2007;370:1358–69.
5. Ministry of Health and Family Welfare, July 2011-June 2016. Government of the People's Republic of Bangladesh, Health, Population and Nutrition Sector Development Program (HPNSDP), Dhaka. February 2012.
6. Mitra and Associates and Macro International. Bangladesh Demographic and Health Survey, 2007. Dhaka, Bangladesh, and Calverton, Maryland, USA: National Institute of Population Research and Training (NIPORT), Mitra and Associates, and Macro International Inc, 2009.

7. Mitra SN, Al-Sabir A, Cross AR, Jamil K.Bangladesh Demographic and Health Survey, 1996–1997. Dhaka, Bangladesh, and Calverton, Maryland, USA: National Institute of Population Research and Training (NIPORT), Mitra and Associates, and Macro International Inc, 1997.
8. Mitra SN, Ali MN, Islam S, Cross AR, Saha T. Bangladesh Demographic and Health Survey, 1993–1994. Dhaka, Bangladesh, and Calverton, Maryland: National Institute of Population Research and Training (NIPORT), Mitra and Associates, and Macro International Inc, 1994.
9. Mitra SN, Kamal GM. Bangladesh Contraceptive Prevalence Survey-1983: Final Report. Dhaka, Bangladesh: Mitra and Associates, 1985.
10. Mitra SN, Lerman C, Islam S. Bangladesh Contraceptive Survey-1991: Final report. Dhaka, Bangladesh: Mitra and Associates, 1993.
11. Mitra SN. Bangladesh Contraceptive Prevalence Survey-1985: Final report. Dhaka, Bangladesh: Mitra and Associates, 1987.
12. NIPORT, Mitra and Associates, MEASURE DHS, ICF International. Bangladesh Demographic and Health Survey, 2011.
13. NIPORT, ORC Macro, John Hopkins University, ICDDRB. Bangladesh Maternal Health Service and Maternal Mortality Survey, 2001.
14. NIPORT, USAID, Australian Govt. Aid Program, UNFPA, MEASURE Evaluation, ICDDRB. Maternal Mortality and Health Care Survey. Summary of key Findings and Implications, 2010.

7

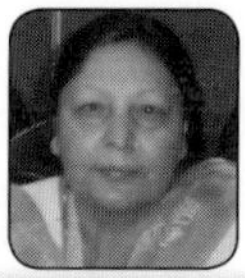

Initiative and Innovations for Safe Motherhood in Nepal

Ashma Rana

INTRODUCTION

Lying between China and India, Nepal stretches over 147,181 sq km grossly in mountainous (75%) terrain having Mt Everest, the tallest peak in the world along with the eight of the ten tallest peaks >8000 m adding to its credit. On the other hand, the steep mountainous topography is viewed less favorable for the accessibility.

Half (50.40%) of the total 30 million female population have women of reproductive age group 15 to 49 years (52.61%) and in this same women of reproductive age group 18 percent have completed secondary school, although the female literacy rate is 52 percent; 17.5 years is the median age for marriage and 5 percent girls <15 to 17 are married and accounts for the marriage of one-third of adolescent girls [15–19]. To the result, 23 percent had given birth before 18 while 48 percent had given birth by the age of 20. Report indicate that 58 percent and 36 percent women in 15 to 49 years had antenatal care (ANC) or were delivery by skilled provide Nepal demographic health survey (NDHS 2011).

This is the health scenario as of today, although two decades ago around 1993 safe motherhood in Nepal was born from the initiative of Nepal Government, Department of Health, were all set to improve reproductive health issues in making pregnancy safer. And to overcome the dreaded speculation of women dying from pregnancy related condition quoted as high as 1/32 for Nepalese women in comparison to women in a developed country, having probability of 1/10,000.

Every country is concerned for the safety of its citizen and more so for women and that too during pregnancy, which has anticipated 5 to 15 percent risk of running into complication. Nepal needs to worry more because of poor economy, education and lack of adequate road transport and problems of air lift during nonpermissible weather, mandating the need to strengthening the health facility services. The country has 14 zones, 75 districts with total health Institutions under Ministry of health and population (MOHP) (4396), hospitals 103 (district, zonal, regional, subregional, ayurvedic, central); primary health centers (209); health post 699, subhealth post (3129); ayurvedic health institutions (29).

INTRODUCING SAFE MOTHERHOOD "BEGINNING TO DATE IN NEPAL"

- Safe Motherhood Program was initiated in 1997
- Nepal Safer Mother Project funded by DFID aimed to work in 3 Districts (Kailali, Surkhet and Baglung) from 1997, and depending the result, proposed to expand the services to other districts in second phase of the project for a total duration of 6 years.
- Three comprehensive and four basic emergency obstetric care (EmOC) facilities were established in an area where adequate EmOC services were previously lacking. From 2000 to 2004, met need for EmOC improved from 1.9 to 16.9 percent; the proportion of births in EmOC project facilities increased from 3.8 to 8.3 percent; and the case fatality rate declined from 2.7 to 0.3 percent.
- National Safe Motherhood Plan (2002–2017).
- Support to the Safe Motherhood Program (SSMP 2006–2008 was) a 5-year DFID-funded program that worked directly with the Government of Nepal (MoHP) to sustain the National Safe Motherhood Program through Nepal National Safer Motherhood Project.
- The revised Safe Motherhood and Neonatal Health Long Term Plan (SMNHLTP 2006–2017).
- Similarly, endorsement of revised National Blood Transfusion Policy 2006.
- The policy on skilled birth attendants (SBA) endorsed in 2006 deploying specifically identifies doctors and nurses/ANMs with lifesaving skill.

The Government of Nepal with Family Health Division (FHD), Ministry of Health and Population (MOHP) aimed to create an environment where the women could have access to obstetric care wherever and whenever they most require it.

- NSMP (1997–2004) worked with MOH to reduce maternal mortality and also supported to develop NSMP.
- The overall goal of the Nepal National Safe Motherhood and Newborn Health second Long-Term Health Plan (1997–2017).

- Long Term Plan (2001–2017)
- (NSMNH-LTP) 2006–2017: The revised National Safe Motherhood and Newborn Health Long Term Plan.
  - To improve maternal and neonatal health and survival especially among poor and socially excluded communities.
  - Reduction in the maternal mortality ratio to 134 per 100,000 live births by 2017.
  - Legalization of abortion; recognition of the significant levels of mother to child transmission of HIV/AIDS.
  - Skilled Birth Attendants (SBA) to 60 percent by 2017.
  - Increase in the number of deliveries in a health facility to 40 percent by 2017.
  - Met need for emergency obstetric complications will be increased by 3 percent each year.
  - Met need for cesarean section by 4 percent each year.

KEY ISSUES IN MAKING SAFE MOTHERHOOD PROGRAM SUCCESSFUL

Safe motherhood umbrella for promoting birth preparedness and complication management readiness including awareness raising and improving the availability of funds, transport and blood supplies, encouraging institutional delivery, expansion of 24-hour emergency obstetric care services (basic and comprehensive) at selected public health facilities in every district.

Steps taken to make pregnancy safer:

- *Birth preparedness package and MNH activities at community level:* Family Health Division (FHD) continued support for expansion and maintenance of MNH activities at community level.

  Birth preparedness package:
  - Jeevan Suraksha Flip Chart
  - Jeevan Suraksha Card
  - Matri Suraksha Chakki (MSC) Misoprostol.

  Government of Nepal approved PPH education and distribution of Matri Suraksha Chakki (MSC) (3 tab or 600 microgram of misoprostol by FCHVs) for prevention of PPH from 8 months of pregnancy onwards as a precautions, should delivery occur at home and was instructed to be orally swallowed after the delivery of the placenta.

  Birth preparedness also facilitated women to make small save money for use in time of need.

  Educated about nearby SBA/health facilities and to be familiar with local transport in case if need or emergency and also arrange for blood donors.

Apart from this, iron from 3 completed months of pregnancy, 2 doses TT, albendazole: one tablet at 4 completed month of pregnancy. Self-care in pregnancy and postpartum period (food, rest, no smoking and no drinking alcohol).

Or knowledge for danger signs in pregnancy, delivery and postpartum period also imparted.

Several external development partners (EDPs) such as NFHP II/USAID, UNICEF, UMN, RHDP/SDC, Care Nepal and Plan Nepal supported FHD in maintenance of BPP in the existing 41districts (25 Government of Nepal and 16 partners) and in expansion of revised BPP in 30 districts (25 by Government of Nepal and 5 others).

- **Rural ultrasound program** piloted in two districts Mugu and Dhading have successfully trained staff nurse detect to malpresentation and placenta previa, and this has been helpful.

  The preliminary finding shows the increment in ANC cases and trained nurses use a portable ultrasound.
- **Human resource:** A total of 1,342 ANMs and 25 staff nurses have been recruited on local contract to support 24-hour delivery services in PHCCs and HPs. Nine MDGP/Gynecologists were recruited locally in nine districts for CEOC services. This has resulted in increased number of cesarean section in these districts.

  National Academy of Medical Sciences (NAMS) has now initiated one-year Diploma course in gynecology and obstetrics, who after their studies are supposed to serve community, CEOC sites.

  Family Health Division has been coordinating with NHTC to provide SBA training to doctors and staff nurses and ANM SBA training, from 2007, a total of 2535 SBAs have been trained.

  And 27 doctors (Medical Officer) are trained in advanced SBA for performing cesarean section.
- **Emergency referral fund** of ₹ 200,000 has been allocated to be used in need for each of 14 total districts: (Bhojpur, Khotang, Sunsari, Rasuwa, Manang, Mustang, Dolpa, Humla, Jajarkot, Mugu, Rolpa, Rukum Bajhang, and Darchula). Table 1 enumerates the obstetrical complications where emergency cases assistance in provided to women.
- **Safe abortion services (SAS)** or also known as comprehensive abortion care (CAC) has been in all the 75 districts of Nepal, through 477 listed sites by certified/trained provider (doctors and nurse) for nonsex selective abortion resulting after unwanted or unplanned pregnancy, and medical abortion.

  Currently IPAS is supporting 23 manual vacuum aspiration implementing districts and even ANM have been trained including 297 providers.

Table 1 Complicated cases: outlined for benefit of NRs. 3000

- Severe pre-eclampsia/eclampsia
- Instrumental delivery
- Multiple delivery
- Rh Negative
- Requiring blood transfusion for hemorrhage [(APH) and (PPH: Retained placenta MRP or uterine exploration)]
- Puerperal sepsis, admission longer than 24 hours with IV antibiotics for sepsis
- Postabortion management

- **Aama Program (four components):**
  1. *Safe Delivery Incentive Program (SDIP)*: Initiated in July 2005, a cash incentive immediately given on institutional delivery (NRs. 1,500 in mountain, NRs. 1,000 in hill and NRs. 500 in Terai region).
  2. *Free institutional delivery care (mid-January 2009)*: A payment to the health facility (HF).
     - *Normal delivery:* NRs. 1,000 to 1500 (HF < 25 bed; HF ≥ 25 beds).
     - Complicated deliveries NRs. 3,000 (Table 1);
       NRs. 7,000: C-Sections /Surgery (Laparotomy)
       (i) Ectopic pregnancy;
       (ii) Uterine perforation on or rupture (abortion/obstructed labor)
  3. Incentive to Health Worker ₹ 200 for home delivery
  4. Incentive to women for four antenatal clinic (ANC) visits (4, 6, 8 and 9 months of pregnancy).

ACHIEVEMENTS

There is decline in maternal mortality to 170 per hundred thousand live births, TFR is decreasing and contraceptive prevalence is increasing (Fig. 1, Tables 2 and 3). The rapid decline in MMR is because unacceptably very high MMR in the outset, still the figures are higher than most countries of the world. Nepal is in the track of achieving MDG goal.

At least 4,573 to 7,623 trained SBAs (doctors and nurses) were estimated for 60 to 100 percent coverage of all births to be attended by an SBA by 2012 and 7,000 SBAs were expected to be trained until 2015 but so far 3 to 4,000 have been trained. Table 2 reveals improvement in obstetric health services in Nepal.

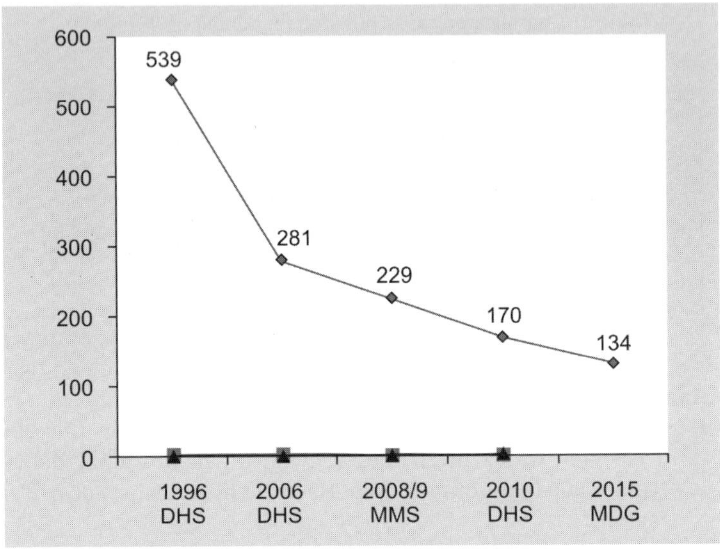

Fig. 1 Trends in maternal mortality ratio in Nepal

Table 2 Increase in obstetric health services in Nepal

- *ANC visit:* 1 (83%) and 4 (57%)
- PNC visit 51%
- Institutional delivery 44%
- SBA conducted delivery was 44%
- *CEOC:* 177 (54 + 123)
- *BEOC:* 151 [(hospital) 42 + 111(PHC)]
- *BC:* 1121 [PHC (75) + HP (573) + SHP (473)]

Table 3 Target set by Nepal and achievements goal 5A

MDG impact indicator	*Achievement*					*Target*	
	1991	*1996*	*2001*	*2006*	*2009*	*2010-11*	*2015*
Maternal mortality ratio	539	539	415	281	229	170	134
Total fertilty ratio	5.3	4.6	4.1	3.1	2.9	3.0	2.5
Adolescent fertility rate (15–19 years)		127	110	98	96.53	89.63	70
CPR (Modern method)	24	26	35	44	45.1	48	67

Limitation: Human resource:

- *OB/GYN specialist:* 350
- *Doctors:* 1457 (total doctors >15,000)
- *Nurse/ANM*: 16,467/17,759
- Paramedics/Health Assistant (7491)
- Village Health Worker (3190)
- *FCHV*: 48,897 and MCHW (3985)
- Ayurvedic doctor (394), Baidhya (360)
- Doctors/Nurse ratio; 1 Doctor: 18,439 Nurses; 1 Nurse for 4,987 Patients
  [*Source:* State of world population 2009 UNFPA]
- *According to WHO 2013:* Per every 1000: Community Health Worker 0.63; Nurses 0.46; Doctors 0.21. Table 3 shows the achievement of Nepal in reductions of MMR, TFR and increase in usage of contraception.

Questions and Concerns

- Sustainability of AMA program
- Appropriate location of health facility [within the public domain: Primary health center (PHC), health post (HP), subhealth post (SHP)]
- Referral mechanism
- Timely supervision, use/misuse of the equipment
- How to reach special groups
- Integration with SRH/FP
- Monitoring and evaluation
- Poor reporting and recording.

Major Challenges in AMA Suraksha Policy and Program

- CEOC/BEOC—making it functional
- Human resources—train/in place/transfer
- Equity access/demand/need
- Flow and monitoring of fund
- Sustainability—tapping local resources
- Involvement of private/medical colleges health facilities
- Tertiary level hospitals are too busy.

CONCLUSION

Nepal has demonstrated that despite significant topographic, financial and cultural/traditional barriers to availability and access of maternal health care, significant progress has been possible because of excellent policies and plan, effective leadership, well-motivated and dedicated cader of health workers and female community health volunteers, active participation by the local community, engagement of the private and NGO sector and generous support of the development partners.

Effective gains can be made and success can be sustained through, enhancing monitoring and evaluation Capacity, effectively managing human resource challenges, addressing geographic and social remoteness and marginalization. Integrating reproductive health services in a comprehensive manner, addressing general poverty and malnutrition, better coordinating with other sectors.

ACKNOWLEDGMENTS

I am grateful to Professor Sudha Sharma, Former Secretary of Health and Dr Kiran Regmi, presently Director of Family Health Division, Department of Health.

BIBLIOGRAPHY

1. Challenges for reducing maternal mortality in Nepal, experience of 3 districts, Kailali Surkhet and Baglung. Nepal safer motherhood project; a part of HMGN Safer Motherhood Programme, Joyace Abbott, 2009.
2. Goodburn L, Basnet I, Sharma S. Sustainable monitoring of Nepal National Safe Motherhood Programme; 2001.
3. National policy on skilled birth attendant, supplementary to National Safe Motherhood Programme 1998; FHD, DOHS; 2006.
4. National safe motherhood programme and new born health: a long term plan 2002-2017; FHD, DOHS; 2006.
5. National Safer Motherhood Plan: 2002-2017. FHD,DOHS, HMGN; 2002.
6. Nepal demographic and health survey; 2011; Government of Nepal, MOHP.
7. Nepal population report 2011, Government of Nepal, MOHP.
8. Safe Motherhood Innovation Project: Adventist Development and Relief Agency (ADRA) and Britain Nepal Medical Trust (BNMT).

8

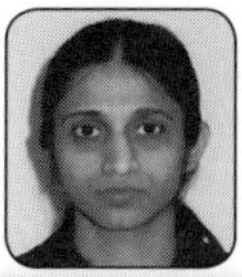

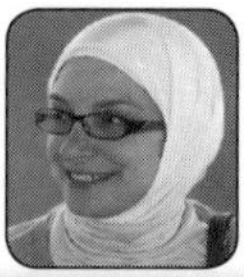

Trends and Concern for Safe Motherhood in Developed World

Padma Munjuluri, Leila Fahel

INTRODUCTION

About 800 women die everyday from complications of pregnancy and childbirth. Ninety-nine percent of these losses happen in the developing world. The World Health Organization (WHO) has set the Millennium Development Goal 5 (MDG5) with an aim to improve maternal health by reducing the maternal mortality ratio (MMR) by three quarters between 1990 and 2015. Although this target remains far from reaching, the total number of maternal deaths decreased from 543,000 in 1990 to 287,000 in 2010. This global decline could be due to an overall improvement in health systems and their accessibility along with a rise in female education. The decline was mainly observed in the developing countries that started with a high MMR. The picture varied for the developed nations: while some countries dropped their MMR further, others seem to have stalled or risen in recent years. Although maternal mortality remains a rare event in the developed world, its impact on the family, community and society cannot be overstated. Over the last century, registers of maternal deaths have helped developed nations to determine the magnitude of the problem, analyze the trends and develop strategies for improvement and prevention of maternal morbidity and mortality. The causes of death are known and most are avoidable but the trends vary nationally and even regionally. This chapter gives examples of various changes and initiatives in the developed world at the pre-conceptional, antenatal, intrapartum and postnatal stages to improve maternal safety.

DEFINITION

WHO defines maternal death in the International Statistical Classification of diseases and related health problems, 10th revision (ICD-10) as: "*The death of a woman while pregnant or within 42 days of termination of pregnancy, irrespective of the duration and site of the pregnancy, from any cause related to or aggravated by the pregnancy or its management but not from accidental or incidental causes."* Maternal deaths are classified as direct or indirect based on their causes. Direct maternal deaths are those resulting from obstetric complications of the pregnant state. Indirect maternal deaths are those resulting from previously existing diseases, or from diseases that developed during pregnancy and that were not due to direct obstetric causes but aggravated by physiological effects of pregnancy. Because of improvements in technologies and life-sustaining procedures, increasingly more women survive adverse outcomes of pregnancy and delivery beyond the 42 days. Such late maternal mortality up to 365 days is now included in the definition employed in countries with advanced civil registration systems.

REPORTING

Although most of the developed countries have held maternal death registers for decades, the use of different reporting methods have made monitoring and comparing maternal deaths difficult. Maternal mortality is reported in ratios (number of maternal death per 100,000 live births), rates (number of maternal deaths per 1000 women of reproductive age), or lifetime risk (takes into account the probability of becoming pregnant and the probability of dying as a result of that pregnancy cumulated across a woman's reproductive years). Moreover, maternal death data is estimated using one or a combination of the following: vital registration data, sibling history data, deaths in household and national and subnational verbal autopsy. Due to underreporting and misclassification of cause of death, the numbers of deaths due to pregnancy and its complications remain underestimated in most developed countries (Atrash et al). Data from death certificates is not sufficient and linkages to national health care registers and inclusion of pregnancies not ending in live births is paramount to ascertain the magnitude of pregnancy related deaths (Deneux-Tharaux et al). The MMR in Sweden between 1988 and 2007 was 64 percent higher than previously reported when death certificates were reviewed and linked to national registers (Esscher et al).

Severe maternal morbidity and near misses are fifty times more common than maternal deaths (Callaghan et al). Incorporation of data on near misses into maternal death enquiries has been shown to strengthen these audits by allowing for more rapid reporting, more robust conclusions, comparisons to be made with maternal deaths, and reinforcing lessons learnt (Hall et al). It also allows better understanding of the progression between severe morbidity to death and establishing the needs to step up to critical care. The UK Obstetric Surveillance System has been surveying a range of rare conditions in pregnancy since 2005 and its data has been incorporated into the latest reports of the confidential enquiries into maternal death changing its scope from 'why mothers die' to 'saving mothers' lives'.

PRECONCEPTION COUNSELING

As nearly 50 percent of pregnancies are unplanned, all women in the reproductive age group may benefit from promoting their health pre-pregnancy. This includes eating healthy, exercising more, reaching a healthy weight, decreasing alcohol intake, quitting smoking and using illicit drugs (CDC). Women should be assessed regarding their mental wellbeing and history of domestic violence at every opportunity. One in four women are at risk of domestic violence in their lifetime and 30 percent of this abuse starts in pregnancy and existing abuse may get worse during pregnancy or after childbirth. Preconception counseling (PCC) is even more beneficial in women with preexisting medical conditions like epilepsy, cardiac disease, diabetes...etc. These women should be informed about the risk of their illness on the pregnancy and vice versa, their disease should be well controlled and medications reviewed. Opportunistic advice should be given as part of routine consultations and if pregnancy is not planned, a safe contraceptive method should be offered. They should also be provided with sufficient knowledge to make informed consent about their fertility plans. This could be provided by their family doctor and/or specialist(s) and often a multidisciplinary team needs to be involved in optimizing the care. The uptake of pre-conceptional counseling (PCC) is still generally low in the developed countries. For instance, in the UK, only 38.2 percent of women with type 1 diabetes and 24.8 percent of women with type 2 diabetes had PCC documented. Professional and public awareness are being raised by colleges and charities.

- 'Recommendations to improve preconception health and health-care' (2006), 'Show your love campaign', by the Center for Disease Control in the United States (http://www.cdc.gov/preconception/index.html).
- *CEMACE and NICE guidelines in the UK* on sex education, family planning, and availability of safe and accessible abortion services.

The use of contraception plays a key role in reducing unwanted pregnancies and therefore, the lifetime risk of maternal death. In high income countries where family planning clinics are easily accessible and services often free, the uptake of contraception remains low amongst women from low socioeconomic groups, ethnic minorities and teenagers. Young adolescents (less than 15 years old) face a higher risk of morbidity and mortality in pregnancy and childbirth compared to older women (WHO). Sex education has been instituted into school curricula in some developed countries secondary to the rise of teenage pregnancies in the sixties. It starts in the primary school in the Netherlands where one of the lowest rates of teenage pregnancies in the world. In the United Kingdom until 2011, sex education was not mandatory and was opposed by faith-based schools. The use of "abstinence only" campaign in the United States has been shown to be ineffective in preventing teenage pregnancy and could be contributing to the continuing rise (Stranger-Hall et al). A review done by the National Campaign to prevent teenage pregnancy in the US showed that sex education discussing contraception was not associated with an increase in sexual activity. With the trend of declining age at first intercourse and delay in starting their families, teenagers need be educated regarding their sexual and reproductive options, different choices of modern contraception including the long acting reversible contraception methods and how to access safe abortion services if unintended pregnancies happen. This should be provided in a youth-friendly setting while ensuring their confidentiality.

ANTENATAL

Strategies to Decrease Mortality Secondary to Early Pregnancy Complications

In the latest CEMACE report, the death rate from ectopic pregnancy has almost halved compared to the previous triennium. This drop could be due improvement in technology such as more sensitive urine pregnancy tests and clear referral pathways to early pregnancy assessment units with easy access to transvaginal scans. However, substandard care was found in 54 percent of the deaths. The report recommends that gastrointestinal symptoms such as diarrhea and vomiting could be early symptoms of ectopic and that a pregnancy test needs to be performed on all women in the reproductive age group presenting with abdominal pain. Patients with suspected ectopic pregnancy should be given verbal and written advice about when to seek help if their symptoms worsen.

Interventions to Decrease Maternal Deaths in Minority Ethnic Groups

While there is no relationship between ethnic group and the cause of death, observational studies in Western countries have shown that black women and women from minority ethnic groups have a significantly higher risk of maternal death than their white counterparts. This could be explained by poor access to care, difficulties with communication (communication failure and inadequate translation services) and substandard care provision. Several heath policies have been introduced to engage these women in a better way including providing link and bilingual workers and better translation services in areas with large groups of a certain minority background, setting up specialist multidisciplinary clinics to address specific problems in a group (e.g. high rate of HIV or female genital mutilation), etc.

Risk Assessment at Every Encounter and Specialist Referral

With the overall improvement in health systems, more women with complex congenital and/or chronic conditions are reaching the reproductive age. Risk assessment at booking, referral to specialist teams, and good communication between different healthcare professionals is essential in optimizing maternal health. Inquiries and audits in high income countries continue to show substandard care in understanding, recognizing and referring serious medical or mental health problems in pregnancy. Guidelines and protocols have been devised to help healthcare professionals identify and manage different clinical problems. For instance, the PRECOG (Pre-eclampsia Community Guideline) was published in the UK in 2001 and provides a simple assessment tool to identify women at risk of developing pre-eclampsia at booking and factors relating to pre-eclampsia that require referral for specialist input. Another example to highlight is cardiac disease; it is the leading cause of indirect deaths in many high income countries. Many cardiac symptoms that happen in pregnancy could be mistaken for physiological changes in pregnancy and junior doctors should have a low threshold for further investigation of pregnant or recently delivered women who complain of chest pain that is severe, or radiates to the neck, jaw or back, or is associated with other features such as agitation, vomiting or breathlessness, tachycardia, tachypnea, orthopnea or acidosis.

INTRAPARTUM

Emergency Skills Training

The use of simulation-based training and 'skills and drills' has gained popularity in modern obstetric training. It provides an opportunity to improve technical skills, rehearse and learn from mistakes in simulated emergency cases that happen infrequently, e.g. shoulder dystocia, umbilical cord prolapse, vaginal breech delivery, maternal cardiac arrest and eclampsia. There is growing evidence that simulation training significantly increases midwives' and doctors' knowledge (Crofts et al) and improves performance. Evidence exists for a positive impact of training in obstetric emergencies, although the majority of the available evidence applies to evaluation at the level of participants' confidence, knowledge or skills rather than at the level of impact on clinical outcomes (Calvert et al). In order to help retaining the skills acquired during simulation training, several studies have suggested yearly training for providers to demonstrate competency after initial training.

National modified early obstetric warning score (MEOWS): These charts are required in all pregnant or postpartum women who become unwell and require either obstetric or gynecology services. This will help in the more timely recognition, treatment and referral of women who have, or are developing, a critical illness during or after pregnancy. It is equally important that these charts are also used for pregnant or postpartum women who are unwell and are being cared for outside obstetric and gynecology services, for example, emergency departments. Abnormal scores should not just be recorded but should also trigger an appropriate response

Reproductive health education among people, risk approach in antenatal care, availability of skilled personal in emerging situation and sound referral system makes the full circle for safe obstetric services (Fig. 1)

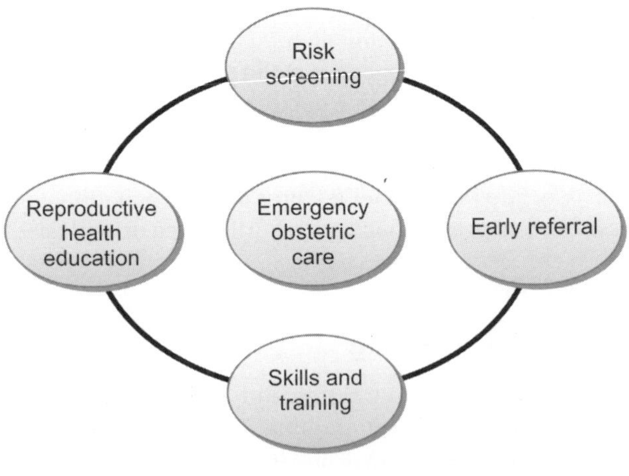

Fig. 1: Safe obstetric care delivery system

POSTPARTUM

Early recognition and referral: Risk assessment and early referral when sepsis of the genital tract is identified is the key to prevent avoidable deaths in postpartum period. Sepsis is the leading cause of the direct deaths in the last triennium.

Back to basics: Lack of clinical knowledge and skills among some doctors, midwives and other health professionals, senior or junior was one of the leading causes of potentially avoidable mortality. This was not only the case when distinguishing the signs and symptoms of potentially serious disease from the commonplace symptoms of pregnancy in primary care or the emergency department but also once a woman was admitted to hospital. There were a number of healthcare professionals who either failed to identify that a woman was becoming seriously ill or who failed to manage emergency situations outside their immediate area of expertise and did not call for advice and help.

Oates et al, 2011 emphasized on red flag symptoms and signs that should prompt health professionals in the community for urgent referral to hospital (Table 1).

SUMMARY

The maternal mortality rates in the UK have been reduced greatly in the last two centuries, particularly in the last 70 years. Probably the better education of women has led to smaller families at a younger age, and the wider use of contraception, including the pill, has probably allowed better spacing of families. Further, there is a background of better health and nutrition of women in Britain, particularly since the Second World War (Chamberlain G, 2006).

The introduction and continuation of the self-audit of confidential enquiries into maternal deaths started in 1952 and has contributed

Table 1 Red flag signs and symptoms

- Pyrexia > 38°C
- Sustained tachycardia > 100 bpm
- Breathlessness (RR > 20; a serious symptom)
- Abdominal or chest pain
- Diarrhea and/or vomiting
- Reduced or absent fetal movements, or absent fetal heart
- Spontaneous rupture of membranes or significant vaginal discharge
- Uterine or renal angle pain and tenderness
- The woman is generally unwell or seems unduly anxious, distressed or panicky.

to greater understanding of maternal deaths. Systematic reporting, analysis and lessons to learn have proven to steadily reduce the maternal mortality in the UK.

The key components for ongoing reduction in maternal mortality are health education for women, risk identification and appropriate referral to the secondary units. Multidisciplinary emergency obstetric care with regular skills training is the way forward to achieve the safe motherhood globally.

BIBLIOGRAPHY

1. Atrash HK, Alexander S, Berg CJ. Maternal mortality in developed countries: not just a concern of the past. Obstet Gynecol. 1995;86(4 Pt 2):700-5.
2. Calvert KL, McGurgan PM, Debenham EM, Gratwick FJ, Maouris P. Emergency obstetric simulation training: How do we know where we are going, if we don't know where we have been? 2013;13. doi:10.1111/ajo.12120.
3. Chamberlain G. British maternal mortality in the 19th and early 20th centuries, J R Soc Med. 2006;99(11):559-63.
4. Crofts JF, Bartlett C, Ellis D, Hunt LP, Fox R, Draycott TJ. Management of shoulder dystocia: skill retention 6 and 12 months after training. Obstet Gynecol. 2007;110(5):1069.
5. Crofts JF, et al. BJOG. 2007;114:1534-41.
6. Deneux-Tharaux C, Berg C, Bouvier-Colle MH, Gissler M, Harper M, Nannini A, Alexander S, Wildman K, Breart G, Buekens P. Underreporting of pregnancy-related mortality in the United States and Europe. Obstet Gynecol. 2005;106(4):684-92.
7. Esscher A, Högberg U, Haglund B, Essën B. Maternal mortality in Sweden 1988-2007: more deaths than officially reported. H Acta Obstet Gynecol Scand. 2013;92(1):40-6.
8. Kirby D. Emerging answers: research findings on programs to reduce teen pregnancy. National Campaign to Prevent Teen Pregnancy; 2001.
9. Oates, et al. BJOG. 2011;118(51):18-23.
10. Stanger-Hall K, Hall D. Abstinence-only education and teen pregnancy rates: Why we need comprehensive sex education in the US PLoS One. 2011;6(10):e24658.

9

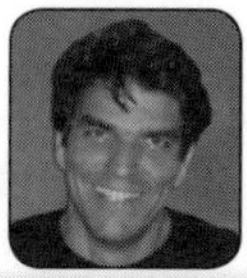

Agency is the Missing Piece in the Safe Motherhood Initiative

Terek Meguid

It always seems impossible, until it is done.

—Nelson Mandela[1]

The Safe Motherhood Initiative (SMI) was initiated more than 25 years ago and has been described in this book very well elsewhere[2]. The purpose of this chapter is to look at determinants for the initiative and its successes and failures without repeating the statistics[3,4] over and over again.

What need to be recalled though are the outrage and the sense of enormous shame about the situations of mothers and expecting mothers that lead to the SMI. It was clear that a great injustice against mothers, children and their families was being allowed to prevail throughout the poorer countries of the world.[5]

In accordance with the Zeitgeist of the 70s and 80s of the last century and following the 1978 Alma Ata Declaration on Primary Health Care (PHC),[6] the solution to this injustice was initially sought in 'empowerment' of the women and their families themselves and later, as happened with PHC, in producing concepts and guidelines that should ensure safe pregnancy and delivery. These concepts and guidelines, the latest is the concept of Comprehensive Emergency Obstetric and Neonatal Care (CEmONC),[7] subsequently dominated the SMI. This top-down approach has its practical and philosophical advantages as well as limitations and drawbacks.

In order to appreciate these, it helps to think of the river to Safe Motherhood as one that has calm and slow and steep and rapid stretches and traveling on that river requires different skills at different stations of the journey. For this reason alone, a 'one fits all' 'magic bullet' approach is problematic.

The different stretches of the river are, amongst others, a situation where there are enough health facilities with enough healthcare workers of all cadres and one where this is not the case. Another aspect is, for both situations, whether those services are adequate and irrespective of the answer to this question whether all the women who need them are using them? This last paragraph can also been summarized with the AAAQ acronym that has been used to describe the Right to Health.[8] This is defined as a service that needs to be *Available, Accessible, Acceptable* and of *High Quality*.

It might help to put the metaphor of the river into a table to show what each of the qualities mentioned above might mean in a given situation (Table 1).

It should be clear from (Table 1) that it is impossible to put all variables into one equation or table in all circumstances. For this reason alone, it is necessary for each stretch of the river, or for each situation to get a clear picture of what is going on there at this point in time (here and now).

The general concepts or principles are interrelated, clear and independent of a given situation. For instance are the concepts of availability, accessibility and acceptability interrelated. A health center might be in the district of the patient but not accessible to her because it asks a user fee that is too high for this particular patient, but not for most other patients. Is this, then a situation where the three A's apply? The answer is yes and no. It seem to be available, accessible and acceptable for most patients but not for all. Obviously, there are numerous possible reasons other than user fees that can make a service inaccessible, not the least discrimination against certain groups of patients, such as adolescents and others, for instance.

All the different aspects of care need to come together and context is everything. It is simply impossible to achieve good results, or to judge a given situation correctly without taking the context into consideration, something global concepts and guidelines cannot do. What they can do, and what SMI has done, is to provide general principles, concepts and ideas that can subsequently be modified and applied. The sounder those principles and concepts are the better, but even the best evidence need to be applied in the appropriate situation. For this reason, researching and improving has to be an on-going, never finished, task of SMI.

The most difficult part of the AAAQ acronym to define is Quality. We have not yet defined clearly and universally what we mean by high quality of care.[9] Part of it, is obviously included in what is usually compiled in statistics under the well-known indicators such as maternal mortality ratio (MMR), case fatality rates (CFR), perinatal mortality rates (PNMR) and so on.[10]

Table 1: *AAAQ*–Acronym for quality of health care (available, accessible, acceptable and quality)

	Available	*Accessible*	*Acceptable*	*Quality*
Patient/Client	Willing to come	Able to come	Feeling respected	Trusting the service
• Health Center • District Hospital • Central Hospital	Numbers per population per geography	• Physical access (roads, ramps) • Economic access (fees)	• Culture and Customs • Gender and expertise mix of health workers • Architecture, Privacy • Acceptable by clients versus authorities	• Medical technical • 'Empowerment' • Conscious of human rights • Number of health workers • Level of expertise of health workers • Measured by biomedical indicators?
Doula	Exist	Allowed to be with expecting mother	• Wanted by mothers • Wanted by health workers	Integrated in service
• Midwife • Doctor • Specialist	Numbers	Attitude, experience	Gender mix	• Audits and continuous professional education • Certification
Family/ Husband	Willing to be involved	Allowed	Possible to physically be present	Welcomed, part of the focus of attention
• Equipment • Drugs • Consumables, etc.	Adequate amounts and appropriate mix of items	No extra limitations (fees)	As under health center heading	Genuine, durable, reliably available

Development of guidelines and evidence to tackle specific clinical situations has been shown to work and to increase therefore the quality of care and are very important technical tools to help SMI to achieve its goals.[11] When employed in the right way and in the right situation, they do influence the indicators in the way we want them to go.

While these indicators do represent important aspects of quality of care, they are not able to catch the whole spectrum of what high quality of health care to human beings should entail.

This leads to the 'empowerment' aspect of the SMI. One of the most striking aspects of maternity wards in most poor countries is their veterinary feel to them. It is as if most patients are not treated as human beings but are only 'appreciated' as problems. Not so much as persons who have a problem but as being the problem themselves. Strictly following clinical technical guidelines enhance this and actually dehumanize patients further.

The context within which this does or does not happen matters because it sustains the status quo and constitutes poor quality of care, even if some health indicators seem to improve. Alternatively, it could be the starting point to achieve sustainable high quality of care. The point here is to work towards sustainable change, change that leads to a situation that will last, and that cannot and should not come through means that actually demean patients. This is not only problematic from a moral point of few but also from a practical one because only a patient care system that has the patients at the center and heart can be sustained through the patients. This will only be possible, if and when the patient is seen and respected and as actively involved as possible.

'Empowering' the patients is not possible for any healthcare system. What is possible however is to disempower the patients and that is the rule rather than the exception in most, of not all, maternities in those countries suffering most of high MMRs; but by no means only in those. Empowerment can only be done by the powerless[12] and the health-care system can assist here. That was the original message from Alma Ata, which has quickly been reversed through endless vertical health programs. The way, the system can assist is to create space for the patients and her family to express herself. This can only happen, if and when the system stops to disempower the patients and starts to create those spaces and sees it as its task to help patients to become their own agents.

Depending on where we are in a given situation we might not be able to provide for this, simply for example, because there are absolutely too few health workers for too many patients.[13] This too is unfortunately more rule than exception and is what needs to be tackled.[14] But if the situation is such that there are enough people on the ground, then this can and should be done. The fact that this will require a change in thinking about the basic relationship between patients and health worker, even the most basic way most health workers think about their professions, does not make this easy.[15]

The tragic bind, we are in is that those patients who need agency the most are those who are most likely to lack it; the poorest of the poor. What makes matters worse is that they depend on maternal healthcare systems that are also heavily, scandalously, understaffed, underequipped and underfunded, and therefore not only not able to provide that kind of care, but actually imposing care to their patients that will only disempower them further.

For this reason, it is of the utmost importance to change the mind-set of health workers and those thinking and deciding around issues of safe motherhood to think further than we have up to this point in time.

This is a complex issue but essentially quite simple at the same time. A paradox; not unlike childbearing itself, which is at the same time the most natural thing to do and has endless possibilities to go wrong and become a disaster for all involved. As every good midwife knows the quality of care for her patients, all three or more, requires her to listen not only for and to the fetal heart but also to all that comes from mother, baby(s) and family. Each delivery is unique and familiar at the same time and the health worker needs to combine those two and apply this to the individual situation at hand at that particular moment.

These simple facts tend to become complex and complicated to those not involved in clinical care (any more), who engage in writing guidelines, conducting research and organizing initiatives only. It is up to the clinicians of all levels to use those guidelines and concepts, in a way that serves the patients at a given situation best; and it is up to those not involved in clinical care anymore to stay in touch with what is actually happening on the ground.

The biggest danger for the future of SMI and maternal health care in general lies in the ability and possibility to disempower the mothers and families in our care, making it impossible for them to develop agency and or not listening to the voices of those patients who do have agency.

For those reasons, all involved in SMI need to be as open towards one another, including and especially towards the patients, to fully use the experiences and insights of all; patients, researchers and clinicians.

After more than two decades of SMI mixed results[16] may be seen as being partly the result of failing to involve the patients and clients actively in this through nurturing their agency. From this follows that this is an aspect that needs to be actively incorporated into the thinking around planning facilities for mothers, their children and families. More importantly, it needs to be incorporated into running those facilities and programs and into a modern understanding of what health care should be all about.

While we need to continue to lobby and convince those in control of funds and policies to ensure to increase the number of health facilities, including especially health workers, we need to ensure at the same time that the quality of service provided there is high. And we need to define a high quality service, in the broadest terms, as a service that sees the patient(s) and her family as being the very center of all efforts to assist. This then has to mean that the patient's agency needs to be nurtured, allowed and welcomed at the very least.

REFERENCES

1. Lagendijk J. It always seems impossible until it is done by Nelson Mandela. Today's Zaman; 17 July, 2011.
2. Vikram Sinai Talaulikar, S Arulkumaran: Global and Historical Perspective of Safe Motherhood Initiative—A small Beginning and a Long Journey. Jaypee Brothers Medical Publishers, New Delhi; 2014.
3. Hoyler M, Finlayson SRG, McClain CD, Meara JG, Hagander L. Shortage of doctors, shortage of data: A review of the global surgery, obstetrics, and anesthesia workforce literature. World Journal of Surgery. 2013;13(11).
4. Bustreo F, Harris Reguejo J, Merialdi M, Presern C, Songane F. From safe motherhood, newborn, and child survival partnerships to the continuum of care and accountability: Moving fast forward to 2015. International Journal of Gynaecology & Obstetrics. 2012;119(S1):s6-s8.
5. AbouZahr C. Safe Motherhood: a brief history of the global movement 1947-2002. British Medical Buletin. 2003;67(1):13-25.
6. WHO. Alma Ata Declaration, 1978. WHO *http://www.who.int/hrp/NPH/docs/declaration_almaata.pdf* (accessed 15 November 2013).
7. Dao B (Ed). Guidelines for In-Service Training in Basic and Comprehensive Emergency Obstetric and Newborn Care. Jhpiego, Maryland, 2012.
8. Hunt P, Gray T (Eds). Maternal Mortality, Human Rights and Accountability. Routledge, Oxon, 2013.
9. Kitson A, Marshall A, Bassett K, Zeitz K. What are the core elements of patient-centred care? A narrative review and synthesis of the literature from health policy, medicine and nursing. Journal of Advanced Nursing. 2013;69(1):4-15.
10. Bhutta ZA, Chopra M, Axelson H, Berman P, Boerma T, Bryce J, Bustreo F, Cavagnero E, Cometto C, Daelmans B, Francisco A de, Fogstad H, Gupta N, Laski L, Lawn J, Maliqi B, Mason E, Pitt C, Requejo J, Starrs A, Victora CG, Wardlaw T. Countdown to 2015 decade report (2000-10): taking stock of maternal, newborn and child survival. Lancet. 2010;375(9730):2032-44.
11. Akker, T van den. Medical mirrors: maternal care in a Malawian district. PhD-thesis, Vrije Universiteit, Amsterdam, 2011.
12. Lewis DL, King. A Biography, 3rd edn. University of Illinois Press, Champaign; 2013.
13. Combs Thorsen V, Teten Tharp AL, Meguid T. High rates of burnout among maternal health staff at a referral hospital in Malawi: a cross-sectional study. BMC Nursing. 2011;10:9.

14. Boseley S. Health worker shortage is a truly global crisis. The Guardian, 18 January, 2011.
15. Illich I. Medical nemesis: the Expropriation of Health. Calder & Boyars, London, 1975.
16. Tita AT, Stringer JS, Goldenberg RL, Rouse DJ. Two decades of the safe motherhood initiative: time for another wooden spoon award? Obstetrics & Gynecology. 2007;110(5):972-6.

Section II

India

"There is only one journey,
going inside yourself"

Chapters

10

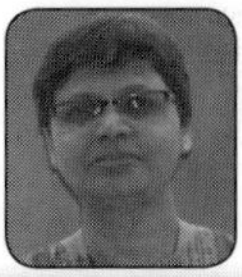
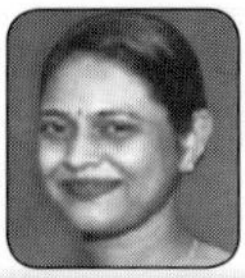

Safe Motherhood in India: Historical Perspective

Sadhana Gupta, Hema J Shobhane

Symbolic rearrangement of the past is an unavoidable aspect of all human attempt to make sense of present.

INTRODUCTION

Historical review of safe motherhood issues in an ancient yet ever young and changing country like India is challenging task. It walks through phases of glory, wisdom as well pain and healing touches of our people.

India is a unique country on this planet. It has been, is and will be not only the place of highest spirituality and philosophy, but also science and technique with wisdom and vision. Despite numerous attacks, invasion and threats, India has been able to retain its treasure of intellectual, natural and economic wealth. It is single country of live and developing civilization of 5000 years with strong democratic governance, values of equality and compassion. It may also be the only country where motherhood and mother is valued as power, eternal force and source of life.

Yet today we have to think hard and act harder to ensure safe journey to life of mother and newborn in course of pregnancy in our country.

A retreat in Indian history in context of women especially maternal health in different phases will help us to see our attempts, failure, and success in right context and frame.

VEDIC AND BUDDHA PERIOD AND AYURVEDA

Ayurveda is conventional method of medicine in India, continued, educated and practiced till present time. By definition Ayurveda implies—knowledge of life. Its origin is traced far back to Vedic times about 500 BC.

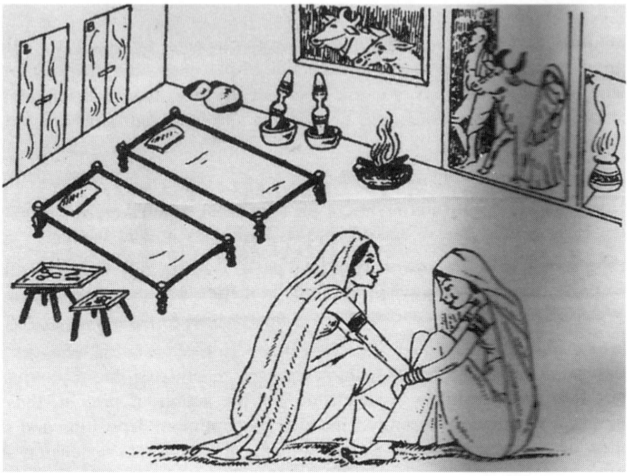

Fig. 1 Preparation for place of child birth—arrangement for warmth, ventilation and attached bathroom—image from ancient India

Ayurveda defines obstetric as separate branch and advices precisely about diet, nutrition, rest, daily routine and precautions in pregnancy. It also specifies the cleanliness, isolation, room temperature, availability of skilled birth attendant and even attached toilet for preparation of delivery (Fig. 1). To some extent it supersedes modern medicine as it understands that mother and fetus are two interdependent yet independent body and soul. It emphasizes on good thoughts and peaceful mind of mother for healthy and worthy newborn.

It appears that maternal health was quiet good in Vedic period, as many scripts tell the story of empowered, healthy mother of many children and hardly any tale of death during child birth.

Ayurveda developed to much height during Buddhist time and schools and hospitals were made during Ashoka (226 BC) and other Buddhist king. Charak and Sushruta are considered father of Indian medicine and surgery respectively and mention asepsis, and even surgical aspect of obstetrics.[1,2]

UNANI–TIBB SYSTEM—MUGHAL PERIOD

There were series of invasion and attack from 12 to 15th century by Muslim rulers, which greatly effected status of women, cultural values including old health system. Unani-Tibb system was introduced and entrenched in certain towns and cities like Delhi, Agra, Hyderabad, Lucknow.[3]

Though from this period there was sharp decline in women's status and health, as probably for sake of protection women were forced to live inside house and deprived of education and decision-making in family society. Scripts of this era tell about numerous stories of women dying in child birth and critically ill women.

MODERN SYSTEM OF OBSTETRIC MEDICINE

Pre-independence Period

Though so-called dark and turbulent years when gradually Mughal rules declined, many small state rules emerged and disappeared and finally East India Company and English Government became formal ruler of India.

It that era of global imperialism there were radical changes in world order. Western world developed research in medicine, and organized medical system. A lot of wealth and resources from their ruled continent like India and neighboring countries facilitated it. Some how, with force of natural laws, the benefit of science and organized health facility reached Indian people also. Beside English rule was like a shock to Indian continent, which reshaped the thought and action of Indian people.

Many radical acts and rules for women empowerment were made with initiative of visionary leader in Indian renaissance like Raja Ram Mohan Rai, Gopalkrishna Gokhale, Mahatma Gandhi. Few of them are ban on Sati system, child marriage act, acceptance of widow marriage, and emphasis on women education. Beside it may be the only freedom struggle of any country and civilization where women took part emphatically in immense number. Mahatma Gandhi called for women to come out of their homes, think and act independently and contribute to country wealth. It is again to be appreciated that Indian people were always the part of administration and political governance and facilitated many public system including maternal health.

Few of landmarks of safe motherhood initiative before independence are as follows:[4,5]

- *1885*: An association for medical aid by the women of India was established by centers of Dufferin. Still we have many district women hospital in name of Dufferin Hospital.
- *1918*: Lady Hardinge Health School was started in Delhi offering health visitor cause.
- *1921*: Lady Chelmsford League was formed in India for developing maternity and child welfare services.

- *1931*: Indian Red Cross Society established Maternal and child Health Bureau in association with Lady Chelmsford League and Victoria Memorial Scholarship Fund and coordinated the Maternal and Child Work throughout the country.
  - Madras (Chennai) was the first city to set-up a separate section for maternal and child welfare in public health department under charge of an Assistant Director of Public Health.
- *1938*: Indian Research Fund Association was established which formed a committee to investigate the incidence and cause of maternal and infant morbidity and mortality. Mudaliar Committee with Sir A Ramasamy Mudaliar as key person presented revolutionary report which pointed facts which are still the key factor for today's maternal and child health for most of the developing and poor world. These are:
  - Institutional midwifery services were limited
  - Maternal and child welfare centers are poorly equipped and staffed
  - Untrained dais mostly handled deliveries.
- *1946*: Bhore Committee stated in its report that India was facing the problem of high maternal and infant death. It recommended emphatically that measures for reduction of sickness and mortality of mother and child should have the highest priority in health development program of India. The golden statement was first stated by Bhore Committee that these deaths are preventable with help of organized health services. Bhore Committee was also first in the world to give word and idea of primary and universal healthcare.

Charitable Hospital and Institution

India may be one of the few countries where from the beginning health and education are in principle supposed to be given to all irrespective of their status and religion. Ramkrishna Mission, Vivekanand Clinic and Hospital and series of charitable hospital in all zones always played an important role in imparting good hygienic care to mother and child.

Post-independence Period

India gained total independence from British Rule on 15th August 1947. It also received a major geographical, economical and emotional trauma in form of partition and division. However, Indian Government and Constitution gave deep thought for universal, affordable, accessible health for all. Many National Program were formulated to fight against Smallpox, Malaria, Tuberculosis, Blindness, Maternal and Child Health

Programs constituted a major share of its health and population policy. Here is chronological order of MCH Programs in postindependence India.

- *1952*: With recommendation of Bhore Committee, primary health centers (PHC) were set-up in each and every part of India to provide universal and essential healthcare to all.
- *1953*: India was the first country in the world to launch National Family Planning Program which introduced concept of small family norm and availability of free contraceptive. From 1953 to 1976 family planning program has been one of the top priority programs by Government of India. Initially it was incentive based target oriented approach. In April 1976, country framed National Population Policy. The disasters of forced sterilization campaign in 1976 lead to major Congress defeat in 1977 election. In June 1977, the new government framed a new population policy ruling out compulsion and coercion for the future. The ministry was renamed family welfare committee. Constitution made amendment for population control and family planning on voluntary basis and involvement of local people in family welfare program at gross root level to accelerate the pace of family welfare program.
- *1970*: All India Hospital Postpartum Family Programs were started.
- *1972*: Medical Termination of Pregnancy (MTP) Act was introduced and abortion was legalized in sets of condition to make abortion safe for women at safe place, by qualified provider.
- *1976*: MTP Act was further liberalized so that majority of women can access to safe abortion services.
- *1977*: Multipurpose health worker scheme was launched to encourage community people involvement for various health issues.
- *1978*: India was signatory to Alma Ata Declaration in 1978 joint WHO UNICEF conference. Primary healthcare approach was accepted for health for all by 2000 AD.
- *1983*: Maternal and child health and family welfare services were integrated under National Health Policy.
- *1985*: A separate department of women and child development was set up under the newly created Ministry of Human Resource and Development. Universal immunization program was launched.
- *1987*: A worldwide "Safe Motherhood Campaign" was launched by World Bank.
- *1992*: The universal immunization, oral rehydration therapy and safe motherhood program were integrated under Child Survival and Safe Motherhood (CSSM) Program. This year infant milk substitute, feeding bottle and infant food (Regulation of production, supply and distribution) Act 1992, came into force. It was achieved through very

hard and consistent work and research based advocacy by Indian Academy of Pediatrics (IAP) and Breast Feeding Promotion Network of India (BPNI) against the milk powder and child food industry.

- *1995*: International Conference on Population and Development in Cairo recommended implementation of unified Reproduction and Child Health (RCH) Program. India was one of the signatories of this movement. In 9th Five Year Plan RCH program integrated all related program of our 8th Five Year Plan. The concept of RCH is to provide need based, client oriented, demand driven, high quality integrated service. RCH phase I focused on essential antenatal care and risk approach. Soon the limitation of essential healthcare for prevention of maternal death was understood. In RCH phase II program the emergency obstetric care facility was taken in account with creation and revitalization of first referral unit at periphery with facility of emergency obstetric care including cesarean section, blood availability and newborn care.

  National Maternity Benefit Scheme (NMBS) was launched by Ministry of Rural Development. Under NMBS scheme pregnant women from below poverty line (BPL) were entitled to cash assistance of Rs. 500/- for up to two births, disbursed 8 to 12 week before delivery.
- *1996*:
  - Pulse polio immunization; the largest single-day public health event took place
  - Family planning program made target free from 1st April 1996
  - Prenatal Diagnostic Act (Regulation and Prevention of Misuse) Act 1994, came into force from January 1996.
- *2000*: Government of India implemented more detailed and comprehensive National Population Policy to promote family welfare.
- *1995–2000*: The three delay model was conceptual model which indentifies three delays in management of obstetrical complication at community and facility level. Identification of this model helped program coordinator to understand determinants of maternal mortality.
- *2005*: Government of India, Ministry of Health and Family Welfare launched the National Rural Health Mission (NRHM) with a strong commitment to reduce maternal and infant mortality, ensure population stabilization, maintain gender balance, provide universal access to public health services, prevent and control communicable and noncommunicable disease and revitalize local health traditions.

National Maternity Benefit Scheme

The Government of India has long recognized its poor performance in maternal and child health and, in August 1995, the National Maternity Benefit Scheme (NMBS) came into effect as a component of the National Social Assistance Program (NSAP) to be implemented by the Ministry of Rural Development. Under the NMBS, pregnant women from below the poverty line (BPL) families were entitled to cash assistance of Rs. 500 for up to two births, disbursed 8 to 12 weeks before delivery. Based on reports and complaints that the scheme was not achieving its goals, it was modified into what is now *Janani Suraksha Yojana* (JSY) and is one of the principal planks of the National Rural Health Mission.[3] The objectives of the JSY are to reduce maternal and infant mortality through increased delivery at health institutions. The JSY implementation guidelines say, "While the NMBS is linked to provision of a better diet for pregnant women from BPL families, the JSY integrates the cash assistance with antenatal care during the pregnancy period, institutional care during delivery and immediate postpartum period in a health center by establishing a system of coordinated care by field level health worker."[4]

Janani Suraksha Yojna

It is one of the most revolutionary and innovative schemes started by Government of India under NRHM. The innovative and unique features of JSY are as follows:[6,7]

- It integrates cash assistance with antenatal care, institutional care and immediate postpartum care
- It establishes a system of coordinated care by field level health worker
- Postnatal care and visit for breastfeeding, contraception and vaccination must also be provided by link healthcare worker.[8,9]

The RCH II program is the key vehicle under the umbrella of the flagship NRHM to address maternal and child health challenges in India. One of the key interventions under the RCH II program is the JSY, along with other evidence-based interventions on the demand and supply-side to address maternal and child mortality.[10] JSY scheme has shown its impact in form of marked rise in institutional delivery among beneficiary women, utilization of health services by women belonging to below poverty lines and scheduled caste women.[11-13]

The impact is more in low performing states, but due to global economy changes scenario even best performing state like Kerala now has to address its population's growing demand for high quality and specialized care in a way that protects the integrity of its public health system and the social equity it has worked so hard to achieve.[14-16]

Voluntary and Professional Organization

Many voluntary and professional organization are working in India for family welfare and maternal and child health services. Family Planning Association of India, Family Planning Foundation, Population Council of India, Public Service International (PSI), Indian Medical Association (IMA), Federation of Obstetrical and Gynecological Society of India (FOGSI) and Indian Academy of Pediatrics (IAP) are actively providing technological and organizational support for reproductive maternal, newborn, child and adolescent health. At the international level, United Nation Fund for Population Activities (UNFPA), US Agency for International Development (USAID), Population Council, PATH, PATH Finder, and UNICEF are few recognized international agencies who are assisting in research, services, training, information and implementation program in field of Maternal and Child Health and Family Planning in India.

Safe Motherhood Day

Prime Minister of India launched 11th April 2009 as Safe Motherhood Day, which is birthday of Kasturba Gandhi, wife of Mahatma Gandhi, father of nation. On this day government and private hospitals, professional organizations and media organize different activities and programs to sensitize the people for issue of safe motherhood.

Sample Registration System

Survey data on maternal mortality ratio (MMR) is available from report of Registrar General of India (RCI-SRS) at three year interval. The latest available data of MMR for period of 2007 to 2009 is 212/100,000 live birth, and infant mortality rate (SRS 2011) is 44/1000 live birth.[17]

According to Maternal Mortality Estimation Inter Agency (MMEIG) group WHO, UNICEF, UNFPA, World Bank—India is ranked 126 out of 180 countries.[18] There is wide discrepancy in data collected from global agencies like WHO, UNICEF and UNFPA, and from country-based studies. It requires proper methodology, credibility, large inputs and transparency. Professional bodies like IMA, FOGSI can help in planning long-term and continued process of correct reporting each and every case of maternal death and severe acute maternal morbidity.

TRENDS IN MATERNAL MORTALITY IN INDIA

The multiple policies and programs run by central, state government and nongovernment organization have been enabled to keep the issue of maternal and child health in main frame and context. It itself is a big achievement where people as well officials do not accept now any maternal death as natural. Kerala, Tamil Nadu and Maharashtra have already achieved MDG goal to MMR less than 109/100,000 live birth. Andhra Pradesh, West Bengal, Gujarat and Haryana are close to target (Table 1 and Fig. 2).

It is also to be emphasized that low performing states are showing decline rate of 18 percent in maternal mortality ratio and thus they are on right track. Southern states had better performance from the beginning due to many factors like matriarchal society, women education, and land

Table 1 State-wise maternal mortality ratio in India

India and major states	*MMR 2004–06*	*MMR 2007–09*
Indian total	254	212
Assam	480	390
Bihar/Jharkhand	312	261
Madhya Pradesh/Chhattisgarh	335	269
Odisha	303	258
Rajasthan	388	318
Uttar Pradesh/Uttarakhand	440	359
EAG and Assam subtotal	*375*	*308*
Andhra Pradesh	154	134
Karnataka	213	178
Kerala	95	81
Tamil Nadu	111	97
South subtotal	*149*	*127*
Gujarat	160	148
Haryana	186	153
Maharashtra	130	104
Pubjab	192	172
West Bengal	141	145
Other	206	160
Other subtotal	*174*	*149*

Maternal mortality ratio measures number of women aged 15–49 years dying due to maternal causes per 1,00,000 live births.

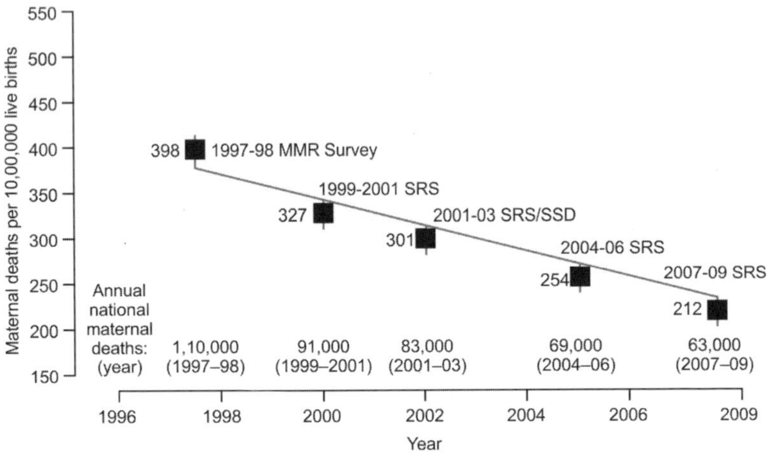

Fig. 2 Trends in maternal mortality ratio in India

reforms. Beside, all political struggle and turbulence right from Mughal era to independence struggle and pang of partition were mainly faced by heartland of people. With result that they were deprived of money investment in British rule and also faced socioeconomic crisis and chaos in neo-independent India. However, currently whole of the country and all participants in women's health are today working towards reaching MDG goal throughout the country.

MAJOR CHALLENGES FOR SAFE MOTHERHOOD TO ALL IN MODERN INDIA

Despite positive development and program for safe motherhood, the present political, economic, sociocultural scenario pose major challenges before Indian people. These challenges require recognition, introspection and hard decisions. Few of these challenges are as follows:

- *To reach the unreached people and provide accessible, affordable quality care for mother and child:* Mammoth industrialization, rapid urbanization, massive destruction of natural resources have marginalized the rural people, scheduled tribes, women and old people in families from main stream of development. Moreover corruption in all sectors eats up major chunk of government expenditure in health and other programs. Medical person do not wish to live and work in villages and small towns as they feel left out in career and level of living. Till now there is no compulsory accountability of educated youth as well adult for their fellow people. Facing this challenge need compassion, vision and determination.

- *To fill in the gaps between triple systems of healthcare:* Today India have three tier of health delivery system—one is public health system which is over burdened with many programs, understaffing and loose administration. Yet *Public Health System* has presence and action in smallest town and village of country. Activation and improvement in infrastructure of public health system has great potential in delivering universal quality obstetric care. NRHM and JSY are pro-people programs and made positive impact in all states. *Small scale private sector* is another tier of health delivery system, where personalized care of varying quality is given at moderate expenses. It has grown in last twenty years and filled the gap between demand and need of obstetric care to some extent. Up to 30 to 50 percent of health facilities are delivered through small scale private sector in few states. Government of India has also proposed many programs for public private partnership with varying responses in different states. Unfortunately recently like all small scale industries, small clinics and nursing homes are threatened by many rules and regulations which favor big corporate sector. *Corporate sector* is the third tier of health delivery system which has grown very fast in India, with exuberantly high charges and glittering advertisement of technology and facilities.

  How to improve public health system, how to survive small scale private sector and how to monitor and regulate corporate sector is a big question for today's Indian health delivery system.
- *Lack of human resources:* There is acute shortage of skilled human resource be it doctors or nurses in India in proportion of population. Due to information technology (IT) and sudden, unexplained high salary in that sector the choice of medicine as career for youth suddenly declined. Moreover the global fast communication and involvement of corporate sector in health hastened brain drain from small to big cities and from developing countries to developed world. Today a good proportion of students, who study medicine at very nominal fees run after job in developed countries. The experienced skilled doctors from even prime government institutions are going for jobs in corporate sector. Final result is the rural, poor and middle income families are not able to receive quality healthcare, and they are compelled to do out of pocket expenses and become more financially compromised. It is the challenge which has to be faced with honest introspection of medical fraternity and political governance.
- *Double system of medical education:* The double system of medical education has also created marked confusion not only on issue of quality education but also the mind set of medical persons. The wide and unexplained disparity in fee structure of government and private

medical colleges, lack of transparency in entrance criterion in private set up are the few major issues of concern. Moreover autonomous bodies like Medical Council of India frame and work is according to criteria and standard of developed world for recognition of graduate and postgraduate medical seats. Consequently the government medical institution due to less funds, fall short of some technological lacuna with reduction of student's seats. In already serious shortage of doctors in country, many bright, hard working youth are deprived of potential medical career. Settling and solving the dual system of medical education is one of the burning concerns of today and require political will and determination.

CONCLUSION

India has traveled a long and tough journey of 5000 years and experienced height of excellence, richness, and independence to lows of slavery, poverty, and invasion. The most remarkable and astonishing fact about India is that it has always survived with its soul, intellect and wisdom. India has regained independence 66 year ago, it has reformed, redefined its goals. Being a vast country of extreme diversity of geography, language, culture, and people with rich democratic values, its challenge are unique. Maternal and child health is one of such challenges.

This chapter clearly shows that Indian people, government, professional organization have been always on the right track. Indian people as well leaders showed vision and openness with changing times. We are strongly committed to dignity and safety of mother and child health. Our plan and policies reflect the need, desire and aspiration of our people. Modern world is again facing challenges of global economic imperialism, environmental threats, brain drain, rapid urbanization and industrialization. In principle, in laws, in policy we are one of the few countries where equality, care and concern of underprivileged are our main concern. Maternal health statistics is improving on all issues, few states have already achieved MDG Goal, few are in queue and EAG states are showing sharp decline.

Commitment of each and every person is the need of today. Get involved, spread in world, and denote time, treasure and talent. One preventable death is one to many.

There can be no greatness without simplicity, truth and compassion—

Leo Tolstoy—*War and Peace*

REFERENCES

1. Jaggi OP. Indian System of Medicine, Atmaram and Sons; 1973.
2. Gokhale BV. Swasth Hind; 1960;4:165.
3. Banerjee JN.Indian Jr. Med Edu. 1966;5:79.
4. Jump up the Newsletter of the Partnership for Maternal, Newborn and Child Health 2. January 2006. ISSN 1815-9184.
5. Neelam Kumari, Shivani Sharma, Preeti Gupta. Midwifery and Gynecological Nursing. (Jalandhar): S Vikas and Company (Medical Publishers); 2010.
6. Implementation of Government Food and Livelihood Schemes in India's poorest districts—a report of a rapid survey, October 2007.
7. Janani Surakasha Yojana (JSY)—a brief on its features and parameters-Modified 2005.
8. UNICEF 2009 State of the World's Children report. Available at http://www.unicef.org/sowc09/report/report.php.
9. National Rural Health Mission-2nd Common Review mission, Kerala: 25th November to 2nd December, 2008.
10. Kerala: A Clash of Health and Wealth. Global Envision, the confluence of global markets and poverty alleviation. Available at http://www.globalenvision.org/tags/kerala.
11. Satish Kumar Chauhan. Impact of JSY on maternal healthcare in India, Lambert Academic Publishing; 2012.pp.87-8.
12. Salient Features of the First Phase of the Reproductive and Child Health Program (RCH I). Reproductive and Child Health Phase II. Available at mohfw.nic.in/NRHM/RCH/Background_new.htm.
13. District Level Household and Facility Surveys (DLHFS). Available at http://www.jsk.gov.in/dlhs3/kerala.pdf.
14. Ibid. Lahariya C. "Cash Incentives for Institutional Delivery" Linking with Antenatal and Post Natal Care May Ensure 'Continuum of Care' in India," Indian Journal of Community Medicine. 2009,34 (1):15-18.
15. Is there hope for South Asia?" BMJ. 2004;328:777-78.
16. Franke R. Lessons in Democracy from Kerala State, India. University lecture transcript, Montclair University; 1999.
17. Survey data on Maternal Mortality Ratio (MMR) is available from the Report of Registrar General of India Sample Registration System (RGI-SRS) at three year for the period 2007-09. New Delhi, Dec 11, 2013.
18. MMEIG (Maternal Mortality Estimation Inter-Agency Group-WHO, UNICEF, UNFPA, World Bank) report titled "Trends in Maternal Mortality: 1990-2010".

11

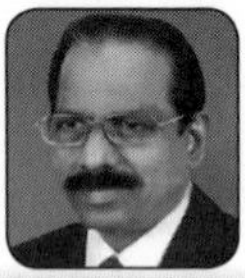

Maternal Death Statistics: A Stepping Stone

PK Sekharan

"Maternal death audit goes beyond counting numbers to listen and tell the stories of the women who died so as to learn lessons that may save the lives of other mothers and babies, as well as aiming to improve the standard of maternal health overall"

—Professor Gwyneth Lewis

INTRODUCTION

The aim of obstetric care is to get a healthy mother and a healthy baby at the end of the pregnancy. Unfortunately, tragedies do strike every now and then and we lose the most important member of the family—The mother; it is more tragic as it is mostly preventable. For reducing maternal mortality, the first and most important step is to have an accurate statistics from every part of the country. This is important for the government, the society at large and for the health care providers to take remedial measures in reducing maternal mortality in the country.

Pregnancy is a normal, healthy state, yet it carries serious risks of death and disability. Often repeated statement that, "half a million young women die every year as a result of complications arising from pregnancy and delivery" is a shocking reality! For every woman who dies, many more suffer from serious conditions that can affect them for the rest of their lives. Each year, approximately eight million women suffer pregnancy-related complications[1]. Each death or long-term complication represents an individual tragedy for the woman, her partner, her children and her family. The impact of such a tragedy on the health workers who cared for her, cannot be overemphasized.

DEFINITION

Maternal Death

The death of a woman while pregnant or within 42 days of termination of pregnancy, irrespective of the duration and site of the pregnancy, from any cause related to or aggravated by the pregnancy or its management but not from accidental or incidental causes (ICD-10, WHO).

Pregnancy-related Death

It is defined as the death of a woman while pregnant or within 42 days of termination of pregnancy, irrespective of the cause of death. This is to facilitate the identification of maternal deaths in circumstances in which cause of death attribution is inadequate.

Maternal Mortality Ratio

The number of maternal deaths during given time period per 100,000 live births during same period.

Maternal Mortality Rate

Is the number of maternal deaths in given time period per 100,000 women of reproductive age of 15 to 49 years.

Maternal Deaths can be Further Subdivided into Direct, Indirect and Coincidental Maternal Deaths

A direct obstetric death results from obstetric complications of pregnancy, from interventions, omissions, incorrect treatment, or from chain of events resulting from pregnancy, labor, delivery, or postpartum conditions. An indirect obstetric death results from pre-existing disease (e.g. diabetes, cardiac disease, malaria, tuberculosis, HIV) or a new disease that develops during pregnancy and is unrelated to pregnancy-related conditions, but is aggravated by the physiologic effects of pregnancy (e.g. influenza). The coincidental maternal deaths are deaths from unrelated causes which happen to occur in pregnancy or the puerperium (Road traffic accedents). Late maternal death is the death of a woman from direct or indirect obstetric causes, more than 42 days, but less than 1 year after termination of pregnancy.

Lifetime Risk of Maternal Death

The lifetime risk of maternal death takes into account the cumulative probability of dying as a result of pregnancy across a woman's reproductive years. It is calculated by multiplying the maternal mortality rate by the length of the reproductive period (approximately 35 years).

NEED FOR MATERNAL DEATH AUDIT

Maternal death audit is essential for every country to know the magnitude of the problem of maternal mortality, at what point during pregnancy and childbirth do women die, why do they die, where do maternal deaths take place, what are the inequalities in the risk of maternal death, and what else do we need to know about maternal mortality. This is important to plan strategies in reducing maternal mortality in every country. The approaches for maternal death audit should go beyond counting the number of cases of death but understanding why they happened and how they can be prevented. It is just not counting the number and calculating the ratios, but to draw conclusion and to formulate recommendations. Acting on the results of these studies offers an opportunity for all involved in planning and providing services for pregnant women to make a real difference to their lives.

WHY MOTHERS DIE?

- Is it because they are unaware of the need for care, or unaware of the warning signs of problems in pregnancy?

Or

- Is it because the services do not exist, or are inaccessible for other reasons, such as distance, cost or sociocultural barriers?

Or

- Are women dying because the care they receive is inadequate or actually harmful?

Answers to these and other important questions about why women die during pregnancy and childbirth will enable health professionals and authorities to act on remedial steps.

HOW TO GET THE DATA ON MATERNAL DEATH?

Civil Registration System

In countries where there is robust civil registration of births and deaths, routine registration of births and deaths will provide accurate data on maternal deaths where coverage is complete with cause of death identified with standard medical certificates.

Household Surveys (Sisterhood Method)

This method obtains information by interviewing a representative sample of respondents about the survival of all their siblings.

Census

A national census, with the addition of a limited number of questions, could produce estimates of maternal mortality.

Verbal Autopsy

This approach is used to assign cause of death through interviews with family or community members, where medical certification of cause of death is not available.

Reproductive-age Mortality Studies (RAMOS)

This approach involves identifying and investigating the causes of all deaths of women of reproductive age in a defined area/population, by using multiple sources of data (e.g. interviews of family members, civil registrations, health-facility records, burial records, traditional birth attendants).

MATERNAL DEATHS WORLDWIDE

It is estimated by different world organizations that an estimated 287,000 maternal death occurred all over the world in 2010, which is showing a 47 percent reduction over a 20 year period from 1990. Two regions of the world, sub-Saharan Africa (56%) and Southern Asia (29%), accounted for 85 percent of the Global burden (245,000 maternal deaths) and two countries of the world, India at 19 percent (56,000) and Nigeria at 14 percent (40,000) account for one-third of maternal deaths occurring all over the world. The global MMR in 2010 was 210 maternal deaths per 100,000 live births, down from 400 maternal deaths per 100,000 live births in 1990.[1-5]

As per the 2008 estimates, the lifetime risk of maternal death was highest in Afghanistan (1 in 11) followed by sub-Saharan Africa (1 in 31), and lowest in developed countries (1 in 4300).[2]

We are not in a position to confirm or dispute the statement that India contribute to a fifth of the total maternal deaths world over nor we are sure of our maternal mortality ratio is 210/100,000 or higher as we do not have the correct figurers.

CIVIL REGISTRATION SYSTEM IN INDIA

Registration of births and deaths was made compulsory by an act of parliament in 1969. Headed by the Registrar-General of India who will issue general directions regarding registration of births and deaths in the territories to which this Act extends, shall take steps to coordinate and unify the activities of Chief Registrars of the states in the matter of registration of births and deaths and submit to the Central Government an annual report. The death certificate has to specify the cause of death of a woman if she was pregnant or recently delivered. Other than this, most of the state governments are also trying to have details of maternal deaths through the respective health service systems to be forwarded to the central government for compilation of the national data.

Unfortunately in spite of having the provision of collecting and collating the data on maternal mortality, we do not have an accurate figure of the maternal death in our country. In order to judge the progress we are making towards achieving the millennium development goal-5 (MDG-5) we should have the data and develop recommendations for providing quality maternity care to all.

Millennium Declaration

The United Nations Millennium Declaration, signed in September 2000, commits world leaders to combat poverty, hunger, disease, illiteracy, environmental degradation, and discrimination against women. The MDGs are derived from this declaration. Each MDG has targets set for 2015 and indicators to monitor progress from 1990 levels. Several of these relate directly to health. The fifth MDG aims to improve maternal health, measured by the maternal mortality ratio, with a target of reducing the MMR by 75 percent between 1990 and 2015, (109/100,000) and achieving universal access to reproductive health by 2015.

For tracking the progress we are making towards achieving the millennium development goal-5 (MDG-5), we must have a reliable mechanism for assessing the number and the cause of maternal death in our country. Unfortunately, we do not have such an accurate data and the government depends on the sample survey system conducted by the Registrar general of India.

SAMPLE REGISTRATION SYSTEM IN INDIA

Largest demographic survey in the country covering about 1.4 million households and 7.01 million population in 7597 sample units across 35 States/UTs. As per the target set by MDG-5, India has to reduce the MMR to 109/100,000. Report of the Sample Registration System published by the Registrar General of India for 2007 to 09, the maternal mortality ratio is 212/100,000. This figure is derived from a sample of 436411 deliveries and 926 maternal deaths in India.[6] As per the SRS an estimated 63,000 maternal deaths has occurred in India for the year 2009 and facts from 926 deaths may not tell the story.

CONFIDENTIAL REVIEW OF MATERNAL DEATHS

A confidential enquiry into maternal deaths can be defined as a systematic multidisciplinary anonymous investigation of all or a representative sample of maternal deaths occurring at an area, regional (state) or national level which identifies the numbers, causes and avoidable or remediable factors associated with them. Through the lessons learnt from each woman's death, and through aggregating the data, confidential enquiries provide evidence of where the main problems in overcoming maternal mortality lie and an analysis of what can be done in practical terms, and highlight the key areas requiring recommendations for health sector and community action as well as guidelines for improving clinical outcomes. **—Gwyneth Lewis.**[7]

The solution of this problem is to start the confidential review of maternal deaths in every state and compile it as the national data.

Confidential enquiries into maternal deaths (CEMD) was started in England and Wales as early as 1954. Such intervention has helped to accurately assess the cause of death in a given case with identification of preventive steps. South Africa is one of the few developing countries with a national confidential inquiry into maternal deaths which was started very early. More than fifty countries in the world are having the system of confidential review of maternal deaths. Acting on the findings and recommendations of the committee, these countries could reduce their maternal deaths.

State Level Maternal Death Review Committees

We should start the State level audit of the maternal deaths in all the states of our country. A confidential systematic multidisciplinary investigation of all maternal deaths occurring in every state to be initiated and should be forwarded to the central government to bring out the national report and recommendations periodically. The audit should be conducted by body of professionals having enough experience to draw evidences and to form conclusion and recommendations.

What FOGSI can do?

FOGSI with its strength of nearly 25,000 obstetricians all over the country can do a great job of conducting the maternal death audit at the district and state level which could be then used to have the national data. All the obstetric and gynecological societies under the Federation can group into state level bodies to coordinate this activity with the help of the state governments to start the state maternal mortality review committee. The state level committee can be constituted by having senior members, both from government and private facilities. They should give their services voluntarily and free of any cost. There should be government orders empowering the committee to carry out the work and making available all the records, both from government and private facility.

Confidential Audit

Anonymity and confidentiality should be strictly maintained at all times in the review process. The name and identity of the patient and the name of the hospital and the staff involved in the management of the case should be kept secret from the enquiry team. The aim is not to find fault with, but to suggest remedial action to avoid such deaths and to suggest change in practice guidelines if necessary and to formulate service requirements by the policy makers. Published reports should focus on ways to improve the system and not single out particular errors that have been committed. This enables those who cared for the woman to have the confidence to provide an unbiased and frank account of the actual circumstances, and any deficiencies, surrounding her death without any fear of punitive action. Thus, a more realistic picture of the precise events and any avoidable or remediable factors in the care she received can be obtained. They provide data on individual cases, which when aggregated together can show trends or common factors for which remedial action may be possible. Before publication, the contents will need to be carefully reviewed to avoid breaches in confidentiality and misuse of information.

Legal Protection

It is necessary to have laws to protect those investigating maternal deaths from civil and professional liability. Laws are also needed to protect the information gathered during the investigation from disclosure and use in subsequent lawsuits (confidentiality). Identities of the women whose deaths are being investigated, their families, and the health care professionals involved in their care will be kept confidential. Data collection forms, case summaries, review meetings, and any reports or dissemination of results should not contain personal identification. Death review report should not be used to blame individuals or institutions, or to punish persons or groups. Once the analysis and findings are finalized, all the documents must be destroyed.

Importance of Government Action

State governments should make rules and regulations for mandatory reporting of maternal deaths to the enquiry committee. State and National data on maternal death audit provide information and recommendation for health planners and ministers to change or develop policies and to raise investment levels in health care. The involvement of the health authorities and the government leads to professional clinical guideline development, dissemination, implementation and audit. The findings can be used to develop national or regional maternal health care programs as well as providing facilities like blood bank facilities. The confidential enquiry into maternal deaths should be the responsibility of the Ministry of Health and it should be mandatory for the state committees to report to the center periodically as decided-yearly, with their recommendations. The findings and recommendations are to be put into action so that the large percentages of avoidable deaths are prevented. The maternal death audit is just not finding the number and ratios, but to put the lessons learned into action to reduce the maternal mortality.

Findings and Recommendations should be put into Action

The purpose of the enquiry is to act upon the recommendations of the committee. The results will determine what the main causes of death are and whether there are any avoidable or remediable factors in the care provided to the women. The enquiry enables practitioners and health planners to learn from the errors of the past. The committee should be able to focus not only on clinical issues, but should also address the underlying socioeconomic and demographic factors that contribute to maternal mortality, such as poverty, malnutrition or geographical location. It provides evidence of where the problems are, and highlights the areas requiring recommendation for health sector and community action as well as clinical guidelines. The enquiry forms a baseline against which the success of changing practice can be monitored.

KERALA MODEL

The ten obstetric and gynecological societies of Kerala has formed a state body known as the Kerala Federation of Obstetrics and Gynecology

(KFOG) and is coordinating the academic activities in the state. The maternal fetal medicine committee of KFOG has started the maternal death review in the state in 2004 under the initiative and leadership of Professor VP Paily. With the help of the Government of Kerala and with the cooperation of all the members of KFOG, we are able to carry on with this project and we have published two reports for the year 2004 to 2005 and for 2006 to 2009 with conclusion and recommendations for management of specific obstetric problems.[6-9] The publication of next report for 2010 to 2012 is in progress. Comparing to other parts of India, Kerala is having a lower level of MMR of around 50/100,000 for the last five years and obstetric hemorrhage and hypertensive disorders of pregnancy are the leading cause of maternal death.

WHAT ALL OF US PRACTICING OBSTETRICS CAN DO?

Conduct maternal death audit of the hospital periodically-monthly review, quarterly review or yearly review and draw conclusion and learn lessons as to why the particular woman died, what action could have changed the outcome, what the family members, the society or the health provider has to do to prevent such deaths. This audit again should be confidential and not to find fault with individuals, but to improve the outcome. One should analyze maternal mortality rate in a particular obstetric problem, for example, eclampsia—the need for change in practice—the use of magnesium sulphate and early delivery. In cases of PPH the advocacy of active management of third stage, and use of very cheap and effective condom tamponade.

The sample survey conducted by FOGSI by collecting the data from its members has given a ratio of 353/100,000 for the year 2005 to 2006 and 257/100,000 for the year 2009 to 2011.[10] The major cause of maternal death continues to be obstetric hemorrhage and hypertensive disorders of pregnancy. The SRS by the Registrar general of India for the year 2007 to 2009 has shown an MMR of 212/100,000. We have to work hard to achieve the goal of MDG-5 (109/100,000) in the coming two years (Table 1).

Table 1 Federation of Obstetric and Gynaecological Societies of India (FOGSI) maternal mortality survey : PK Sekharan

Year	*2005–2006*	*2009–2011*
No. of deliveries	12,53,696	19,73,068
No. of maternal deaths	4420	5084
MMR	353/100,000	257/100,000

It is important to have multidisciplinary team approach for developing protocols for managing complicated cases.

Participating in these studies builds on the natural altruism of individuals or teams of health care professionals who are prepared to freely give their time and effort in order to learn lessons to help save women's lives.

REFERENCES

1. WHO/UNICEF/UNFPA, Maternal mortality in 2000: estimates developed by WHO, UNICEF and UNFPA. Geneva, World Health Organization; 2004.
2. Trends in maternal mortality: 1990 to 2008 Estimates developed by WHO, UNICEFF, UNFPA and The World Bank. http://www.who.int/reproductivehealth/publications/monitoring/9789241500265/en/index.
3. Beyond the Numbers: Reviewing maternal deaths and complications to make pregnancy safer, WHO; 2004.
4. Estimates of maternal mortality worldwide between 1990 and 2005: an assessment of available data. Lancet. 2007;370:1311–9.
5. Trends in Maternal Mortality:1990 to 2010 WHO, UNICEF, UNFPA and The World Bank estimates, © World Health Organization, 2012.
6. Special Bulletin on Maternal mortality in India 2007 to 2009, sample registration system, office of Registrar General, India, June, 2011.
7. BJOG Volume 118, Supplement 1, March 2011; Saving Mothers' Lives, Reviewing maternal deaths to make motherhood safer: 2006–2008.
8. Why Mothers Die-Kerala 2004–2005 Ed. V P Paily, Kerala Federation of Obstetrics and Gynaecology, 2009.
9. Why mothers die-Kerala, VP.Paily, K Ambujam, Betsy Thomas, (Eds) Kerala Federation of Obstetrics and Gynaecology. 2012.
10. PK Sekharan FOGSI Maternal Mortality Survey of India. Unpublished data.

12

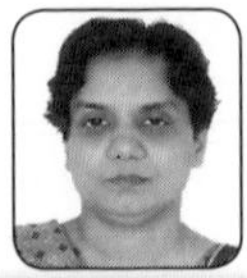

Maternal Death Audit: Necessity and Complexities

Asmita Rathore, Neelam Yadav, Abha R

INTRODUCTION

Motherhood is aspiration of most of the women but this physiological life affirming process is associated with risk of morbidity and mortality. Maternal mortality is an indicator of status of women in the society, their access to health care and adequacy of health care system to respond to their needs. Of the eight United Nations Millennium Development Goals, the goal of reducing maternal mortality is the one that remains the furthest from reaching its targets.[1-3]

Medical audit is a quality improvement process that seeks to improve patient care and outcomes through systematic review of care against explicit criteria and the implementation of change and then to reaudit to ensure that these changes have an effect.[4,5] The application of same to maternal mortality can bring about the targeted improvements.

NECESSITY OF MATERNAL DEATH AUDIT

According to WHO, important causes of maternal death globally are hemorrhage 34 percent, obstructed labor 11 percent, eclampsia 16 percent, unsafe abortion 18 percent, infection 21 percent.[6] Maternal deaths can be averted but for the 'three delays'—delay in decision to seek professional care, delay in reaching the appropriate health facility, and delay in receiving care after arriving at a hospital.[7] Tackling and averting this trio of delays will help the world as India to reduce the burden of maternal mortality.

A number of different types of information and actions are needed to reduce maternal mortality. The information required includes data related to the magnitude of the problem and who is affected by it (levels/numbers), information explaining the factors that directly cause or contribute to the death (determinants) and they can provide indications on practical ways to rectify the problems or potential solutions (interventions), information to base the plans and assess the implementation (monitoring). All these types of information can draw attention to the problem of maternal mortality (advocacy). A key requisite for success is commitment to act upon the findings.

Maternal death audit is an important tool. It is used in many countries worldwide as a strategy to reduce maternal mortality. According to WHO, reducing maternal mortality is not just an issue of development, but also an issue of human rights with universal coverage and targeting excluded group.

In the United Kingdom, confidential enquiries into maternal death (CEMD) were driven by a desire to improve care and a great many people are involved. CEMD reports showed a fall in maternal deaths due to abortion from 153 in 1952 to 54 to one in 1994 to 99, attributable to the legalization of abortion. Between the same periods, maternal deaths from hemorrhage fell from 188 to nine because of oxytocic injections, ultrasound diagnosis of placenta previa, and improved intensive care. Death due to thromboembolism, which remains an important cause of maternal mortality, fell from 138 to 46 over this same 40 years period. In the triennium 2006 to 2008, 261 maternal deaths occurred in the UK with overall maternal mortality rate of 11.39 per 100,000 maternities. Direct deaths decreased from 6.24 in 2003 to 2005 to 4.67 per 100,000 maternities in 2006 to 2008 ($p=0.02$). This decline is predominantly due to the reduction in deaths from thromboembolism and, to a lesser extent, hemorrhage.[8]

In United States of America, American College of Obstetrics and Gynecology (ACOG) has kicked off their new "MOMS" program—Making Obstetrics and Maternity Safer.[9] This program can be easily incorporated into practices and their lobbying on Capital Hill has resulted in Maternal Health Accountability Act of 2011, which requires each state to establish a maternal mortality review committee. ACOG has developed Educational Bulletins and Committee Opinions dealing not only with clinical care but also with quality and safety approaches to protect patients. Last but not least, ACOG makes the Voluntary Review of Quality Care Task Force available to hospitals attempting to advance their clinical safety standards.

The Nepal Safer Motherhood Project adopted an 'all inclusive' approach with the aim of saving the maximum number of women's lives.[10] In 2004, a study measuring the utilization of emergency obstetric care (EmOC) found that the principal users of services were high caste women. WHO enforces lower caste people to exercise there right of health and use these emergency facility. Higher income states to assist lower income states to reduce maternal mortality.

In Sri Lanka, the country has faced years of internal conflict, and more than one-third of Sri Lankans live below the poverty line. Yet political commitment to providing health care to women in clinics and hospitals, and in their homes, has resulted in the reduction of the country's maternal mortality rate by 87 percent in the past 40 years.[11] The front line of this maternal health system is a cader of midwives assigned to every district in Sri Lanka to provide basic home care for expectant and new mothers. In addition, Sri Lanka expanded its system of hospitals and clinics and encouraged women to visit these facilities during pregnancy and for childbirth. Today, 99 percent of pregnant women in Sri Lanka receive four or more prenatal visits and give birth at a health facility.

Thus, to reduce maternal mortality, it is critical to determine the levels and causes of maternal mortality but knowing only levels is not enough. Further information is needed on where things are going wrong and what can be done to rectify them. Policies based on right kind of information can reduce maternal mortality even in resource-poor settings.

How is Maternal Death Audit Performed?

Maternal death audit is the process of identification, notification, quantification, determination of causes and avoidability of maternal death and using this information to implement interventions to reduce maternal mortality. Flow chart 1 shows maternal death audit cycle.[12]

Flow chart 1: Maternal death audit cycle and review team

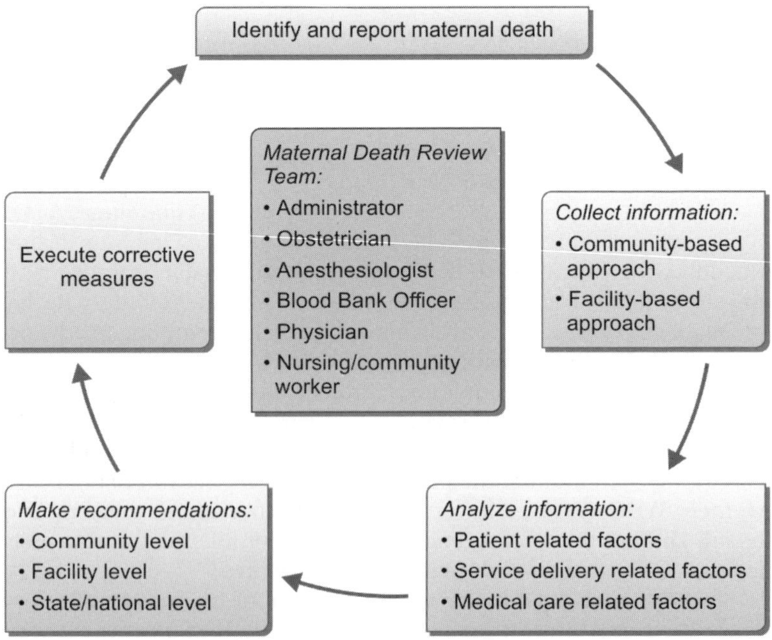

Steps of maternal death audit are:

- Identify and reporting maternal death
- Collect information about the maternal death
- *Analyze information:* Periodic data analysis, recommendations
- Findings into action: Action plan, dissemination
- *Evaluation* and reaudit.

Identifying Maternal Death

Defining maternal is the prerequisite to identify maternal death.

Maternal death is defined as the death of a woman while pregnant or within 42 days of termination of pregnancy, irrespective of the duration and site of the pregnancy, from any cause related to or aggravated by the pregnancy or its management but not from accidental or incidental causes.[13] They are further subdivided into direct as those are unique to pregnancy and resulting from conditions or their complications or management during antenatal, intrapartum or postpartum period. Indirect maternal deaths are those occur due to pre-existing diseases or disease developing during pregnancy but not due to direct obstetric cause, but aggravated by physiologic changes during pregnancy, e.g. heart disease, etc. ICD-10 has introduced 2 new terms related to maternal death. One is pregnancy related death which is defined as death of woman during pregnancy or within 42 days of delivery irrespective of cause of death. This definition allows maternal death to be defined and identified even if cause cannot be determined and is useful in countries with low levels of medical certification of cause of death and where significant number of maternal deaths occur outside medical facilities. Late maternal death is defined as the death due to direct or indirect obstetric causes occurring after 42 days but before one year of termination of pregnancy. This helps to include women who had complications of pregnancies but survived more than 42 days. This definition is commonly used in countries where MMR is low.

Maternal deaths can be identified from health facility by review of hospital record or reporting by health care provider when death occurs in facility. Civil registration systems like vital registration or census data can also be used to identify maternal death. Accuracy of identifying and compliance with reporting should be complete. The difficulty commonly occurs for deaths outside medical facility or in community and may be identified from vital data registration systems. Deaths in community can also be identified by population surveillance or house hold surveys.

Generating Information

Different strategies can be used to identify why mothers die. The sources of information can be case records, information obtained by interview of health care providers, patient relatives.

The data to be collected should be decided beforehand and tools used should be simple and validated for local use.

The different approaches are described to generate the information about maternal death at different level and each level can assess different types of issues. They are:

- Community based approach
- Facility based approach
- Confidential enquiry into maternal death.

Community-based Approach

It finds out cause of maternal death and factors at personal, social and community level which contributed death. It is also known as verbal autopsy. It is generally used for a woman who died outside the facility but may also used in some cases of deaths occurring in facility to complete the gaps in information.

The verbal autopsy consists of interviewing people who are knowledgeable about the events leading to the death such as family members, neighbors and traditional birth attendants. Cases are identified by community health workers or trained birth attendants (TBA). The interviews may be structured, semistructured or open ended. The most important factor for success of community-based audit is willingness of family of deceased women to participate and sensitivity of interviewer to extract information. Interviewers should be trained properly to collect the information sensitively.

Its advantage is that it gives opportunity to ascertain cause of death in women dying outside facility and social and personal factors contributing to death can be judged. The family and community participation gives an opportunity to get their views on health care services and sensitizing them. The disadvantage is that cause ascertainment may not be accurate, the judgment about contributory factors is subjective, dependant on participation of family-community which needs to sensitively tackled at that point. Early pregnancy deaths may be underreported and indirect causes are over reported.

Actions based on community based surveys may be directed in improving community awareness and knowledge by introducing or refocusing health education messages as well as reconfiguring local services to make them more acceptable, accessible and available in addition to modifying clinical practices.

Facility Based Approach

For deaths occurring in facility, in-depth investigation around the cause of death is conducted. If necessary, community-based audit can also performed to supplement the information. This process enables more complete picture to be obtained and may be more acceptable as some form of procedure to review maternal deaths already exist in many facilities. Data should be collected by sensitized and trained people in predesigned formats. It is important the health care providers at facility are open in sharing the information. The quality of case notes available is important determinant of information available on which final recommendations will be based. The disadvantage is that it may generate large volume of information which is difficult to manage, need for committed skilled professional to conduct the process and supportive hospital managers to carry out corrective measures. It does not provide any information of deaths in community. It can consider both clinical and nonclinical aspects of patient care, can bring about beneficial changes in local practices but may not be applicable to wider level.

Confidential Enquiry into Maternal Death

It is systematic multidisciplinary anonymous investigation of all or representative sample of maternal deaths at regional or national level. It identifies number, causes and avoidable factors in maternal death. It provides most complete picture of maternal deaths on wider geographical area, results can be generalized and widely disseminated. These are generally instituted by close political commitments and thus improve coordination between government and health service providers. Most important limitation of this method is need for regular statistical infrastructure and trained healthcare providers in each facility to give accurate information. It is more resource-intensive, focuses more on medical factors and sociodemographic factors are undermined, may be more complex and time consuming in situations with large number of maternal deaths. These are generally conducted at regional or national level. They can effect policy and guideline development resulting in wider impacts. The confidential enquiries in maternal deaths (CEMD) in UK is the best example of successful maternal death audit.

Analyzing Information

The data generated should be analyzed by assessors, which are generally medical professionals, to identify cause of death, whether its avoidable or not, presence of specific avoidable factor related to personal factors of the patient, service delivery or quality of care.

The objective of maternal death audit is to identify factors contributing to maternal death and target interventions to correct the avoidable factors. From point of view of targeting corrective measures the avoidable factors are classified as:

- *Patient related:* Women may be unaware of need of care or warning signs of pregnancy or availability of health care services. Social issues like concern for women's health, financial resources can affect utilization of health services. The realization that women are important part of society and ignoring pregnant women health is loss of two lives are important. The corrective measure can targeted to improving information, education, counseling (IEC) campaign and dissemination of information regading availability of health facilities.
- *Health service delivery related:* The factors like nonavailabiltiy of health services or barriers to access like cost, distance or sociocultural problems are important contributors to maternal death. The knowledge about these factors in a particular area can result in directed interventions to correct deficiencies by taking specific measure like setting up more first referral unit (FRU) in rural areas.
- *Quality of medical care related:* Adequacy of health care has great impact on survival of woman after she reaches health facility. Prompt assessment of women on arrival, availability of expertise and equipment, ensuring quality care is important. It is important to ensure that medical care provided is not harmful. Corrective measures can be refering the case at appropriate time if not managed at lower center.

Both quantitative and qualitative analysis of data should be done to find out factors responsible for maternal death.

Translating Findings of Audit into Action

Learning lessons is important. The information obtained by above methods should be used to improve maternal health outcomes by appropriately analyzing and acted upon.

They should result in recommendations for change which are effective, simple, affordable, feasible and locally adaptable. It should direct health care professionals to modify their practices in evidence-based manner. The prime objective of this exercise is to promote interventions to reduce maternal deaths without which such expensive and labor intensive process is futile. The proposed interventions may be at level of community, health service issues or clinical practice. The recommendations should be widely disseminated to all stakeholders from community to policymakers. The leadership to execute to these changes is important.

Evaluation

Closing the audit loop by evaluating impact of recommendations made is vital step in maternal death audit. It should ideally be a continuous process as the factors affecting maternal death are dynamic and recommendations will change with time and changing environment like sociodemographic variables, infrastructure, advances in medical technology and their accessibility to general population. Both efficiency and effectiveness of interventions should be evaluated.

COMPLEXITIES IN MATERNAL DEATH AUDIT

The maternal death audit is associated with many complex issues existing in different situations.

First and most important problem is identifying maternal death. Identifying maternal deaths is extremely difficult especially where vital registration systems are weak. With many deaths occurring in community without supervision of health care provider the reporting may be incomplete. The data from death registry may not correctly identify maternal death due to improper information on death certificate. Cause of death on medical certificate is important identifying deaths. Few developing countries have facilities of certification by medical personnel. The capability of medical personnel to correctly identify cause of death is another limitation. In many deaths especially the indirect deaths, early pregnancy may be missed.

Incomplete data is another limitation in conducting audit and finding true picture of causes and avoidable factors. The quality of case records is the most important determinant of effectiveness of such exercise.

Typically, medical records capture only the immediate, biological causes of maternal deaths. The personal, familial, sociocultural, economic and environmental factors contributing to these deaths are left out. Sensitization of health care providers in obtaining and recording these data is important.

Lack of awareness amongst health care providers regarding importance of reporting and auditing maternal deaths especially in primary care setting is not uncommon. Even in secondary and tertiary care setting where significant number of maternal deaths occuring due to indirect causes may be in department not sensitized to intricacies of pregnancy thus reporting may be incomplete and auditing may not be meticulous.

Fear amongst health care provider about the apprehension that true reporting of deficiencies and inadequacies may result in punitive action is an important factor which prevents audit. The basic principle of maternal death review is nonthreatening environment in which factors are described and analyzed. Confidentiality and anonymity can encourage openness and getting true picture of situation. The information obtained should not be base for punitive action and participants should be assured that whole purpose of this exercise is to learn from past experiences and use to prevent future deaths. The approach of problem-solving instead of blame-fixing should be encouraged. In countries like UK enquiries in maternal death have been confidential without putting blame on any individual and delivered good results in terms of finding avoidable problems and directing policies to solve them.

The legal and ethical framework of country should be kept in mind. The culture and customs can significantly impact process of investigation which should be sensitive. Autonomy and privacy should be respected. The law of the land can influence access to information, protection or environment of workers (immunity and confidentiality) and utilization of information obtained.

The recommendations based on these audits should be actionable and dissemination of recommendation to end users is vital for good results.

Poor governance and action plan execution is an important limitation in efforts to reduce maternal mortality. Lack of political commitment and poor budget allocation can make the whole exercise of maternal death audit futile.

Indian Scenario

The current estimated maternal mortality ratio in India is 212 per 100,000 live births[14] with about 67,000 maternal death per year. MMR vary widely in different states of India with Kerala having minimum value of 81 and Assam recorded highest of 390. The huge difference is due to various factors like difference in access to emergency obstetric care, uptake of antenatal care, levels of anemia in addition to education levels of community.

In order to accelerate the pace of decline of MMR to achieve MDG of 100 by 2015, Government of India (GOI) has accepted maternal death review (MDR)[15] as the strategy and has recommended facility and community based approaches for MDR which would help in identifying the gaps in the existing health care delivery systems and prioritize plan for intervention strategies and to reconfigure health services.

Community-based MDR using a verbal autopsy format are recommended for all deaths that occurred in the specified geographical area, irrespective of the place of death, be it at home, facility or in transit where as Facility Based Maternal Deaths Reviews will be taken up for all government teaching hospitals, referral hospitals and other

Flow chart 2: Guidelines of Government of India (GOI) for maternal death review (MDR)

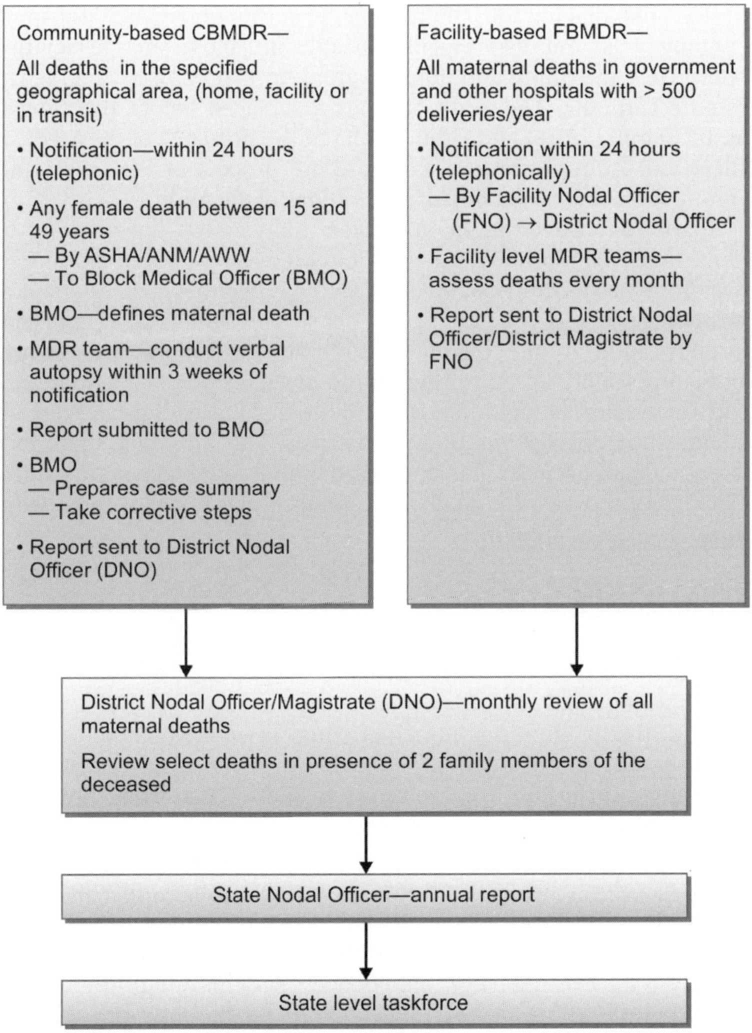

hospitals (District, Subdistrict, CHCs) where more than 500 deliveries are conducted in a year. MDR teams will conduct annual analysis of maternal deaths to understand causes of death and formulate appropriate response. Flow chart 2 shows summary of the Government of India guidelines for MDR in India.

The maternal death audit may tell about the problems like poor distribution of first referral units (FRUs), unnecessary referrals, poor quality of care, delay in accessing emergency transport, obstetric first aid not provided before referral, etc. and help to formulate possible solutions like making FRUs functional, ensuring emergency transport by setting up an ambulance facility, establishing blood storage facilities at the PHCs, providing additional training to PHC staff in emergency obstetric care, etc. The audit findings are placed before the Arogya Raksha Samithi (ARS) and Gram Sabha in the presence of the Medical Officer and Administrator to facilitate the process of PHC staff and community taking ownership of the findings of the Audit.

Apart from Government initiatives many NGOs are working to reduce maternal mortality. Independent Maternal Mortality Audit Cell (Swatantra Matra-Mratyu Samikshak Dal) has been set up in Allahabad, Kaushambi, Fatehpur, Pratapgarh districts to undertake maternal mortality audit in the region.[16] Academic institutions are already conducting facility-based reviews and one such study of 296 maternal deaths at tertiary center in New Delhi found that the leading causes were hepatitis, hemorrhage and puerperal sepsis. They observed that more maternal death occur in medicine ward than in obstetrics wards at the facility[17] and most of the death were nonpreventable as women were critically sick at admission.

CONCLUSION

To conclude, most of the maternal deaths can be avoided with good health care and preventive measures. The maternal death audit is a maternal surveillance and response system that includes maternal death identification, reporting, review which tell us the public health importance of specific maternal health problems and guide appropriate interventions to reduce maternal mortality. Aspects of the structure, processes, and outcomes of care are selected and systematically evaluated and changes are implemented at an individual, team, or service level and further monitoring is used to confirm improvement in health care delivery. The current convergence of factors including political wills, technical innovation and financial resources provide an ideal opportunity to make such system reality.

REFERENCES

1. The Millennium Development Goals Report 2011. New York: United Nations; 2011.
2. Trends in maternal mortality: 1990 to 2008. Geneva: World Health Organization; 2010.
3. Lozano R, Wang H, Foreman KJ, Rajaratnam JK, Naghavi M, Marcus JR, et al. Progress towards Millennium Development Goals 4 and 5 on maternal and child mortality: an updated systematic analysis. Lancet; 2011;378:1139–65 doi: 10.1016/S0140-6736(11)61337-8 pmid:21937100.
4. National Institute of Clinical Excellence, Principles of Best Practice in Clinical Audit. London: NICE; 2002. (ISBN 1-85775-976-1).
5. Main E, Cawthorn S. What is Clinical Audit?. Evidence Based Medicine, Hayward Medical Communications; 2002.
6. WHO World Health Report 2005.
7. Maine D, Rosenfield A, Wallace M, et al. 'Prevention of Maternal Mortality in Developing Countries: Programs, Options and Practical Consideartions' Official Background paper for Safe Motherhood, Nairobi; 1987.
8. Centre for Maternal and Child Enquiries (CMACE). Saving mothers' lives: reviewing maternal deaths to make motherhood safer: 2006–08. The Eighth Report on Confidential Enquiries into Maternal Deaths in the United Kingdom. BJOG. 2011;118(Suppl. 1):1–203.
9. The American College of Obstetricians and Gynaecologist's Making Obstetrics and Maternity Safer Initiative; 2010.
10. Safe Motherhood Policy, Family Health Division, Department of Health Services, Ministry of Health, Government of Nepal; 2007.
11. Senanayake H, Goonewardena M, Ranatunga A, et al. Achieving Millenium Development Goals 4 and 5 in Sri Lanka. BJOG. 2011;118-[supple 2]–78–87.
12. Beyond the numbers: Reviewing maternal death and complications to make pregnancy safer, WHO, Geneva, 2004.
13. Maternal Mortality in Central Asia, Central Asia Health Review (CAHR), A Review of Progress in Maternal Health in Eastern Europe and Central Asia, UNFPA, 2 June 2008.
14. Maternal and Child Mortality and Total Fertility Rates—Sample Registration Survey, Office of Registrar General of India, 7th July 2011.
15. NRHM 2005–2012: Maternal Death Review-Guidebook, Maternal Health Division Ministry of Health and Family Welfare, Government of India, Nirman Bhawan, New Delhi.
16. Maternal mortality audit cell in four districts, Kapil Dixit, TOI, 3 Aug 2013.
17. Goswami D, Rathore AM, Batra S, et al. Facility based review of 296 maternal deaths at tertiary centre in India: Could they be prevented Journal of Obstetrics and Gynaecology Research. 2013;39(12):1569-79.

13

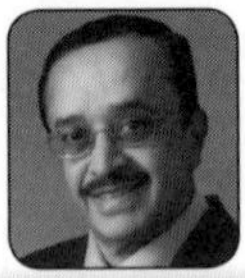 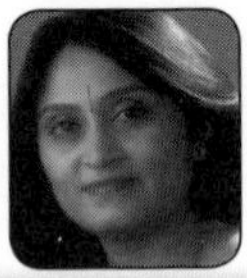

Maternal Health Statistics: An Experience from Eclampsia Registry

Sanjay Gupte, Girija Wagh

INTRODUCTION

Statistics are important to give us an overview of the health parameters in any context. They help us assess the prevalence of the entity in perspective, the occurrence and recurrence and the magnitude. In addition it helps us to assess the impact of any treatment or remedial measure undertaken and association with any demographic, environmental or other factors. It therefore is an important quantification to judge the health status of any population. Documentation of these health events are important and then only can one analyze and draw conclusions.

THE CONTEXT—NATIONAL ECLAMPSIA REGISTRY

Inception

The contribution of hypertension in pregnancy to the maternal mortality and grave morbidity is well established. Hypertension in pregnancy not only is a multisystem disorder it also occurs as a result of multifactorial etiological factors and therefore it is identified to be difficult to treat or prevent. But eclampsia can be certainly prevented and this has been understood from the experiences in the United Kingdom where they have been able to control this devastating pregnancy disease considerably. On looking closure we realized that this was due to the proper documentation of each such case through the eclampsia registry. Ten years of this registry in place has helped them nearly eradicate the condition in entirety and avoid deaths due to pre-eclampsia. The UKOSS, i.e. UK Obstetric Surveillance System helped reduce maternal mortality due to pre-eclampsia.

Taking cue from this we realized the need of such a registry to understand the eclampsia much more. The purpose was to quantify, understand the demographics, to analyze the data, learn from this analysis the prevalence and the strategies that can be planned to reduce the occurrence of this condition. The registry is a web based registry and many enthusiastic members regularly report and help us with the inputs. What is more important is that it has given us a lot of insights into understanding the health status of these patients.

The registry was initiated to help evaluate the incidence and the prevalence. The limitation of course is the fact that we have access only to the members of the FOGSI who would participate voluntarily. But all the same we felt that this would be a valuable sample survey to be able to understand the treatment practices, inculcate the habit of reporting and documenting. It also has helped to pool the data for statistical analysis to base our understanding and plan measures for better health care delivery.

Methodology

The methodology was simple. The reporter had to fill two forms. One was a case form which gave the details of the case and the monthly form which gave the monthly delivery statistics which was restricted only to pregnancy hypertension. This was made simple in order to increase the ease of reporting. The registry was initially launched in 2008 and would encourage both the web as well as postal reporting. The registry was launched with modified format to make it simpler to report in 2012. We therefore will be quoting here the observations as per the both these formats in this article.

The reporters are essentially all FOGSI members and therefore gynecologists. The reporting centers were predominantly private set ups (62%) and 32 percent were institutional facilities while very few (6%) were from rural health centers. We feel that the incidence and prevalence would definitely change if all the facilities especially in the rural settings participate.

Observation

The registry in its initial format has a report of 134775 delivery cases out of which 2554 had eclampsia. Thus the prevalence observed in the registry is 1.9 percent while the national sample surveys in the past have mentioned it to be 1 to 5 percent. The prevalence of pregnancy with hypertension was reported to be 8.3 percent (n = 11266) with the prevalence of preeclampsia being 11.71 percent with a total of 15784 cases.

The 3428 had severe preeclampsia and 1090 imminent eclampsia. Thus reflecting the scale of the presentation and the problem at hand.

It was observed that the disease afflicts the young women rendering them morbid and 79 percent of women were in the age group of 21 to 30 years and what was appalling was that 16 to 17 percent were form the adolescent age groups of 16 to 19 years of age. This is the reflection of the social reality of still existing teenage marriages and their consequences. The disease essentially is the disease of the primigravidas as 81 percent of the mothers were pregnant for the first time. 16.51 percent were multiparas while 2.2 percent were grand multiparas.

We know the disease initializes in the first trimester with deficient trophoblastic invasion and reflects only later. We also have started realizing the need of reversing the triangle of care of antenatal services and concentrating on interventions such as nutritional and anemia corrections during the earlier parts of pregnancy. The patients of eclampsia as per the registry had predominantly sought care in the second and the third trimester (90% : 49%, 40% respectively). Very few (10%) had sought antenatal care in the first trimester. The details of the contents of the care were not analyzed and this can be an important area to be evaluated probably through retrograde analysis.

The presenting symptoms in eclampsia can be varied and the most common symptom reported in our group of patients was headache, nausea, vomiting and very few had epigastric pain and giddiness. What was most remarkable that 55 percent had no presenting complaints. This implies that the disease presents silently and the clinician has to be vigilant. The patients reported in the registry significantly had postpartum convulsions (78%) with 9 percent antepartum and 13 percent presenting with intrapartum convulsions. This calls for a very close vigilance during the postpartum period and continued eclampsia prevention measures even after delivery like monitoring, antihypertensive medication and magnesium sulfate.

Out of the reported cases 50 percent had more than one convulsion before being admitted and 13 percent even more than 4. The duration between the onset of confusion and admission in the reporting facility was found to be more than 4 hours in 32 percent of the cases while 72 percent reported between 1 and 4 hours. The facts revealed from this is that referral and transit therapy needs to be enhanced and also the access to the facility may not be easy in these situations. After admission 22.7 percent patients had convulsions while 78 percent received effective care and did not have seizures.

It was observed that only 44 percent patients had received magnesium sulfate before admission, 29 percent received nifedipine while 11 percent received diazepam. Looking at the magnanimity of the problem the need to train the health care personnel in delivering magnesium sulfate in the right dose and without fear is hugely felt.

The early onset pre-eclampsia (EOPET) is surely a grave disease and 35 percent of the mothers reported with onset of pre-eclampsia between 28 to 34 weeks of gestation while 42 percent had hypertension starting after 34 weeks. Thirty-five percent of patients had hemoglobin between 7 and 9 /dL while 4 percent had severe anemia of less than 7 gm/dL. LDH levels and platelet counts have been identified as important laboratory investigations to estimate the gravity of the disease and to help guide us about the existence of HELLP. It was observed that nearly 40 percent of the eclamptics did not undergo LDH and 13 percent did not undergo platelet estimations. This did not for standardization in evaluation protocols of these patients.

Changing Trends in Obstetric

After 2012 till date we have a little changed analysis as the data was collected in a newer format to understand some more facts. The 46575 deliveries were reported with 798 cases of eclampsia with a prevalence of 1.7 percent which is nearly the same as the past three years which implies that we need to work fast to curb the menace. The prevalence of pregnancy hypertension continues to be 9 percent and that of pre-eclampsia 5 percent. Early onset pre-eclampsia (EOPET) is of concern as 42 percent had onset of hypertension before 34 weeks while 55 percent were reported to have hypertension after 34 weeks. Twenty percent of the patients were referred by general practitioners, 15 percent by public health centers while 30 percent by other doctors and 35 percent of the patient were self-referred. Nine percent patients had epilepsy while 4 percent had family history of hypertension. There is a significant improvement in the care delivered with 96 percent receiving antihypertensive treatment and 99 percent receiving magnesium sulfate. The Pritchard's regimen is more popular with 70.8 percent patient getting this while 7 percent were offered Zuspan's regimen and 20 percent cases were treated with low dose regimen. Nifedipine is a popular antihypertensive agent and methyldopa next in the line of preference followed closely by labetalol. 1.3 percent patients also received Atenolol in spite of it not being recommended antenatally. Out of the 98 patients of eclampsia analyzed for complications 30 percent were shifted to ICU care stressing the need of obstetric HDU. One percent died, 14 percent had abruptio placentae, 10 percent postpartum hemorrhage, 7 percent pulmonary edema, 6 percent status elampticus and 1 percent magnesium toxicity. Twenty percent had HELLP syndrome while 3 percent adult respiratory distress syndrome and 4 percent had ARF.

Lessons Learnt

Standardization of laboratory assessment and continuum of care word in postpartum period is essential. Increasing awareness for early antepartum care, preventive strategies like magnesium sulfate and antihypertensive medications and training there into all health care providers is essential. Preventive measures for fluid monitoring and postpartum hemorrhage are to be practiced. Epilepsy, early marriages, anemia continue to be important issues requiring aggressive care. Hypertension targeted antenatal care and public awareness programs essential.

Please join hands one and all and register today at *www.ner-fogsi.in* and become the valuable NER reporter.

14

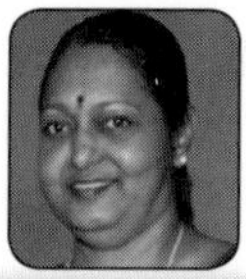

Severe Acute Maternal Morbidity

Arulmozhi Ramarajan

MATERNAL HEALTH PYRAMID AND THE CONCEPT OF SEVERE ACUTE MATERNAL MORBIDITY

Pregnancy is a physiological event designed for the perpetuation of the species. A pregnancy may be thought of as being uncomplicated, complicated, severely complicated or life-threatening. Accordingly, outcomes may vary from a normal, uncomplicated delivery of a healthy infant, to small complications and easy recovery, to severe complications, 'near-miss' or even death (Flow chart 1).

Conceptually, severe morbidity or near-miss during pregnancy represents part of a continuum between the extremes of good health and death (Fig. 1). It is that stage where organ dysfunction and organ failure have occurred. When this stage is reached, then the woman is literally in the jaws of death, and may survive, if medical intervention and luck

Flow chart 1 Pregnancy: Continuum between extremes of good health and death

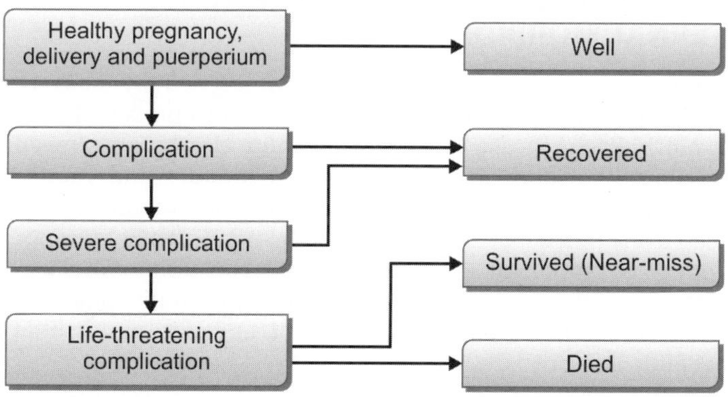

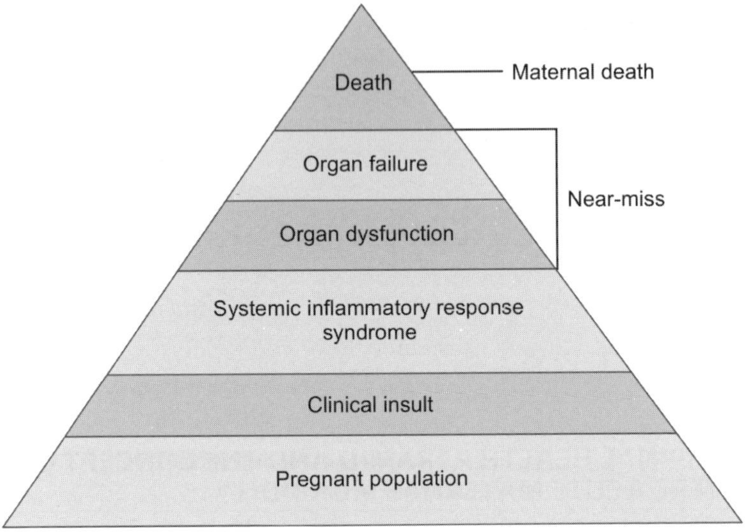

Fig. 1 Maternal health pyramid

are in her favor. Maternal health and safe motherhood are clearly more than the avoidance of maternal death. As maternal deaths are becoming fewer, the focus is slowly shifting from maternal mortality to severe morbidity, and near-miss appraisal is emerging as the new yardstick to assess the quality of health care. The World Health Organization defines direct obstetric morbidity[1] as resulting from obstetric complications of the pregnancy states (pregnancy, labor and puerperium) from interventions, omissions, incorrect treatment, or from a chain of events resulting from any of the above.

MAJOR CONTRIBUTORS TO SEVERE ACUTE MATERNAL MORBIDITY

The majority of our maternal deaths are caused by hemorrhage, hypertension and sepsis. These are almost always preceded by severe acute morbidity. At least 90 percent of these deaths are preventable (Flow chart 2). Good antenatal care can identify and modify risk factors that lead to severe morbidity; appropriate emergency obstetric care can avert mortality. Sometimes death strikes like lightening: as in amniotic fluid embolism, anesthetic mishaps, thromboembolic events, etc. These, however, are but a small part of our mortality figures. These conditions are difficult to predict or prevent, and give us very little time to treat effectively.

Flow chart 2 Progression of severe acute maternal morbidity to mortality

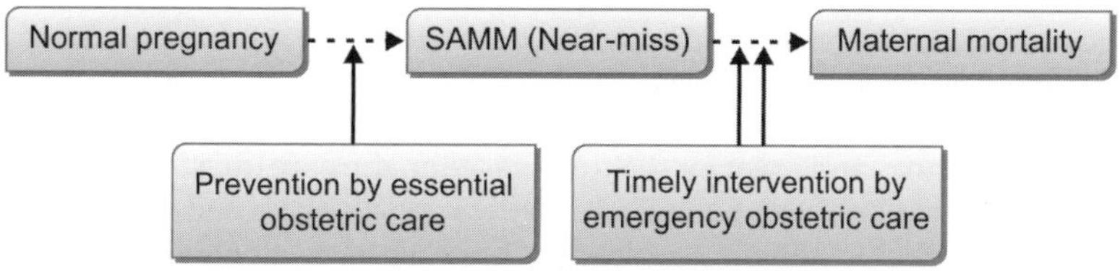

Hemorrhage

Hemorrhage contributes to nearly 60 percent of maternal deaths. Timely and efficient management of hemorrhagic emergencies can save million of mothers. Antenatal correction of anemia, active management of third stage of labor, and effective management of postpartum hemorrhage are measures that can bring down deaths due to hemorrhage. High-risk pregnancies such as those with severe anemia, placenta previa or malpresentation, can be managed better in institutions with operation theaters (OT), high dependency unit (HDU), intensive care unit (ICU) and blood bank facility. Obstetric interventions can contribute to additional blood loss and thus increase morbidity: induction of labor, augmentation, operative vaginal deliveries and cesarean deliveries must be performed for valid indications only. Even episiotomy should be 'indicated' and not 'routine'.[2]

Hypertension

Pre-eclampsia and eclampsia are significant contributors to maternal and perinatal mortality and morbidity. Pre-eclampsia usually occurs during the second half of pregnancy and causes complications in 2 to 8 percent of pregnancies.[3] Eclampsia accounts for more than 50000 maternal deaths each year.[4] Overall, 10 to 15 percent of maternal deaths are associated directly with pre-eclampsia and eclampsia in low-and middle-income countries.[5] While pre-eclampsia itself is not preventable, eclampsia can be prevented/treated by using injection magnesium sulfate.

Sepsis

Sepsis contributes to death in two situations: unsafe abortions (12%), and mismanaged labor (11%). Apart from the acute morbidity, sepsis can cause chronic ill health, infertility and chronic pelvic pain, which will affect the quality of life for the woman. Access to contraception, institutional deliveries and the practice of asepsis can prevent much of the morbidity and mortality caused by sepsis. In this era of easy access to antibiotics, no woman should suffer, or die due to sepsis.

CASE STUDIES

Severe acute maternal morbidity (SAMM) situations are not far and few in actual practice. They are everyday occurrences. Detailed here are some near-misses that happened in our institution. While there is always a sense of victory and relief for the treating team, the core question is: could this complication have been prevented? As we analyze and understand each near-miss situation, we will grow more sensitive to preventing such events. Identifying and modifying risk factors for obstetric morbidity is a major part of antenatal care.

Essential obstetric care: 'Peacetime Preparation' for a safe delivery.
Emergency obstetric care: 'Wartime Works' to save lives.

SAMM 1: Dysfunctional Labor Leading to Atonic and Traumatic Postpartum Hemorrhage (PPH)

A full-term primigravida in labor for several hours was referred to higher center for delivery. On admission, she was found to be exhausted, vital signs stable, uterus acting well, fetal heart sounds regular, cervix fully dilated, caput ++, vagina hot and dry. A diagnosis of obstructed labor was made. She was taken up for an emergency cesarean section, under spinal anesthesia. Baby was extracted and placenta removed. Patient had atonic PPH which was effectively controlled with injection Oxytocin 10 units IM and injection. Prostodin 250 mcg IM. Though the uterus was well contracted, there was brisk welling of blood in the lower segment, and attempts to control the bleeding with sutures failed. The urine draining in the tube was now blood stained. On closer examination, it was noted that the left corner of the uterine incision had extended down up to the bladder. A senior Obstetrician was called in, the tear in the lower segment was repaired, and the uterine incision closed in two layers. Hemostasis was satisfactory. The integrity of the bladder was checked and abdomen closed. Clear urine was draining by the end of the operation. The patient required transfusion of 3 units of packed RBCs.

Severe Acute Maternal Morbidity

She did recover, but after going through several hours of labor, much exhaustion, an emergency cesarean, blood loss, and transfusions. Drained of all energy, she was not able to take care of the newborn baby effectively. Bonding and breast feeding have been delayed. The psychological trauma and the financial drain for the family can very well be imagined. Boxes 1 and 2 summarize the effective intervention and preventive techniques for SAMM.

Box 1 What saved her?

- Emergency cesarean section
- Being a second-stage cesarean section, extension of uterine incision was anticipated, traumatic and atonic PPH promptly managed
- Timely blood transfusion and antibiotic cover
- Close monitoring and appropriate management in the high dependency unit (HDU).

Box 2 What could have prevented SAMM?

- Assessment of CPD in a primigravida by an experienced caregiver
- The use of a partograph for monitoring the progress of labor to identify tardy progress or non-progress earlier, enabling earlier transfer to a higher center
- Avoidance of multiple vaginal examinations and futile attempts at delivery in dysfunctional or prolonged labor.

SAMM 2: Septic Incomplete Abortion

A 19-year-old girl with missed period underwent pregnancy termination in her village. An untrained nurse offered to 'clean the uterus' secretively and at low cost. Two days later, the girl was taken to the Medical College Hospital in a moribund state with high fever, severe pain in abdomen and vomiting. She was pale, dehydrated and could hardly speak coherently. On repeated interrogation, she divulged the history of having undergone an abortion in her village. Pelvic examination revealed a tender, bulky uterus, products of conception in the cervical canal, and a pelvic abscess of size 8 cm × 6 cm. Her hemoglobin was 6.8 gm%, total WBC count was 18,400. She was put on intravenous fluids, broadspectrum antibiotics, given blood transfusions and supportive therapy; a digital evacuation of products of conception was done and the pelvic abscess was drained. She was discharged 8 days later, but it took her several months before she regained energy and enthusiasm to get back to her original bubbly self.

Severe Acute Maternal Morbidity

She is alive and back with her family. But she is left with more questions than answers about her future reproductive health and fertility. Her chronic pelvic pain will remain as a constant reminder of the ordeal that she went through. Again, the psychological morbidity is immeasurable. Boxes 3 and 4 summarize the life saving and preventive measures for SAMM in this case situation.

Box 3 What saved the girl?

- Quick assessment and resuscitative measures
- Evacuation of the uterus and drainage of the pelvic abscess
- Antibiotics, blood transfusion, comprehensive care.

Box 4 What could have prevented the situation?

- Reproductive health education for the young adults
- Access to contraception, sensitive approach to the problems of young girls
- Awareness and access to MTP services at licensed centers.

SAMM 3: Eclampsia

A-21-year-old primigravida was brought to the hospital in an unconscious state following a convulsion. She was 36 weeks pregnant. The patient's brother, who had accompanied her, said that she had convulsions many times since childhood, and the local doctor was treating her for the problem. They were asked to reach a major hospital this time, because she became unconscious, and also because she might deliver.

On examination, the patient was unconscious, responding to painful stimuli. Her pulse was 68 per minute, BP was 220/120 mm Hg. She had gross pedal edema, abdominal wall edema and facial puffiness. Uterus was 32 to 34 weeks size, fetal heart sounds heard. She was admitted to the high dependency unit, and intravenous (IV) access obtained. Oxygen by facemask was given. Injection magnesium sulfate 4 gm IV stat was given and continued as per prescribed regime. She was taken up for an emergency cesarean delivery. A live 2 kg baby was extracted. Postoperative period was closely monitored. BP on day 5 of delivery was 140/90 mm Hg. She was on nifedipine retard 20 mg bd. She escaped death, and was discharged with her baby on Day 8.

Severe Acute Maternal Morbidity

It was not her fault. Her doctor should have detected hypertension early, and recognized the convulsions as eclampsia. She was fortunate to have reached a tertiary care center just in time to survive. Antihypertensives were continued postnatally till the BP became normal. She is being evaluated for her 'convulsions' that have been happening since childhood. She has been counseled on spacing her next pregnancy and on recurrence risk for hypertension in the next pregnancy. Boxes 5 and 6 summarize the life saving intervention and preventive measures in eclampsia.

Box 5 What saved the patient?

- HDU care
- Injection magnesium sulfate for managing eclampsia
- Decision to perform lower segment cesarean section (LSCS) without delay.

Box 6 Measures to prevent such a situation

- Good antenatal care to identify hypertension early
- Edema and rapid weight gain should alert the caregiver
- Convulsions during pregnancy must be treated as eclampsia unless proved otherwise
- Magnesium sulfate injections must be available in all health facilities, and must be used without fear.

SAMM 4: Acid Aspiration Syndrome

An obese 36-year-old G7P4L4A2 presented at 34 weeks gestation with pain abdomen. Her ultrasound report showed mild hydrocephalus and polyhydramnios. She was admitted and treated for threatened preterm labor with tocolysis; prophylactic steroid injections for fetal lung maturity were given. She was discharged and advised to return for follow-up. However, she returned only with pains at 39 weeks. An elective cesarean delivery for CPD, with tubal ligation, was planned.

At surgery, spinal access was not obtained, and hence GA was given, after much difficulty in intubating. Patient's oxygenation was suboptimal, and the fetal heart rate also was 70 to 80 per minute. The anesthetist requested a quick extraction of the baby, which would also facilitate better maternal ventilation. A 2 kg baby with hydrocephalus and midline facial defect was delivered. About 6 liters of amniotic fluid was drained. Uterus closed, hemostasis achieved. There was no PPH in spite of gross polyhydramnios. However, the maternal oxygen saturation remained low, and hence tubal ligation was deferred and abdomen closed.

Patient was shifted to the ICU for ventilatory and inotropic support. She developed acute respiratory deficiency syndrome (ARDS) secondary to aspiration pneumonia. Meropenem, linezolid and levofloxacin were started to fight any sepsis. Low molecular weight heparin was given for thromboprophylaxis. Over the next 24 hours, she suffered two episodes of cardiac arrest, and was revived. She stabilized on day 3, was extubated on day 4 and transferred out of the ICU on day 6. She was discharged on day 12.

The baby had hydrocephalus, midline facial defects and it was decided not to actively resuscitate.

Severe Acute Maternal Morbidity

A most unanticipated situation and a rare complication: truly a bolt from the blue for the obstetrician. The family also finds it difficult to understand why and how something went so terribly and so suddenly wrong. Awareness, ICU care and team management saved her life.

Some Points to Ponder

- Obesity compounds problems in any given situation. Maternal obesity hinders proper imaging of the fetus in the anomaly scan; it increases the possibility of developing gestational diabetes mellitus and contributes to thromboembolic complications. It is a risk factor for shoulder dystocia at delivery; obesity adds to the woes of the anesthesiologist, especially when it comes to emergency inductions in-term gestations. With increasing childhood obesity, we will see more and more obese pregnant women.
- The relative safety of regional anesthesia over general anesthesia is well established, particularly, in pregnant women. Caution should be exercised in accepting requests for general anesthesia for cesarean delivery. Emergency obstetric care is like a wartime work and we need intensive care facility, focused team work, good communication and documentation (Box 7).

  Essential obstetric care is peacetime preparation where close focussed antenatal care and family planning—play pivotal role in preventing life-threatening complication (Box 8).

MATERNAL MORTALITY VIS-A-VIS SEVERE ACUTE MATERNAL MORBIDITY

- For every mother who dies, 20 to 30 more others suffer SAMM.
- Understanding SAMM will contribute to improvement in obstetric care. SAMM audits help us to analyze practical issues and ground realities thread-bare. The survivors of SAMM have literally escaped death to teach us to make pregnancy safer.

Box 7 Emergency obstetric care: Wartime works

- The patient was directly shifted from the operation table to the ICU bed, with the team ready for ventilation and cardiovascular support
- The collective effort of a committed team that included the obstetrician, the anesthetist, the intensivist, a senior physician, residents and staff of the ICU
- Good communication among team members and with the immediate family regarding patient status and the efforts taken; proper documentation of events.

Box 8 Essential obstetric care—Peacetime preparation

- The gross and lethal fetal anomalies should have been identified by a standard anomaly scan (Sub-standard care)
- This lady could not keep up follow-up visits as advised (Socio-economic constraints)
- She presented at term, with a hydrocephalic fetus and gross CPD that necessitated a cesarean delivery (Operative deliveries carry higher morbidity)
- Access to contraception would have averted the 7th pregnancy for this woman.

Table 1 Case fatality ratios (2011)[2]

Country	*Case fatality ratio*	*Percentage*
France	1:222	0.45
UK	1:118	0.85
India	1:11	9.09
S Africa	1:5	20

- Maternal mortality ratio (MMR) is currently used world over to assess the quality of healthcare services. With the decline in the number of maternal deaths, it has become difficult to derive meaningful conclusions that could have an impact on quality of care using maternal mortality data. The emphasis has recently shifted to severe acute maternal morbidity (SAMM), as an adjunct to maternal mortality reviews.[6] Audits of severe maternal morbidity should be complementary to maternal mortality reviews. Near-miss is the new yardstick to measure healthcare standards across the globe.
- Maternal death to near-miss ratio indicates the proportion of critically ill patients who died due to suboptimal level of care for life-threatening situations. This is referred to as the 'Case Fatality Ratio' and is a sensitive measure of the standard of obstetric care. The incidence of severe maternal morbidity ranges from 0.07 to 8.23 percent, the case-fatality ratio from 0.02 to 37 percent.[7] There is a huge difference between case-fatality ratios in developed and developing countries (Table 1). Reasons include delay in seeking help, lack of access to a health facility, nonavailability of drugs or transport and inadequate or inappropriate intervention.

RISK FACTORS FOR SEVERE ACUTE MATERNAL MORBIDITY

Near-miss does not always happen unannounced. There exist certain clues to its possibility, and these are the 'antenatal risk factors' that one should look for, to avert a near-miss situation. When there are risk factors, the problem may develop insidiously and intensify, to blow up at an unexpected moment. A classic example would be that of pre-eclampsia going on to eclampsia. Or it could be just round the corner, to strike at the time of labor: undiagnosed CPD or malpresentation leading to rupture uterus is not uncommon; prolonged or dysfunctional labor with ruptured membranes is an ideal setting not only for PPH but also for sepsis-related morbidity. Even when there is no risk factor, it can strike like a bolt from the blue, like in cases of accidental hemorrhage or amniotic fluid embolism.

Extremes of maternal age, hypertension and diabetes, malnutrition and anemia, unwanted or unplanned pregnancies, absent antenatal care, social exclusion, poverty and domestic abuse, are all risk factors to be looked for during antenatal care. Going by this list, nearly every pregnant woman is at risk for a near-miss event. The antenatal care is largely about screening for risk factors that are likely to lead to complications during pregnancy and delivery.

THE WAY FORWARD—MATERNAL NEAR-MISS REVIEWS

Unlike mortality reporting which is associated with a sense of shame, blame, guilt, and fear, near-miss is generally reported with a sense of having achieved something great-saving life. Therefore collecting near-miss data is easier than collecting mortality statistics. An outcome-audit of severe acute maternal morbidity would be a useful adjunct to an assessment of maternal deaths, and would concentrate on the management of morbidity once it has occurred.

For meaningful research, we need a database to work on. In relation to SAMM, we need to know how many are happening, why, when and where they are happening. For this, each and every one of us must record and report our near-miss cases to our professional body, FOGSI. The 'National Eclampsia Registry' of FOGSI was initiated in 2009, in an effort to build a national database relating to one of the causes of maternal morbidity, that is, pre-eclampsia/eclampsia. Safe Motherhood Committee (2011–2013) of FOGSI has formed the database for severe acute maternal morbidity cases and trying to do it online (Annexure). Annexure shows the database for near-miss cases. A 'Near-miss Registry' with online reporting will help build our national database on SAMM.

Until there is clarity and consensus on the definition of SAMM and criteria for identification, reporting and large scale audits will be difficult. The inclusion criteria for a maternal near-miss are categorized in three areas: clinical criteria, laboratory-based criteria and management-based criteria. Table 2 summarizes currently accepted inclusion criteria for severe acute maternal morbidity.[8] The goal is that these identification

Table 2 Guidelines for inclusion criteria for near-miss analysis and definitions of severe maternal morbidity

Code	*Category*	*Definition*
1	Major obstetric hemorrhage	Estimated blood loss ≥ 2500 mL or transfused 5 or more units of blood or received treatment for coagulopathy (fresh-frozen plasma cryoprecipitate, platelets) (Includes ectopic pregnancy meeting these criteria)
2	Eclampsia	Seizure in presence of pre-eclampsia
3	Renal or liver dysfunction	Acute onset of biochemical disturbance, urea > 15 mmol/L, creatinine > 400 mmol/L, AST/ALT > 200 u/L
4	Cardiac arrest	No detectable major pulse
5	Pulmonary edema	Clinically diagnosed pulmonary edema associated with acute breathlessness and O_2 saturation < 95%, requiring O_2, diuretics or ventilation
6	Acute respiratory dysfunction	Requiring intubation or ventilation for > 60 minute (not including duration of general anesthetic)
7	Coma	Including diabetic coma. Unconscious for > 12 hour
8	Cerebrovascular event	Stroke, cerebral/cerebellar hemorrhage or infarction, subarachnoid hemorrhage, dural venous sinus thrombosis
9	Status epilepticus	Unremitting seizures in patient with known epilepsy
10	Anaphylactic shock	An allergic reaction resulting in collapse with severe hypotension, difficulty breathing and swelling/rash
11	Septicemic shock	Shock (systolic blood pressure < 80 mm Hg) in associated with infection. No other cause for decreased blood pressure. Pulse of 120 bpm or more
12	Anesthetic problem	Aspiration, failed intubation, high spinal or epidural anesthetic
13	Massive pulmonary embolism	Increased respiratory rate (> 20/min), tachycardia, hypotension. Diagnosed as 'high' probability on V/Q scan or positive spiral chest CT scan. Treated by heparin, thrombolysis or embolectomy

criteria may be used in any setting, regardless of the development status. They should be comparable across settings and over time, and there should be a high threshold for identification of cases in order not to overload the health system with extra work.[9] The development of the near-miss criteria by WHO in 2011 serves as a guideline for evaluating the quality of care for severe pregnancy complications, based on the concept of criterion-based clinical audit.[10]

FOGSI is currently working with the Government of India and six medical colleges in six States across India to develop contextual near-miss definitions and tools with the aim to have these definitions and tools approved by the government and implemented across India.

At this point of time, individual clinicians and institutions can carry out their own near-miss enquiries using appropriate local criteria to identify potential areas for improvements. Without doubt, much more can be achieved by collective action. There have been a few published studies of obstetric morbidity from India.[11-14] Near-miss cases were six times as many as maternal deaths. Hemorrhage, severe hypertension and sepsis were the leading causes of near-miss cases.[15]

SAMM is Preventable, Treatable

Reducing severe morbidity in pregnancy will translate into reduction in maternal mortality. Severe morbidity is largely preventable, and if it occurs, treatable too. Our blueprint for action in this direction should include:

- Prevention and treatment of anemia
- Access to contraception—avoidance of unplanned pregnancies
- Improving awareness and access to safe abortions
- Essential antenatal care for all women
- Training of traditional birth attendants
- Scaling up of emergency obstetric care training
- Achieving 100 percent institutional delivery
- Partographic monitoring of all labors
- Active management of third stage of labor for all women
- Early referral of high-risk women to tertiary care centers, improved transport
- Use of early warning system charts
- Protocols for all obstetric situations including admission, discharge and follow-up
- Making blood and blood components more available through blood storage units
- Making near-miss reporting and audit mandatory

The practical implementation of maternal near-miss concept should provide an important contribution to improving quality of obstetric care to reduce maternal deaths and improve maternal health. Review of women with SAMM and maternal deaths give different information but they complement each other. The study of near-miss maternal morbidity can help improve obstetric care and support the struggle against maternal mortality.

REFERENCES

1. Measuring Reproductive Morbidity. Report of World Health Organization. Unpublished document WHO/MCH/90.4; World Health Organization, 1211 Geneva 27, Switzerland.
2. Ramarajan A. Severe acute maternal morbidity, 1st edn. Jaypee Brothers Medical Publishers, 2011.
3. World Health Organization International Collaborative Study of Hypertensive Disorders of Pregnancy. Geographic variation in the incidence of hypertension in pregnancy. AJOG 1988;158:80-3.
4. Duley L. Maternal mortality associated with hypertensive disorders of pregnancy in Africa, Asia, Latin America and the Caribbean. British Journal of Obstetrics and Gynaecology. 1992;99:547-53.
5. Khan K, Wojdyla D, Say L, et al. WHO analysis of causes of maternal death: a systemic review. The Lancet. 2006;367:1066-74.
6. Senanayake H, Dias T, Jayawardena A. Maternal mortality and morbidity: epidemiology of intensive care admissions in pregnancy. Best Practice and Research Clinical Obstetrics and Gynaecology. 2013;27(6):811-20.
7. Meilė Minkauskienė, Rūta Nadišauskienė, Žilvinas Padaiga, et al. Systematic review on the incidence and prevalence of severe maternal morbidity. Clinics of Obstetrics and Gynecology, Department of Preventive Medicine, Kaunas University of Medicine Hospital, Lithuania.
8. Learning from adverse events: Developing a system for identification and assessment of maternal near misses. Fetal Report to MHS, quality improvement; Scotland.
9. Say L, Souza JP, Pattinson RC. Maternal near-miss-towards a standard tool for monitoring quality of maternal health care. Best Practice and Research Clinical Obstetrics and Gynaecology 2009;23:287-96.
10. Graham WJ. Criterion-based clinical audit in obstetrics: bridging the quality gap? Best Practice and Research Clinical Obstetrics and Gynaecology. 2009;23:375–88.
11. Khosla AH, Dahiya K, Sangwan K. Maternal mortality and 'near-miss' in rural north India. Int J Gynaecol Obstet. 2000;68:163-4.
12. Bang RA, Bang AT, Reddy MH, Deshmukh MD, Baltule SB, Fillipi V. Maternal morbidity during labour and the puerperium in rural homes and the need for medical attention: a prospective observational study in *Gadhchiroli*, India. Br J Obstet Gynaecol. 2004;111:231-8.
13. Datta KK, Sharma RS, Razack PMA, et al. Morbidity patterns amongst rural pregnant women in Alwar, Rajasthan: a cohort study. Health Popul Perspect Issues. 1980;(3):282-92.
14. Chhabra P, Guleria K, Saini NK, et al., Vaid NB. Pattern of severe maternal morbidity in a tertiary hospital of Delhi, India: a pilot study. Tropical Doctor. 2008;38(4);201-4. doi:10.1258/td.2007.070327 © 2008 Royal Society of Medicine Press.
15. Taly A, Gupta S, Jain N. Maternal Intensive Care and 'Near-miss' Mortality in Obstetrics. J Obstet Gynecol. 2004; 54(5).

ANNEXURE

Data collection of case history of maternal mortality and near-miss maternal mortality to improve the quality of obstetric case = FOGSI safe motherhood committee (2011–2013)

S. No.	*Questions*	*Response*	*Answer*	*Comments of Team*
A: Details				
1.	Hospital name			
2.	Date of case extraction	Date:		
3.	Name of women			
4.	Registration No. (if any)	No./ NA		
5.	Antenatal record available in case-notes	Yes: No:		
6.	Date and time of admission	Date: Time:		
7.	Pulse	Rate/minute		
8.	Blood pressure	Systolic mm Hg Diastolic mm Hg		
9.	Alive	Yes: .... 1 No: 2		
10.	Date and time of discharge			
11.	*Dead:* Date and time of death	Date:		
12.	No. of days in the hospital			
13.	Was the woman referred to the hospital from elsewhere?	Yes: .... 1 No: 2		
14.	From where?			
15.	For what reasons?			
16.	Discharge diagnosis			
B: Woman's details				
1.	Age			
2.	Parity	No. of deliveries:		
3.	Gravidity	No. of pregnancies:		

Contd...

Contd...

4.	Maternal complication in previous pregnancy	Yes: .... No:		
5.	Early pregnancy losses	No:		
6.	Live births	No:		
7.	Stillbirths	No:		
8.	Neonatal deaths	No:		
9.	Low birth weight	No:		
10.	Preterm births	No:		
11.	Any others	No:		
C: Obstetric hemorrhage				
1.	When did the hemorrhage start?	Before admission After admission		
2.	At what time of day did the hemorrhage start?			
3.	Was the hemorrhage ante-, intra- or postpartum?	Antepartum Intrapartum Postpartum		
4.	Total estimated amount of blood loss			
5.	Status of clinician who saw the patient on admission	Student midwife Midwife Senior midwife Medical student Medical officer Senior medical officer Specialist obstetrician Other (specify)		
6.	Was an experienced member of staff informed?	Yes:		
7.	At what time was a senior member of staff informed of the hemorrhage?	Time:		

Contd...

Contd...

8.	At what time did a senior member of staff first examine the patient?	Time:		
9.	Was intravenous access achieved?	Yes: No:		
10.	Blood type/Cross match	Yes:		
11.	Hemoglobin/ Hematocrit	Yes: No:		
12.	Was a request made for units of blood?	Yes: No:		
13.	How many units of blood were requested?	Unit:		
14.	Time span between request and availability of blood for transfusion	Hours: Minute:		
Were there any of the following Indications of the need for coagulation tests?				
1.	Placenta abruption	Yes: No:		
2.	Pre-eclampsia	Yes: No:		
3.	Sepsis	Yes: No:		
4.	Transfusion of more than 2 liters of blood	Yes: No:		
Were any of the following tests carried out?				
1.	Bleeding time/ Clotting time	Yes: No:		
2.	Platelet count	Yes: No:		
3.	Was a blood transfusion given?	Yes: No:		
4.	Were intravenous fluids given	Yes: No:		
5.	How many unit and which I/V fluids (crystalloids and/or colloids) given?	Less than 3 liters/ 3 liters or more		

Contd...

Contd...

6.	Was the pulse rate monitored at all in the first two hours after the hemorrhage was recognized?	Yes: No:		
7.	At what intervals was the woman's pulse measured during the first two hours after the hemorrhage was recognized?	15 minutes interval 30 minutes interval Other (specify)		
8.	Was the blood pressure monitored in the first two hours after recognizing the hemorrhage?	Yes: No:		
9.	At what intervals was the woman's blood pressure measured?	15 minutes interval 30 minutes interval Other (specify)		
10.	Was a urinary catheter inserted	Yes: No:		
11.	Was urine output measured at all?	Yes: No:		
12.	Was it measured at least once every hour?	Yes: No:		
13.	Was the patient ever taken to the operating theater because of the hemorrhage?	Yes: No:		
14.	Which operation was performed?	Yes: No:		
15.	What was the date of operation?	Date: Time:		
In the event of antepartum hemorrhage were any of the following examinations conducted?				
1.	Abdominal examination	Yes: No:		
2.	Ultrasound scan	Yes: No:		

Contd...

Contd...

3.	Vaginal examination	Yes: No:		
4.	Was the placental site known (by scan) at the time of vaginal examination?	Yes: No:		
5.	Where was the vaginal assessment conducted?	Operating theatre Labor/maternity ward Other (specify)		
6.	Were oxytocics used in the treatment of the postpartum hemorrhage	Yes: No:		
D: Eclampsia				
1.	Where did the first convulsion occur?	In the hospital In another hospital In a health center/ clinic At home Other (specify)		
2.	Date and time of first convulsion?	DD MM YY Time: MM PM		
3.	Was a management plan formulated for this case?	Yes: No:		
4.	Who formulated the management plan?	Student midwife Midwife Senior midwife Medical student Medical officer Senior medical officer Specialist obstetrician other (specify)		
5.	What was the highest diastolic blood pressure recorded in the case notes?	mm Hg		

Contd...

Contd...

6.	Is it severe hypertension? (severe hypertensive BP on two occasions at least 4 hours apart) > 160/110 mm Hg	Yes: No:		
7.	Was anti-hypertensive treatment given?	Yes: No:		
8.	What was route and dosage of anti hypertensive drug?			
9.	Anti-convulsant used	Yes: No:		
10.	Dose and route of anti convulsant	Magnesium sulfate Diazepam Other		
Were the following measurement taken whilst the woman was receiving Magnesium Sulfate				
1.	Respiratory rate	Yes: No:		
2.	Tendon reflexes	Yes: No:		
3.	Urine output	Yes: No:		
Were the following investigations performed at least once during the woman's in patient stay?				
1.	Bleeding/clotting time	Yes: No:		
2.	Platelet count	Yes: No:		
3.	Urine albumin/ renal function test	Yes: No:		
4.	Liver function test	Yes: No:		
5.	Did the woman labor at the hospital	Yes: No:		
6.	Mode of delivery	Normal: Instrumental: LSCS:		

Contd...

Contd...

7.	Outcome of delivery	Normal: NICU: Still birth:		
Was fluid balance chart maintained?				
1.	Before labor?	Yes: No:		
2.	During labor?	Yes: No:		
3.	Was the blood pressure monitored after delivery?	Yes: No:		
4.	How often was the blood pressure monitored?	At least once every hr. Longer than every hr.		
5.	How long after delivery did this monitoring continue?	< 48 hrs. > 48 hrs.		
6.	Was urine output monitored after delivery	Yes: No:		
7.	How often was urine output monitored	At least once every hrs. Longer than every hrs.		
8.	How long after delivery did this monitoring continue?	< 48 hrs. > 48 hrs.		
Obstructed Labor				
1.	Date and time of the diagnosis of obstructed labor?	DD MM YY AM PM		
2.	Method of documentation of labor	Verbal Clinical note Partogram Paperless partogram		
3.	Was the interval of time between the diagnosis of obstruction and delivery of the fetus	Less than 2 hrs. Two hrs or more		

Contd...

Contd...

4.	Were any reasons given in the case notes for this delay in delivery?	Yes (specify) No (reasons)		
5.	Was a urinary catheter inserted?	Yes: No:		
Monitoring of Obstructed Labor				
1.	Urine output	Yes: No:		
2.	Blood pressure	Yes: No:		
3.	Pulse	Yes: No:		
4.	Temperature	Yes: No:		
5.	Was blood taken for typing and cross matching?	Yes: No:		
6.	Was intravenous access achieved?	Yes: No:		
7.	Were any antibiotics started once obstructed labor was diagnosed?	Yes: No:		
8.	Date and time of antibiotics first started	DD MM YY AM PM		
9.	Detail of doses route and type of antibiotic given			
10.	Mode of delivery	Normal: Instrumental: LSCS:		
11.	Outcome of delivery	Normal: NICU: Still birth:		

15

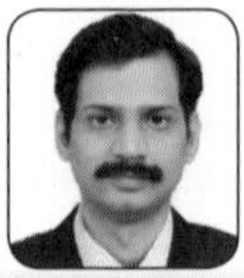

Janani Suraksha Yojana in India: Hopes and Realities

KS Prashanth

INTRODUCTION

Janani Surkhsha Yojana (JSY) was introduced as a part of the National Rural Health Mission (NRHM) in India on 12 April 2005. The scheme encourages delivery, in a government or accredited private health facility, of expecting mothers, irrespective of age, socioeconomic status, and parity, providing conditional cash assistance, at the time of 'institutional' delivery with the support of Accredited Social Health Activists (ASHAs) in JSY implementation identifying pregnant and expecting mothers motivating them for antenatal care, institutional deliveries, and postnatal care.[1]

The program divided states into low-performing (LPS) and high-performing (HPS) depending on the preprogram level of performance. The level of financial assistance was based on the LPS/HPS status and whether the place is rural or urban. In low performing states, the financial assistance for institutional delivery was available to all pregnant women regardless of age and parity who gave birth in a government or private accredited health facility. In high performing states, financial assistance for institutional delivery was only available to women from BPL/SC/ST households, aged 19 years or above and up to two live births for giving birth in a government or private accredited health facility. Further, in all the states/union territories, the scheme provide ₹ 500/- to BPL women, aged 19 years or above and up to two live births, who preferred to home delivery.[1] This was the scheme when it was launched.

The scheme underwent a lot of changes since its inception in terms of the conditionalities mandated for release of payments to beneficiaries, the mode of payments, etc. based on the evaluations of the scheme as well as monitoring visit reports by the GOI teams. Conditionalities associated with parity and minimum age of the mother for institutional deliveries in the high performing states were done away with from May 2013. The details of the financial assistance applicable as of now to the beneficiaries are as indicated in Tables 1 and 2.[2]

WHY INDIA WENT FOR JANANI SURAKSHA YOJANA?

Janani Suraksha Yojana (JSY) is not a stand-alone package or a set of mechanisms whose effectiveness could be subjected to a standard model of impact. Evaluation outcomes cannot be attributed straight away to JSY, alone. It has to be interpreted with the impact of NRHM, the part of which it was launched. This is important in terms of timelines (many studies comparing pre- and post- 2005 to study the impact of JSY) where infact the program was operational only in April 2007, after a lapse of 14 months between launch of the program (from March 2005) and approval of the framework on implementation (to July 2006) and operation of financial year (April-March). The actual time period of implementation of the first phase of NRHM coincided with the 11th five year plan period.[3]

Health is a state subject in India and the state governments spend 65 to 80 percent of the public expenditure on health care. Family planning, disease control and medical education and research are supported by the Central Government. Health financing by the Central Government at the time when NRHM was launched, was limited to a few National Disease Control programmes and the Reproductive and Child Health (RCH) programme.[3]

In the nineties, owing to a fiscal crisis, expenditures in health care by state governments declined significantly. There was no expansion of public health systems capacity, and many states were unable to fill up retirement vacancies. The private sector grew, but its growth was most uneven, concentrated by its very nature, in urban areas. This combination of factors led to a deterioration in the availability of skilled health professionals and a decline in access to health care especially in rural areas. Structural adjustments and the increased need for international financial support led to an understanding of health sector reform which was aligned to the economic reform of these years. The main features of this reform called for the government to focus public health financing on a selective list of health priorities, which had the most favorable estimated ratio of money spent for Disability Adjusted Life Years (DALYs) saved. This in effect meant a focus on reproductive and child health and vertical health programs related to Tuberculosis, HIV/AIDS, vector borne diseases, and blindness control. The remaining health care needs were seen as better addressed through health markets.[3]

Table 1 Financial assistance for institutional delivery

Category of states	*Rural area*			*Urban area*			*Eligibility criteria*
	Mother	*ASHA*	*Total*	*Mother*	*ASHA*	*Total*	
Low performing states	1400	600	2000	1000	400	1400	Available to all women regardless of age and number of children for delivery in government/private accredited health facilities
High performing states	700	600	1300	600	400	1000	Available only to BPL/SC/ST women regardless of age and number of children for delivery in government/private accredited health facilities

Table 2 Financial assistance for home delivery

Category of states	*Rural area*			*Urban area*			*Eligibility criteria*
	Mother	*ASHA*	*Total*	*Mother*	*ASHA*	*Total*	
Low performing states	500	Nil	500	500	Nil	500	Available only to BPL women who prefer to deliver at home regardless of age and number of children
High performing states	500	Nil	500	500	Nil	500	

Further it was considered desirable to expose the public health sector to market like mechanisms. As part of this understanding, the collection of user fees for all hospital services was made a part of financing conditionalities, and public hospitals aimed for cost recovery as a policy objective. In this policy environment most public hospitals withdrew from provision of free drugs and diagnostics, except for select National Disease Control Programs. Also in line with keeping government small there was little effort to fill up vacancies, or expand public health system capacity, especially in the high focus states where there were huge gaps even prior to the nineties. Medical education which until the nineties had been predominantly government run, shifted dramatically into the private sector, and by the end of the decade became predominantly private. Needless to say, left to market forces, medical and nursing colleges set up by private agencies, expanded rapidly in only about four to six of the better developed states in the southern and western part of the country. Similarly, market driven growth led to weak rural health services and primary health care, but in this same period tertiary health care services grew rapidly in the major cities. Government of India thus required a financing mechanism for strengthening public health systems in the states, which was done through the National Rural Health Mission.[3]

National Rural Health Mission (NRHM) tried to address the design considerations of the mission by providing Architectural Corrections so that dysfunctional states make optimum use of the funds allocated and by remaining itself an 'additionality' to the existing RCH, Immunization and Disease Control programmes whose designs were already finalized.[3]

With the back up support of the institutional mechanisms provided by the NRHM, JSY was launched as a demand side financing mechanism for ensuring 'safe delivery', capable of impacting maternal mortality ratio.

JANANI SURAKSHA YOJANA AS A DEMAND SIDE FINANCING IN HEALTH

The concept of demand side financing (DSF) in health originated in response to developing countries' felt need to improve access to and utilization of health services, particularly among the poor. Policymakers in developing countries have come to realize that the utilization and uptake of services has been very low among those who would benefit most from these services, i.e. the poorer and vulnerable sections of the population. DSF was therefore seen as a tool that could improve the utilization of under-used services among the needy and under-served populations by placing purchasing power, as well as the choice of provider (where possible), directly in the hands of the recipients.[4]

Though not often stated explicitly, the main argument cited in favor of DSF is that beneficiaries face mainly financial barriers that prevent them from using a particular service or intervention. The financial barrier argument often extends to geographical distance, so that providing either funds for transport or providing transport itself is also seen as a way to overcome the barriers to access.[4]

Demand is influenced by factors that determine whether an individual identifies illness and is willing and able to seek appropriate health care. The model leads to a demand for health care of a given quality that is determined by individual and community factors as well as the price of medical care and other similar goods. Thus, demand is a function of individual/household factors, community factors, and prices.[5]

Individual (and household) factors include age, sex, income, education and knowledge about the characteristics of, and need for, medical treatment. Community factors include cultural and religious influences and other social factors that affect individual preferences. Price is a complex variable and includes the direct price and distance cost, opportunity (time) cost of treatment—since treatment can be time consuming, and any informal payments made to the facility for commodities or to these staff. Also included are prices for substitute commodities that impact on health (pH), since individuals have some scope for choosing healthy lifestyles, safer employment or better nutrition in order to improve health or reduce the probability of ill health.[5]

The global literature contains many examples of DSF, with different terminologies (output-based aid, conditional cash transfer, consumer-led DSF, provider-led DSF) used for slightly differentiated products. The defining characteristic of DSF—what sets it apart from supply side financing—is the direct link between the subsidy, the beneficiary and the objective of the subsidy. DSF can be consumer-led (vouchers, cash transfers, tax rebates) or provider-led (capitation payment, referral vouchers), and can be provided before or after service utilization. Other examples of recent initiatives on DSF are conditional cash transfers (CCT) which aim to reduce poverty by making welfare programmes conditional upon the recipients' actions (The government transfers the money only to persons who meet certain criteria).[4] India's JSY is a CCT program.

HOW DID JANANI SURAKSHA YOJANA EVOLVE AS A SCHEME?

The JSY was built on two past schemes: the first—a payment of INR 700 for referral transport and the second—a provision of a maternal entitlement (Maternity benefit scheme) of INR 500 during pregnancy, intended to provide support to improve nutritional status[6] previously delivered through Panchayati Raj Institutions (PRIs). These pre-JSY schemes, financed through Reproductive and Child Health (RCH)—phase I programme, were perceived as having failed to achieve the objective. Thus, when RCH—phase II was incorporated into the NRHM, the existing fund was topped up by an additional INR 200, to create the JSY scheme, and to this was added INR 600 as incentive package for the ASHA. However, while deciding the writ petition challenging the discontinuation of NMBS due to introduction of JSY, the Honorary Supreme Court held that the NMBS would continue with the amount be payable to women irrespective of parity and age. In effect, this would mean that the top up over the NMBS would be 700 instead of 200.[7]

While the pre-JSY entitlement for pregnant women was both an enabling and empowering instrument to provide nutrition and transport to the institutions that would otherwise be out of reach, in JSY the dominant position became that of a cash transfer that hinged on whether the women chose to deliver in a institution or not. The incentive was hence expected to trigger a change to the health seeking behavior of the women.

What is the Outcome and What are the Hopes?

As stated before, evaluating JSY has to be in the context of the larger umbrella, which was holding a plethora of schemes, support structures, and institutions that were created to aid implementation of the mission in the states. The success of JSY owes a lot to these schemes, support structures, and institutions viz Programme Management Units at State, District and Block level; Society structure for flexible financing; Financial guidelines for clarity on utilization at peripheral level; Janani Shishu Suraksha Karyakram (JSSK)—ensuring all services free for mothers and children up to 1 year; Government of India guidelines on wuality service delivery for RMNCH+A services, etc. to mention a few. Besides this, there were a lot of innovations and best practices in States like maternity waiting homes, birth companion, boat clinics etc. The Clinical Establishments (registration and regulation) Act, 2010—covering all types and levels of clinical establishments and mandating them to observe minimum standards is a major step undertaken by the Government of India to ensure quality service delivery.

In terms of outcomes, JSY, which is the largest cash transfer programme in the world,[8] has clearly increased the number of institutional deliveries. This increases documented in various surveys, studies and evaluations. In absolute numbers, the number of institutional deliveries has increased from 10.85 million in 2005 to

2006 to 16.15 million in 2012 to 2013 and the C-section as a percentage of this has increased from 9 to 12 percent in the same time period. In the year 2004 to 2006, the MMR of India was 254 and the current figure (2010 to 2012) is 178.[9,10] The question is whether the increase in institutional delivery has resulted in a proportional reduction of MMR and whether the rate of decline is substantial.

Availing JSY was found to be significantly associated with institutional deliveries.[11] Money is of course a powerful incentive to change behaviors.[12] So as to influence behavior, money must be paid in time. The evaluation of JSY done by MoHFW[13] reveals that delayed payments were common and nonpayments in some districts were as high as 55 percent. Similar findings were reported in the CAG report[14] on NRHM as well as studies conducted later also.[15] Irregular fund flows, and local imposition of additional conditionalities like insistence on photographs, 48 hours stay, etc. were found to be the common hindrances to payment of incentive on time. This could probably explain persistent home deliveries to the tune of 40 percent. Adding to this, the 40 percent of women who had home deliveries reported that the messages regarding JSY had not reached them as well. The reasons attributed by the beneficiaries for preferring home delivery were: (i) poor financial condition, (ii) lack of transportation, (iii) nonavailability of facilities and lady doctor at health centers, (iv) traditional taboos and lack of motivation by health workers. Thanks to financial guidelines, regular audit systems, cheque payments and regular feedback through review missions and integrated monitoring visits, the fund flow and utilization has improved a lot, in the last 2 years.

In order to influence the outcome, the women who have availed institutional care must have received quality care. The evaluation of JSY done by MoHFW[13] revealed that 'qualities of care' in institutions were a problem. Practices like use of partogram, active management of third stage of labor, use of injectable antibiotics, oxytocics, magnesium sulfate, neonatal resuscitation, all of which representing life saving skills were not being followed. Along with this, misuse of oxytocics and irrational use of antibiotics and IV fluids were also reported. Lack of association between institutional birth proportions and MMR, is probably/to an extent attributed to/due to the poor quality of care in antenatal, institutional and postnatal care.[16] Compounding to this would be cleanliness, hygiene, housekeeping and behavior of the staff,[15,17] which was also poor.

One possible argument would now be, was it not imperative to lay stress on ensuring quality of care and cleanliness in hospitals before an incentive was given to mothers for opting institutional care for delivery? Between 1992 and 2006, the Ministry of Health and Family

Welfare focused on strengthening the health system infrastructure to better support emergency obstetric care (EmOC) services especially in the public sector. A concerted effort was made to increase capacity for institutional deliveries by upgrading facilities to improve access to skilled birth attendance and EmOC.[18] Key strategies included upgrading community health centers to function as first referral units, creating 24/7 access to health centers for delivery, and training and empowering nonspecialist qualified medical doctors (nonperformance among these trained doctors is a challenge thou) to administer anesthesia for emergency obstetric procedures. In spite of this government investment, national surveys showed that the proportion of institutional deliveries only increased marginally from 26 to 39 percent during that period.[20] Well, then it can be argued that, while it is extremely important to invest in EmOC facilities, developing strategies that increase the use of these services especially among the poor who suffer the largest burden of maternal deaths are equally significant.[21] Most deaths can be avoided by prompt access to EmOC services. But, despite strengthening the supply side (facilities), poor women are still at risk as they face a number of barriers (particularly financial) to access EmOC in the absence of social safety nets and widely prevalent out-of-pocket payment mechanisms.[22]

Government of India is now looking at quality of care quiet comprehensively and has now come up with two important steps—Clinical Establishments (registration and regulation), Act, 2010 and Quality Assurance guidelines, 2013.[23] These initiatives are expected to help clinical establishments ensure 'minimum standards' in India. Important quality assurance/improvement initiatives that were in place during the 1ST phase of NRHM, like the NABH and ISO proved to be resource intensive; while the progress of the former has been limited to a few institutions, the later suffered issues of sustainability as well. Studies from India[24] and many 'integrated monitoring visit reports of GOI' repeatedly indicated poor skill levels and attitudinal problems of health personnel, as the key bottle necks which cannot be addressed by DSF alone, especially in the high focus states. The family friendly hospital Initiative, undertaken by Government of Bihar was a good initiative which tried to address these issues, using an in-house certification model.[25]

Even if we presuppose that women opted institutional care for delivery only motivated by money; and even if they did not receive money on time (or did not receive money at all) they would by and large be happy at the end of the day, if they had not have to spend money on their own. The evaluation of JSY done by MoHFW[13] revealed high out-of-pocket expenditures (to the tune of INR 1028 excluding transport) in many instances. Instances of informal payments make the situation even worse.[15] This is detrimental, since this would defeat the argument that incentive would result in 'change in health seeking behavior'.

Institutional care mandates 48 hours stay in the hospital, which is very important for ensuring clinical outcomes. The evaluation of JSY done by MoHFW[13] reveals that only 14 percent of women reported staying more than 48 hours in the hospital. Since the family was not sure of drop back facility, they choose to go back in the same vehicle which they came in for delivery. This would also have created pressure on the health workers to augment delivery when it was not indicated leading to complications including ruptured uterus. Augmentation of emergency transportation facilities and assured drop back facility under the JSSK would help a lot in addressing this.

If these three findings are still holding good—delayed/nonpayment, poor quality of care and high out-of-pocket expenditure; the community will distance from the hospitals more than as is now, if the incentives are withdrawn and quality of care is not addressed immediately.

If we look at the other important determinants, many of the integrated monitoring visit reports have shown that location and distance costs, lack of emergency transportation facilities are often seen to negatively impact service utilization, which has been reported from other countries also.[25-29] One important thing to note here will be to see how nearer the institutions are to the beneficiary as a result of GOI effort to 'operationalize facilities—FRU, 24 × 7 PHCs and SHCs'? The evaluation of JSY done by MoHFW[13] reveals that increase in institutional deliveries was skewed with only a few institutions taking up the load of this substantial increase. Of the 5830 institutions in the 21 districts studied that should have managed 955,138 deliveries, only 852 or roughly 15 percent (mainly district and block) actually provided institutional delivery services. This would mean that the beneficiaries still have to travel great distances to access health care. But by the end of March 2012 there was 165 percent increase in the number (955–2536) of FRUs, and 500 percent increase in 24 × 7 PHCs (2243–15014). These facilities were expected to have helped a better reach for the beneficiaries and also would have decongested the existing one's.

Another problem beneficiary would have faced would be to identify which institution would be providing the required set of services, say management of complications. The referral system study undertaken by MoHFW showed many instances of 3rd, 4th and 5th referrals and even instances of delays in obtaining life saving treatments due to avoidable procedural steps.[30] Interesting findings have also been reported in the JSY evaluation study on the role of private sector in referral linkage (Box 1).

Box 1 Evaluation of JSY, MoHFW, 2011

The private sector accounted for 12.5 percent of all institutional deliveries. As a first resort for care in complications, the public and private sector were equally sought after. In the first referral there is a significant shift from public to private sector and in the second and third referral, a smaller proportion of patients from private sector gets referred back to the public sector at the higher level—medical colleges and district hospitals.

Another important factor is to look at the role and influence of the motivator for institutional delivery. A study conducted in Madhya Pradesh revealed that only a minority of mothers received support from the ASHA in deciding the place of delivery (17%) or arranging transportation (13%), as these decisions were reported to be taken by husbands or other household members. The study also found that less than half (49%) of the women were accompanied by the ASHA to the hospital; and only 4 percent of mothers received a postdelivery home visit from the ASHA. The behavior of the ASHA could also have been influenced by the feedback from the mothers; since they are living in the same village and have to co-exist peacefully. The evaluation of ASHA programme by NHSRC[31] and integrated monitoring visits indicates that she has not been receiving incentives on time and in some cases ever. At many times, even though she has been receiving incentives, it was not adding up to a significant amount, so as to remain motivated to 'motivate' mothers for institutional delivery.

Now the National Health Mission, under which the NRHM and NUHM will function as sub-missions, will continue the role of motivator (USHA in NUHM) for 'institutional delivery' for JSY.[31]

CONCLUSION

Evidence suggests that poor often benefit less from public spending[32] and poor women in developing countries often do not have adequate access to maternal health services. Both supply-side as well as demand-side barriers are held responsible for the low use of these services.[33] It is known that poorer households face numerous financial and nonfinancial barriers that prevent their access to services, even where services are nominally free.[34] Demand-side barriers are likely to be more important for the poor and other vulnerable groups, where the costs of access, lack of information and cultural barriers impede them from reaping the benefits of public spending.[5]

Family health surveys from India (NFHS-3) showed that many non-BPL households choose to have their deliveries at home, indicating that institutional deliveries are not always a function of economic status. A recent study has shown that maternal satisfaction of services did not depend much on the money, but on the cleanliness of the hospital, attitude of the staff and perceived good care at the hospital.[35]

Ultimately, nations have to understand what are the critical barriers to utilization, to devise effective solutions. If DSF is the choice of financing, the assumption is that financial constraints are key to lower utilization. Where provider incentives are put in, the assumption is that there is reasonable assurance about quality. If consumers are left to choose from a set of providers, it is implicitly assumed that such a set already exists with reasonable quality assurance.[4]

The NRHM-JSY has not only resulted in women increasingly accessing institutional care for delivery, but has resulted also in higher detections of anemia cases (2.5 million in 2008–2009 to 9.7 million in 2012–2013), hypertension (0.28 million in 2008–2009 to 7.5 million in 2012–2013), number of complicated pregnancy cases treated with blood transfusions (25,140 in 2008–2009 to 241,184 in 2012–2013), to mention a few. JSY also resulted in creating demand for service in hospitals and health personnel were expected to make themselves available for providing services.

The use of financial incentives including cash transfers needs to be handled sensitively, especially because it could become political in nature and used as a populist measure without sufficient research into the factors that inhibit demand. Muthu Lakshmi Reddy Maternity Benefit Scheme[36] in Tamil Nadu, launched immediately after the JSY, for instance, offers nearly 4 times the package, which was doubled (INR 12,000) in 2011, the research findings which would substantiate this increase are not known, but there was a change in tenure of 2 governments, which makes an apprehension, whether these schemes are becoming more political than evidence based.[37]

Yet another important determinant that needs to be focused now is the culture and beliefs and life situations of the families. Objection from a family member not allowing the mother to opt for institutional care could be owing to a host of reasons, which needs to be understood and addressed, and one has to withstand the temptation to correlate the outcomes with the monetary values alone.

The high focus States must now focus on implementing basic quality of care parameters in their hospitals before beneficiaries face possible bitter experiences in institutions, which would necessitate larger investments for potential 'change in behavior'.

REFERENCES

1. MOHFW, Government of India. nrhm.gov.in/JSY accessed on 29th December 2013
2. JSY office order: No. Z.14018/1/2012-JSY. Dated 13.5.2013
3. NRHM in the 11th five year plan (2007–2012), Strengthening Public Health Systems, MoHFW, GOI.2012.
4. Demand Side Financing in Health: How far can it address the issue of low utilization in developing countries? Indrani Gupta, William Joe, Shalini Rudra. World Health Report (2010) Background Paper, No 27.
5. Overcoming barriers to health service access: influencing the demand side. Review article. Oxford University Press, 2004 Tim Ensor and Stephanie Cooper, Health policy and planning; 19(2): 69-79.
6. http://planningcommission.nic.in/reports/sereport/ser/maker/mak_cht5c.pdf
7. Supreme Court of India. In Re: State of Bihar WP (C) No. 196 of 2001 at www.righttofoodindia.org.data/2007nov11scorder.doc accessed on 28th December 2013.
8. Lim SS, Dandona L, Hoisington JA, James SL, Hogan MC, Gakidou E: India's Janani Suraksha Yojana, a conditional cash transfer programme to increase births in health facilities: an impact evaluation. The Lancet 2009, 375(9730):2009-2023.
9. HMIS 2012-13, MoHFW, GOI at www.nrhm-mis.nic.in accessed on 2nd January 2014
10. RGI, SRS, 2004-06 and 2010-12 http://www.censusindia.gov.in/Vital_Statistics/SRS_Bulletins/SRS_Bulletins_links/SRS_Bulletin
11. Lim SS, Dandona L, Hoisington JA, James SL, Hogan MC, Gakidou E. India's Janani Suraksha Yojana, a conditional cash transfer programme to increase births in health facilities: An impact evaluation. Lancet 2010;375:2009-23.
12. Morris SS, Flores R, Olinto P, et al. Monetary incentives in primary health care and effect on use and coverage of preventive health care interventions in rural Honduras: Cluster randomized trial. Lancet 2004;364:2030-7.
13. Programme Evaluation of Janani Suraksha Yojana. NHSRC. 2011.
14. Performance Audit of the National Rural Health Mission. Report of the Comptroller and Auditor General of India. March 2008.
15. Are Institutional Deliveries Promoted by Janani Suraksha Yojana in a District of West Bengal, India? Tanmay Kanti Panja1, Dipta Kanti Mukhopadhyay, Nirmalya Sinha, Asit Baran Saren, Apurba Sinhababu, Akhil Bandhu Biswas. Indian Journal of Public Health, Volume 56, Issue 1, January–March, 2012
16. Bharat Randive, Vishal Diwan, Ayesha De Costa. India's Conditional Cash Transfer Programme (the JSY) to Promote Institutional Birth: Is There an Association between Institutional Birth Proportion and Maternal Mortality? June 2013, Volume 8,Issue 6, e67452, at www.plosone.org
17. Integrated monitoring visit reports, MoHFW, GOI available at nrhm.gov.in
18. McCarthy J, Maine D: A framework for analyzing the determinants of maternal mortality. Stud Fam Plan 1992, 23(1):23-33.

19. Shiffman J, Ved RR: The state of political priority for safe motherhood in India. Int J Obstetrics and Gynaecology 2007, 114(7):785-90.
20. http://rchiips.org/nfhs/index.shtml accessed on 12th December 2013.
21. Ensor T, Cooper S: Overcoming barriers to health service access: influencing the demand side. Health Policy and Planning 2004, 19(2):69-79.
22. Ministry of Health and Family Welfare: Government of India. New Delhi: National health accounts, India 2001-2002; 2005.
23. Acharya A and McNamee P. Assessing Gujarat's Chiranjeevi Scheme, Economic and Political Weekly, volume XLIV (48) 2009.
24. P Padmanaban, KS Prasanth, Family Friendly Hospital Initiative, SHS, Bihar, 2010.
25. Ensor T. 1996. Health sector reform in Asian transition countries: study on social sector issues in Asian transition economies. York: University of York, for the Asian Development Bank.
26. Schwartz JB, Akin JS, Popkin BM. 1993. Economic determinants of demand for modern infant-delivery in low-income countries: the case of the Philippines. In: Mills A, Lee K (Eds). Health economics research in developing countries. Oxford and New York: Oxford Medical Publications.
27. Amooti-Kaguna B, Nuwaha F. Factors influencing choice of delivery sites in Rakai district of Uganda. Soc Sci Med 2000;50:203-13.
28. Raghupathy S. Education and the use of maternal health care in Thailand. Soc Sci Med 1996;43:459-71.
29. Referral systems for institutional delivery in Tamil Nadu and Jharkhand. MoHFW, GOI 2011.
30. ASHA – Which way forward...? An evaluation of ASHA programme. NHSRC. 2011.
31. http://nrhm.gov.in/images/pdf/NUHM/Implementation_Framework_NUHM.pdf
32. Makinen M, Waters H, Rauch M, et al. Inequalities in health care use and expenditures: empirical data from eight developing countries and countries in transition. Bulletin of the World Health Organization. 2000;78:55-74.
33. Sachs J. Macroeconomics and health: investing in health for economic development. Report of the Commission on Macroeconomics and Health. Geneva: World Health Organization. 2001.
34. Shakil Ahmed, Nossal Institute and Chris Morgan, Burnet Institute. Demand-side financing for maternal health care: the current state of knowledge on design and impact. Health policy & health finance knowledge hub, number 1, September 2011.
35. Women's perception of quality and satisfaction with maternal health services, PHFI, 2011.
36. Muthu Lakshmi Reddy Scheme, G.O (EPII-1) No. 276 dated 3rd November, 2011.
37. Grossman M. The human capital model. In: Culyer AJ, Newhouse JP (Eds). Handbook of Health Economics: volume 1A. Amsterdam: North-Holland. 2000.

16

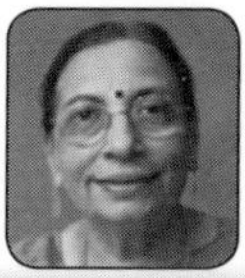 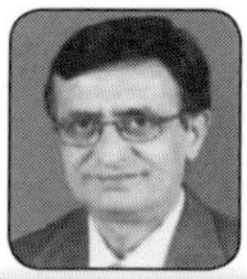

Emergency Obstetric Care Training for Nonspecialist Doctors: A FOGSI Experience

Sadhana Desai, Prakash Bhatt, Ajey Bhardwaj

INTRODUCTION

Maternal mortality ratio (MMR) in India has shown an appreciable decline from 398/1,00,000 live births in the year 1997-98 to 301/1,00,000 live births in the year 2001–03 to 254/1,00,000 live births in the year 2004-06 to 212/1,00,000 live births as per the latest RGI-SRS survey report, released in July 2011. However, to accelerate the pace of decline of MMR in order to achieve the NRHM and MDG goal of less than 100/per 1,00,000 live births and less than 109 per 1,00,000 live births by 2015 respectively, there is a need to give impetus to implementation of the technical strategies and interventions for maternal health. One of the main reasons for the high MMR has been identified as the lack of high-quality emergency obstetric and newborn care (EmONC) in rural areas. Currently, most medical colleges in India prepare specialist physicians as the only providers of EmONC services, catering largely to urban populations. General medical officers, who tend to have limited skills in managing maternal and newborn complications, however, typically serve rural populations.

MATERNAL MORTALITY: A BURNING ISSUE IN INDIA

India has an unacceptably high maternal mortality ratio. Due to its sheer size and population 20 percent of global maternal deaths occur in India. Besides for every maternal death, there are 20 women who suffer severe morbidity so that their lives are not worth living. These women suffer from long-term disability such as chronic pain, vesicovaginal or rectovaginal fistula, impaired mobility and damage to reproductive system leading to infertility or prolapse of uterus. Seventy percent of India's population lives in rural areas where MMR is high due to lack of prompt and adequate treatment.

CAUSES OF MATERNAL DEATHS

Direct Causes

Hemorrhage (postpartum or antepartum) sepsis, complications of unsafe abortion, prolonged or obstructed labor, and hypertensive disorders of pregnancy, especially eclampsia are some of the complications, which can occur at any time during pregnancy and labor and without any forewarning.

These maternal deaths are preventable by evidence-based intervention. A swift and competent emergency obstetric care service using resources effectively can have a significant impact on pregnancy outcome. Figure 1 shows that direct obstetric complications are causes of 75 percent of total maternal death in India. Figure 2 shows major causes of maternal death in India.

Other Problems that Contribute for Increased Maternal Mortality in India

Maternal mortality is not merely a health disadvantage but also a reflection of social and gender injustice. The low social and economic status of girls and women limits their access to education, appropriate nutrition as well as health and family planning services. All this directly impacts pregnancy outcomes. The over-riding causes of high mortality in India are poor access to emergency obstetric care in case of a complication and absence of skilled birth attendant at delivery. Any skilled birth attendant also needs the back-up of a functioning health system, i.e. having minimal infrastructure for managing life-threatening

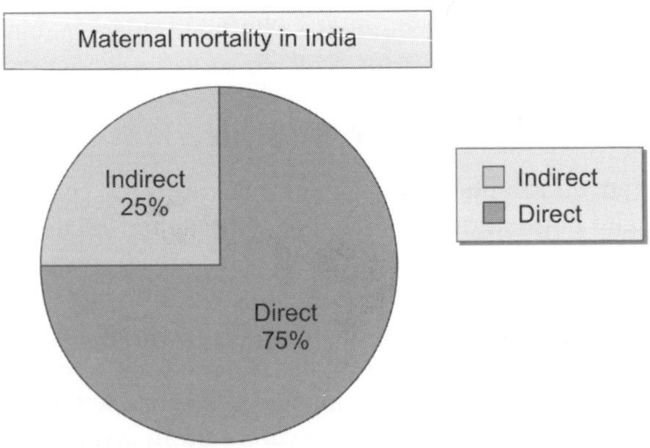

Fig. 1 Direct obstetric causes accounts for 75 percent of maternal death in India

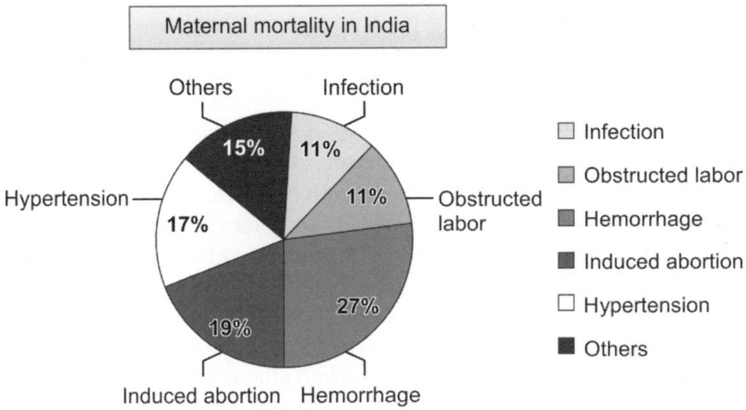

Fig. 2 Causes of maternal death in India

complications in pregnancy and labor like availability of life-saving drugs, safe blood, functioning operation theater with electricity, running water an d anesthetist and 24 hours emergency obstetric care. These infrastructures are lacking in many small towns and villages of India.

Key strategies to save life of pregnant women are:

- Skilled birth attendance at delivery
- Emergency obstetric care
- Timely and effective referral system
- Availability of safe abortion services.

Why Focus on Emergency Obstetric Care?

Over the past several decades, maternal health programs have used antenatal screening to try to identify women at risk for complications. Though useful—these efforts have not succeeded in reducing maternal deaths. It is proved by many studies that many women who develop complications do not have any known risk factors. Once an unpredictable complication occurs, she will require emergency services. As a results 24 hours, quality EmOC services will be required to save a woman who develops life-threatening complications.

There are three types of delays that can affect a woman's chance of surviving an obstetric emergency:

1. Delay in problem recognition and decision-making.
2. Delay in reaching a health facility.
3. Delay in receiving care at healthcare facility.

Having a quality 24 hours EmOC services can prevent the last delay.

Public Health Concept

We have undertaken various public health intervention programs to reduce MMR for last 50 years. Unfortunately, they have not yielded desired results. The emerging Public Health evidences in the field of reduction of MMR tell us a different story. With the exceptions of prevention of anemia, tetanus vaccination, universal availability of safe-abortion services and of course high quality family planning services, none—training of Traditional Birth Attendants, High-risk screening—could significantly reduce MMR. The Public Health studies have clearly demonstrated that:

1. Most critical complications occur amongst low-risk patients.
2. They cannot be predicted or prevented effectively.
3. They have to be managed effectively in time.

The management of critical complications needs high quality, accessible and timely interventions. This forms the basis of emergency obstetric care (EmOC).

It is proved by various studies that organization of such emergency obstetric care proves the cheapest cost—benefit factor to the administration with reference to the estimated maternal death prevented.

DEFINING EMERGENCY OBSTETRIC CARE

Emergency obstetric care is often discussed in terms of basic and comprehensive care that is provided to a woman with obstetric complications.

Basic EmOC—Seven Key Function

In basic emergency obstetric care (EmOC) facility, skilled birth attendant should be able to administer, the seven key functions that is parenteral antibiotics, parenteral oxytocic drugs, parenteral anticonvulsants for pre-eclampsia and eclampsia, perform manual removal of placenta, perform manual removal of retained products, manual vacuum aspiration and perform assisted vaginal delivery.

Comprehensive EmOC

In comprehensive EmOC, the doctors on duty should be able to perform all the functions of basic EmOC and in addition, he should be able to perform emergency cesarean section to save the life of woman. Facilities of safe blood and an anesthetist should also be available in centers having comprehensive EmOC services.

Challenges in Addressing Emergency Obstetric Care in Low Resource Settings

There is a lack of standard guidelines in training doctors and their supervision. There is shortage of continuous supply of drugs and repair of equipment in time. Besides, there is lack of technical and clinical decision-making skills. There is no emergency preparedness. Infection prevention practices are poor and neither enough training facilities nor trainers are available to train non-skilled MBBS doctors in emergency obstetric care.

Quality EmOC poses unusual challenge because EmOC must be available 24 hour. a day, seven days a week to be maximally effective. Therefore, a local doctor must be available and constant efforts must be made to make all the emergency drugs available all the time.

The Federation of Obstetric and Gynaecological Societies of India (FOGSI) and EmOC Program

Emergency obstetric care is an emerging concept of rural obstetrics to reduce maternal mortality and FOGSI is committed to working towards a significant reduction in MMR in the near future by addressing this issue.

The concept of rural obstetrics has developed during the past few years all over the world. The aim is to make basic obstetric life-saving surgery within limited resources accessible to those who have no access to it under existing socioeconomic circumstances.

Current curricula of most medical colleges are generated towards hospital-oriented medicine and cater to urban population while non-specialized doctors are catering population living in rural areas. Most of skilled obstetricians prefer working in urban areas.

This leads to a situation where action needs to be taken to ensure training enough number of human resources/staff providing EmOC in rural India. This should be the key strategy to reduce maternal mortality.

FOGSI–ICOG EmOC CERTIFICATION COURSE

Overcoming Challenges and Difficulties

The Federation of Obstetrics and Gynaecological Societies of India (FOGSI) is a conglomeration of 221 Obstetric and Gynaecological Societies from all over India and comprises of 29060 qualified Obstetricians and Gynecologists working with the aim to improve the maternal health. Besides fellowship and giving continued medical education to its fellow members, FOGSI carries out various activities to improve maternal health and reduce maternal mortality and morbidity of Indian women.

In the year 2006 for the first time in the history of our country, FOGSI/ICOG in association with Government of India (GOI) launched a 5-year program of EmOC (EmONC) certification course as a novel public private partnership. The aim of the public private partnership was to train government MBBS doctors working in first referral units (FRUs) in emergency obstetric care in order to reduce the maternal mortality and morbidity in rural areas.

Being clinicians looking after women, the members of FOGSI always felt the need to contribute towards upliftment of maternal health and wellbeing.

However, this was the first time that a public health platform was available to address this need. This endeavor would not have taken shape without the tremendous support from Professors, Associate Professors and Lecturers from medical colleges of various states where Indian College of Obstetricians and Gynaecologists (ICOG) started EmOC certification course. It is rightly said, "Nothing great is ever achieved without enthusiasm and dedication". The success of this program is mainly due to enthusiastic teachers of EmOC.

A mammoth project like this, related to public health requires experience and FOGSI had none. The difficulties and challenges faced while implementing this program was overcome by the sheer perseverance, ability and dedication of everyone associated with this program.

Dr Dileep Mavalankar from IIM-Ahmedabad guided FOGSI in drafting the pilot project on EmOC and helped FOGSI obtain funds from Macarthur Foundation as well as from averting maternal death and disability (AMDD). It was advocacy of Dr Deborah Maine and Dr Lynn Freedman of AMDD that brought final approval from GOI for joint partnership with FOGSI to train Government MBBS doctors in rural India. FOGSI-EmOC website was only possible due to availability of generous funds from AMDD. Ms Poonam Muttreja and Ms Dipa Nagchoudhury from Mac Arthur Foundation continued financial support not only during implementation of the pilot project but also during the EmOC program implementation with GOI.

Dr Harshad Sanghvi from Johns Hopkins Program for International Education in Gynecology and Obstetrics (JHPIEGO) played a key role by providing a strong technical support to set-up nodal centers as well as 5 master training centers of our pilot project for EmOC training. All the teaching videos prepared by master trainers were reviewed and supervised by Dr Sanghvi.

The Department of Obstetrics and Gynecology of Christian Medical College, Vellore, Tamil Nadu, India, very willingly agreed to train master trainers of this program. JHPIEGO and United Nations International Children's Emergency Fund (UNICEF) already set-up the Vellore center for implementing EmOC training and our task of training master trainers became easy.

The UNICEF provided timely finance support during the financial crisis of the program and United Nations Population Fund (UNFPA) has given guidance to FOGSI during the turbulence while implementing the program.

The whole program would not have been successful but for the very hard work put in by Mr Ajey Bhardwaj of Avni Health Foundation. Mr Bhardwaj is a technical expert on public health who has supervised the program as FOGSI's national coordinator and has liaised between Government of India, State Government officers and FOGSI/ICOG very efficiently.

Dr Himanshu Bhushan, Deputy Commissioner, Maternal Health, Ministry of Health and Family Welfare gave constant support and encouragement. The untiring efforts of Dr Prakash Bhatt as well as all the members of EmOC National Advisory Board have contributed to success of FOGSI/ICOG-EmOC program. All the Presidents and office bearers of FOGSI as well as ICOG Chairpersons during 7 years program encouraged and supported in implementing the program.

TAKING EmOC TO SCALE

FOGSI GOI-EmONC Five Year Goal up to 2011

Government of India had given following targets to be achieved in first five years:

- Setting up and operationalizing four fully functional EmONC "nodal centers" that are routinely preparing EmONC trainers. These training-of-trainers centers, based at premier public medical colleges, will also provide ongoing strengthening, support and certification (through ICOG) of training centers and district practicum sites.
- Setting up and operationalizing 20 fully functional EmONC training centers based in leading public medical schools in the 20 states with the highest MMR. These centers expand capacity to train competent rural EmONC providers by conducting three 16-week courses for a total of 24 participants per year; developing at least 8 EmONC district practicum sites per training center; and maintaining a database of information about training event and service-related quality data.

- 160 district practicum sites providing closely supervised clinical practice for EmONC skills for trainees. These hospital-based sites conduct practica for at least 3 to 4 EmONC candidates per year and maintain high quality EmONC service.
- 2,000 trained EmOC MBBS doctors manning a functional first referral unit providing comprehensive 24/7 EmONC services.

Making the Impossible, Possible

This 16 weeks intensive EMOC program includes training in stages (theoretical and practical), supervised drills and examinations.

In seven years, 6 nodal centers for training master trainers, 34 medical colleges for training MBBS doctors and conducting examinations and 238 district sites for practical training have been set-up (CMC Vellore as a training site already existed before GOI started the program scale-up). A pool of 340 district trainers, 212 master trainers have trained and certified 1363 MBBS doctors across 20 States and One Union Territory.

In first-five years, the achievements of FOGSI were far more than targets set by GOI. Therefore, GOI extended the EmOC program for two more years. Table 1 shows the target achieved by FOGSI.

Nodal Training Centers = Where master trainers from Medical College and District Hospitals are trained.

Table 1: The achievements of FOGSI

Items	*Targets of Government of India (January, 2011)*	*In 5 Years Total numbers (January, 2011)*	*In 7 years Total numbers (August, 2013)*
Nodal Training Centers	4	6	6
Tertiary Training Centers	20	30	34
Master Trainers in Medical Colleges	Nil	168	212
District Hospital Training Centers	160	197	238
District Hospital Master Trainers	Nil	231	340
MBBS doctors trained in EmOC	2000	828	1363

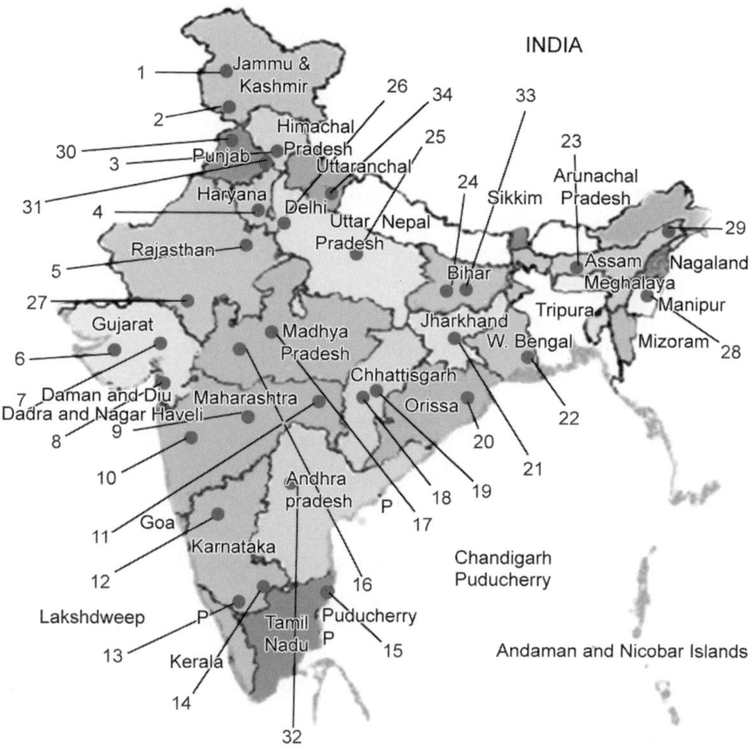

Fig 3 Marking of tertiary training center by 2013 for EmOC program *(for color version see Plate 5)*

Tertiary Training Centers + District Hospital Training Centers = Where a medical officers undergoes 16 weeks EmOC training program. Figure 3 shows marking of Nodal Training Center for EmOC in India.

EmOC Program Impact (2006 – 2012)

We carried out an interim study to understand the impact of our program by analyzing baseline and quarterly database of 74 medical officers in year 2011. This analysis showed clear benefit in performance of EmOC trained doctors as regards management of emergency treatment of hemorrhage, hypertension, abortions and sepsis of in pregnant women that they handled. Data for one complete year before and after training was compared and key findings were encouraging. Clearly, the ability of the MBBS doctors to recognize the signs and symptoms of an emergency improved owing to which the cases were managed within their facilities itself, instead of being referred out to a higher center.

1. An increase in the attendance at the antenatal clinic when pre- and post-training data was compared.
2. After the training the percentage of women with:
    - Hemorrhage treated increased from 1.1 to 1.4 and out-referral decreased from 0.3 to 0.2.
    - Hypertension in pregnancy treated increased from 2.2 to 2.4 and out-referral decreased from 0.5 to 0.3.
    - Women treated for abortions showed a decrease from 2.3 to 2.0 and referral decreased from 0.29 to 0.16 post-training. Better management of the cases during ANC phase led to fewer cases of abortions.
    - Women treated for miscellaneous causes (malaria, hepatitis, cardiac diseases in pregnancy) showed increase from 0.66 to 1.1 and referral slightly increased from 0.14 to 0.16 owing to timely referral.
    - Percentage of women treated for sepsis showed an increase from 0.4 to 0.5 and referral decreased from 0.15 to 0.12.

Given our positive experience with the program implementation, we in the year 2012, again analyzed the impact of EmOC program with a larger sample size. A total of 355 Medical Officers (MOs) trained in EmOC submitted their pre-training and post-training achievement data sets. Out of which we carefully picked 178 datasets, which were complete in all respects and met the criteria of 1 year pre-post-training data. The 2,50,000 datasets from MOs representing 12 States (Bihar, Gujarat, Haryana, Himachal Pradesh, Jammu, Jharkhand, Karnataka, Madhya Pradesh, Rajasthan, Tamil Nadu, Uttar Pradesh, and West Bengal) was analyzed.

Results

- Antenatal care (ANC) coverage at the facility increased (Fig. 4).
- An increase in the number of cases treated for hypertension, hemorrhage, abortions and sepsis and ability to manage complications (Fig. 5).
- Maternal death owing to pregnancy related complications declined (Fig. 6).

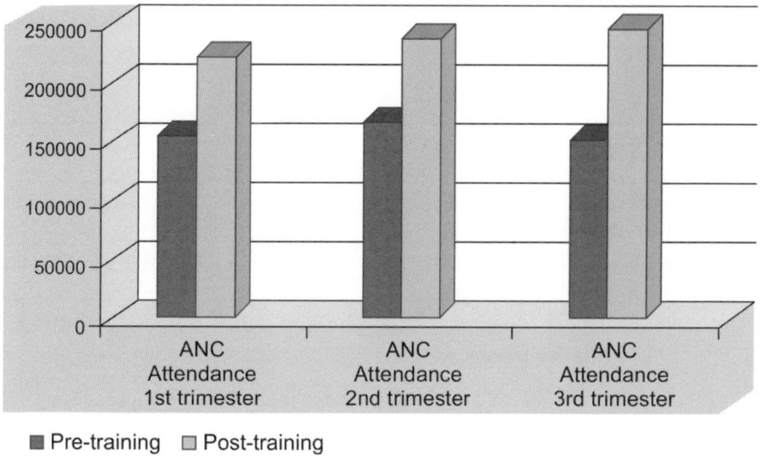

Fig. 4 Differences in antenatal coverage before and after training

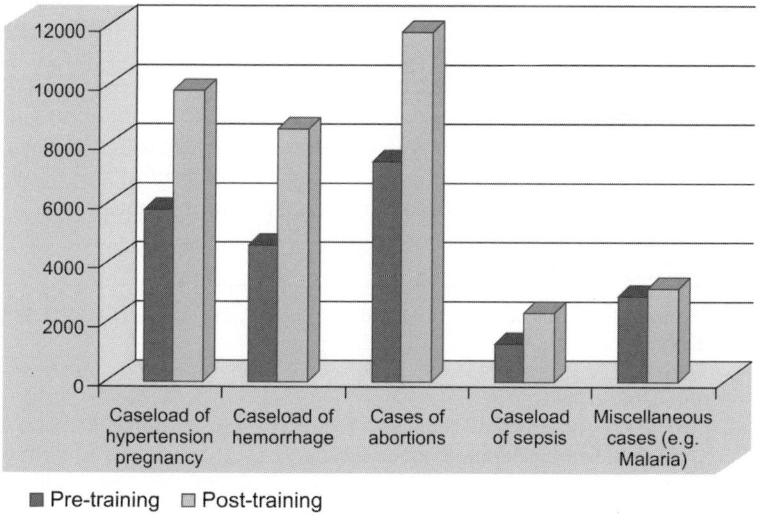

Fig. 5 Difference in cases managed at facility before and after training

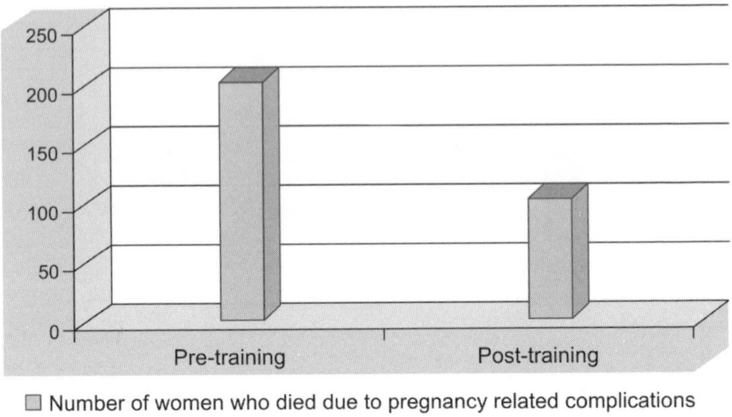

Fig 6 Difference in maternal mortality at facility before and after training of nonspecialist doctors under the EmOC program

CONCLUSION

The Federation of Obstetric and Gynaecological Societies of India (FOGSI) has come a long way in the last 7 years. We have crossed many hurdles and barriers and we have been consistent in our endeavor to keep improving. This has helped us to take the program to its present scale. In our analysis as with any large scale program, few implementation gaps and challenges are still present, but we are confident that the enthusiasm of all associated with the program, we will overcome them and we will continue to work towards reducing maternal mortality in India.

BIBLIOGRAPHY

1. Annual Report of Ministry of Health and Family Welfare–2012-2013. New Delhi.
2. Berwick DM, et al. Curing health care. San Francisco: Jossey-Bass Publishers, 1990.
3. Bruce J. Fundamental elements of quality care: a simple framework. Studies in Family Planning. 1990;21(2):61-91.
4. Engender Health, 2002. Community COPE®: building partnership with the community to improve health services, New York.
5. Engender Health, COPE®: handbook—A process for improving quality in health services, revised edition, New York, 2003.
6. Engender Health, Facilitative supervision handbook. New York, 1999.
7. Engender Health. Cope®: client-oriented, provider-efficient services—A process and tools for quality improvement and other reproductive health services, New York, 1995.

8. Engender Health. Medical monitoring handbook: working draft. New York, 1996.
9. Harper A, Harper B. Team barriers: action for overcoming the blocks to empowerment, involvement and high performance. New York: MW Corporation, 1996.
10. Huezo C, Diaz S. Quality of care in family planning: clients' rights and providers' needs. Advances in Contraception 1993;9:129-39.
11. Imundo LV. The effective supervisor's handbook. New York: AMACOM, 1993.
12. Maine D. Safe Motherhood Programme: Options and Issues. Center for Population and Family Health. Columbia University, New York, 1999.
13. McCaffery J, et al. Performance improvement: Stages, steps and tools. North Carolina: INTRAH, 2000.
14. Ministry of Statistics and Programme Implementation, Government of India, Press note 2006.
15. Thaddeus S, Maine D. Too far to walk: Maternal mortality in context. Social Science Medicine 1994;38(8):1091-110.
16. UNFPA. Maternal Mortality Report update: delivering into good hands. 2004.
17. UNICEF. Guidelines for monitoring the availability and use of obstetric services. 1997.
18. United Nations. 1966. International Covenant on Economic, Social and Cultural Rights. GA Res. 1966;2200A(XXI), 21 U.N. GAOR, Supp. No. 16, U.N. Doc, A/6316 (1966), 993 U.N.T.S. 3(Artile 12.12a, "General Comments on its Implementation"), entered into force Jan. 3, 1976.
19. WHO. World Health Report: Make every mother and child count. 2005.
20. World Health Organization (WHO)/UNFPA/UNICEF/World Bank. Integrated Management of Pregnancy and Childbirth (IMPAC). 2000. Managing complications in pregnancy and childbirth: a guide for midwives and doctors. Geneva: WHO.

17

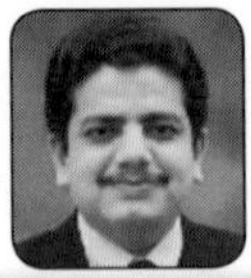

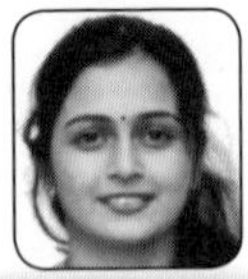

Unsafe Abortion and Maternal Health: Changing Trends and Challenges

Milind R Shah, Meenal A Chidgupkar

INTRODUCTION

World Health Organization defines unsafe abortion as a procedure for terminating an unintended pregnancy either by individuals without the necessary skills or in an environment that does not conform to minimum medical standards or both.[1] Unsafe abortion mainly endangers women in developing countries where abortion is highly restricted by law and countries where although legally permitted, safe abortion is not easily accessible.

Obtaining accurate data for abortions is challenging, and especially so for unsafe abortion. Two-thirds of nations do not have the capacity to collect data, and data collection varies from country to country in both quantity and quality.[2]

In these settings, women faced with an unintended pregnancy often self-induce abortions or obtain clandestine abortions from medical practitioners[3] or by paramedical workers or traditional healers.[4]

By contrast, legal abortion in industrialized nations has emerged as one of the safest procedure in contemporary medical practice with minimum morbidity and a negligible risk of death.[5] In Western nations, only 3 percent of abortions are unsafe, whereas in developing nations 55 percent are unsafe. The highest incidences of abortions that are unsafe occur in Latin America, Africa, and South East Asia.[6]

ABORTION SCENARIO IN INDIA

India pioneered in legalizing induced abortion (Medical Termination of Pregnancy MTP act of 1971) under which a woman can legally avail abortion if the pregnancy carries the risk of grave physical injury, endangers her mental health, when pregnancy results from contraceptive failure in a married woman or from rape or is likely to result in a birth of a child with physical or mental abnormalities. Abortion is permitted up to 20 weeks of pregnancy duration and no spousal consent is required.

According to the ministry of health and family welfare in 1996-1997 about 4.6 lakhs MTPs were performed in the country (MOHFW 1997) against that an estimated 6.7 million abortions per year are performed in other than registered and government recognized institutions often by untrained persons in unhygienic conditions.

WORLDWIDE BURDEN

Worldwide estimates for 1995 indicated that about 26 million legal and 20 million illegal abortions took place every year. Almost all unsafe abortions (97%) are in developing countries and over half (55%) are in Asia. Reliable data for the prevalence of unsafe abortion are generally scarce, especially in countries where access to abortion is legally restricted.[7]

UPGRADING FACILITIES

How safe are safe abortions is always a million dollar question. Abortion providers vary widely in both quantity and quality. Even where abortion is legal, providers may be limited in both number and in skill. There are variation in MTP centers and population served by these centers. seventy to eighty percent of primary health care (PHC) are without MTP facility. Many clinicians have little training for induced abortion. Experience with spontaneous abortion, where the cervix is often dilated, is not analogous to induced abortion. Many clinicians continue to use obsolete instruments, such as the metal curette. Moreover, limited evidence suggests that mid-level clinicians, such as physician's assistants and midwives, are competent to provide not only care of complications[8] but also to perform first-trimester abortions themselves.[9]

Simple, inexpensive equipment is needed for providing abortion services and caring for most complications that occur. Elaborate operating theater set-ups and availability of general anesthesia, required by some bureaucracies as a prerequisite for licensing are inappropriate.[10] Provided that arrangements and transportation (e.g. a jeep-taxi in rural India or a speedboat in Bangladesh) are in place for quickly moving patients to hospitals, if needed, free-standing abortion clinics around the world have achieved an outstanding safety record. Although abortion equipment is simple, it must be available. A major barrier to care in many developing countries is the lack of basic equipment and drugs for all gynecological care.[10] It was interesting to know about one study conducted by FOGSI about center registration. Only 28.8 percent Obs/Gyn got easy registration, 12.7 percent got it after delay by 1 to 7 years, 44.1 percent got difficulties in navigating process and 11.9 percent were unaware of this center registration.[11]

Lack of training, unfamiliarity with treatment options, out-of-stock drugs, broken equipment, sporadic electricity and water, and transportation challenges all threaten the health of women grappling with unsafe abortion.[12] Perhaps the greatest danger of all is indifference—or overt disdain.

The lack of commitment on the part of medical and nursing staff to provide prompt, attentive and emotionally supportive care indirectly dooms women whose lives could easily be saved. Many women who reach medical facilities are met with suspicion and hostility, and their treatment deferred while other more 'suitable' candidates receive medical attention.[12] When dealing with patients in need, judgmental behavior on the part of health care personnel is both medically dangerous and ethically indefensible. Many of them start giving moral advice without knowing facts and files of that scenario.

WHY WOMEN GO TO QUACKS?

It is common myth amongst women and girls that it is very expensive procedure if they go to private sector. They always carry lot of guilt and so tremendous fear and shame and so prefer to seek abortion from quack sitting in dark corner. In rural India, quite few of them are unaware of certified public centers and also have reluctance to go there as they are worried about losing confidentiality. It is also noticed that many public centers have low quality care and more so lack of compassion and courteous interaction. Many colleges and civil hospitals insist compulsion of IUCD insertion or sterilization operation before giving service of abortion which again deprives women from safe abortion facility.

MORBIDITY AND MORTALITY DUE TO UNSAFE ABORTION

Measurement of the worldwide prevalence of abortion related morbidity and mortality is difficult. At a population level, national vital registration system routinely undercounts such deaths. Worldwide, an estimated 68,000 woman die as a result of complications from unsafe induced abortions every year—about 8 per hour.

Worldwide, some 5 million women are hospitalized each year for treatment of abortion-related complications such as hemorrhage and sepsis, and abortion-related deaths leave 220,000 children motherless.[12] The main causes of death from unsafe abortion are hemorrhage, infection, sepsis, genital trauma, and necrotic bowel. Data on nonfatal long-term health complications are poor, but those documented include poor wound healing, infertility, consequences of internal organ injury (urinary and stool incontinence from vesicovaginal or rectovaginal fistulas), and bowel resections. Other immeasurable consequences of unsafe abortion include loss of productivity and psychological damage.[3]

EFFECT OF LAW ON HEALTH

Legalization of abortion can dramatically improve women's health. Several natural experiments reveal the potential. In the USA, for example, the legalization of abortion led to the emptying and then closing of septic abortion wards in major metropolitan hospitals.[14] On a nationwide basis, deaths from illegal abortion nearly disappeared within a few years of nationwide legalization.[15]

The opposite was observed in Romania after abortion was made inaccessible by the dictator Ceausescu. Birth rates remained stable, but maternal mortality rates soared to the highest in Europe. Women resorted to unsafe abortion to control their fertility, and many died. When Ceausescu was deposed and abortion again became accessible, maternal mortality rates plummeted.[14] More recently, Poland severely restricted abortion after decades of easy access. The result has been an estimated 80,000 to 200,000 clandestine abortions annually, women traveling to other countries for service, an increase in the cost of abortion, and no change in birth rate.[15] Clearly, the public health has suffered as a result.

Legalization of abortion, although important, is insufficient. India has had legal abortion on the books for several decades, as has Zambia. However, the 'devil is in the details'. In both countries, numerous impediments to care, ranging from requirement for several doctor's signatures to lack of accessible clinics, prevent most women in need from getting care in a timely fashion.[12] Hence, women continue to rely on unsafe abortion to control their fertility.

Access to safe abortion is also mediated by woman's awareness of the law knowledge which is often poor even in the countries with long standing liberal laws. Misinterpretation about specifies of the law are not uncommon, thus making women vulnerable to poor care, financial exploitation and persecution.

Even where legal abortion is widely available on request misperception about legality of minors having sexual intercourse delay some adolescents from seeking care.

In many cultures perception of legality are affected by stigma attached to premarital or extramarital sexual activity.

PRECONCEPTION AND PRENATAL DIAGNOSTIC TECHNIQUES ACT

The Preconception and Prenatal Diagnostic Techniques (PCPNDT) Regulation and Prevention of Misuse Act 1994 and its amendment in 2002, an Act to provide for the prohibition of sex selection, before or after conception and for regulation of prenatal diagnostic techniques for the purpose of detecting genetic abnormalities or metabolic disorders or chromosomal abnormalities or certain congenital malformations or sex-linked disorders and for the prevention of their misuse for sex determination leading to female feticide and for matters connected therewith or incidental thereto.

It is very important to understand intents of MTP act and PCPNDT Act as one is to prevent unsafe abortion and other is to prevent sex selection. Using one law to fulfill the intent of the other is rather counterproductive and does not help fulfill the objectives of both Acts.

Not all second trimester abortions are sex selective. In fact, while sex determination takes place mostly in the second trimester of pregnancy, 80 to 90 percent of reported abortions take place in the first trimester.

Placing limitations on second trimester abortions and /or increasing unnecessary reporting requirements for abortions will discourage providers from offering abortion services. This may lead uneducated and poor society to unsafe abortions and risk their lives.

The indirect costs of unsafe abortion are substantial yet more difficult to quantify. They include the loss of productivity from abortion related morbidity and mortality on women and household members.

LEVELS OF PREVENTION

Preventive medicine is traditionally viewed in three levels.

Primary Prevention

Includes reduction in the need for unsafe abortion through contraception, legalization of abortion on request, the use of safer techniques and improvement of provider skills.

The developing world has seen a revolution in contraceptive use-from mere 9 percent of couples using any method in 1960-65 to 59 percent in 2003. Nevertheless an estimated 27 million unintended pregnancies happen worldwide every year with the typical use of contraceptives. Six million would happen even with perfect use. An estimated 123 million women have an unmet need for family planning.

Manual vacuum aspiration is safer than sharp curettage, and the WHO recommends vacuum aspiration as the preferred method of uterine evacuation before 12 weeks of pregnancy.

The combined use of mifepristone and misoprostol has become the standard WHO recommended regimen for early abortion as well as second trimester abortions and is better than either drug alone.

Secondary Prevention

Entails prompt and appropriate treatment of complications. This includes timely evacuation of uterus after incomplete abortion. WHO has issued technical and clinical guidelines for the provision of safe abortion care and treatment of abortion complications.

Tertiary Prevention

Mitigates long-term damage. Rapid transfer to a hospital can be lifesaving. Prompt repair of uterine injury could preserve fertility. Acute renal failure and tetanus from unsafe abortions remain important causes of death and lengthy disability. Repair of fistulas in bowel and bladder can end the suffering and can check stigmatization and abandonment that these injuries cause.

PUBLIC HEALTH IMPERATIVE

The burden of unsafe abortion lies not only with the women and families, but also with the public health system. Every woman admitted for emergency post abortion care may require blood products, antibiotics, oxytocics, anesthesia, operating rooms, and surgical specialists. The beneficiaries of access to safe legal abortion on request include not only women but also their children, families and society for present and future generation.

Key Points

- The World Health Organization deems unsafe abortion one of the easiest preventable causes of maternal mortality.
- Data suggest that even as the overall abortion rate has declined, the proportion of unsafe abortion is on the rise.
- Methods of unsafe abortion include drinking toxic fluids; inflicting direct injury to the vagina, cervix, or rectum; or inflicting external

injury to the abdomen. Complications also arise from unskilled providers causing uterine perforation and infections.

- Worldwide, 5 million women are hospitalized each year for treatment of abortion-related complications, and abortion-related deaths leave 220,000 children motherless.
- Data indicate an association between unsafe abortion and restrictive abortion laws.
- Preventing unintended pregnancy, providing better access to health care, and liberalizing abortion laws to allow services to be openly provided can reduce the rate of abortion-related morbidity and mortality.

WHO places access to safe abortion services squarely within the right to quality sexual and reproductive health services, which WHO sees as fundamental to realizing women's basic right to health. It speaks directly to policymakers in calling for the creation of an "enabling environment," so that "every woman who is legally eligible has ready access to safe abortion care." But WHO goes further than that to address law and policy directly. "Policies," it asserts, "should be geared to respecting, protecting and fulfilling the human rights of women, to achieving positive health outcomes for women, to providing good-quality contraceptive information and services, and to meeting the particular needs of groups such as poor women, adolescents, rape survivors and women living with HIV. The respect, protection, and fulfillment of human rights require that comprehensive regulations and policies be in place to ensure that abortion is safe and accessible."

CONCLUSION

Although daunting, the predicament is not without solutions. Preventing unintended pregnancy should be a priority for all nations. Educating women regarding their reproductive health should be incorporated in schools. In nations that are not opposed to contraceptive use, increasing contraceptive services is necessary; this includes providing accurate information choices and proper use of contraceptive methods. Governments and nongovernmental organizations need to find effective ways to overcome cultural and social misconceptions that restrict women from receiving necessary health care.

In nations where abortion is legal, providing women better access to health centers that perform abortions is imperative. Practitioners need to become better trained in safer abortion methods and be able to transfer patients to a medical facility that is capable of providing emergency care when a complication arises. WHO strongly advises that all health facilities that treat women with incomplete abortions have the appropriate equipment and trained staff needed to ensure that care is consistently available and provided at a reasonable cost. In addition, post abortion family planning counseling needs to be an integral part of the service.

Evidence demonstrates that liberalizing abortion laws to allow services to be provided openly by skilled practitioners can reduce the rate of abortion-related morbidity and mortality. However, socio-political and religious obstacles have and will continue to play a role in passing abortion laws. The roles of research, grassroots organizations, health providers, activists, and media are vital in highlighting the importance of relaxing abortion laws. The emotional, physiologic, and financial cost on women and families, as well as the burden on the economic health system, should no longer be ignored.

SUMMARY

Unsafe abortion is a persistent, preventable pandemic and ending this silent pandemic of unsafe abortion is an urgent public-health and human-rights imperative as with other more visible global-health issues throughout the developing world and also in developed world due to restrictive abortion policy. Every year, about 19 to 20 million abortions are done by individuals without the requisite skills, or in environments below minimum medical standards. Nearly all unsafe abortions (97%) are in developing countries. An estimated 68,000 women die as a result, and millions more have complications, many permanent. Important causes of death include hemorrhage, infection, and poisoning. The underlying causes of morbidity and mortality from unsafe abortion today are not blood loss and infection but, rather, apathy and disdain toward women. Legalization of abortion on request is a necessary but insufficient step toward improving women's health. In countries like India, where abortion has been legal for decades, access to competent care remains restricted because of other barriers. Access to safe abortion improves women's health. The availability of modern contraception can reduce but never eliminate the need for abortion. Direct costs of treating abortion complications burden impoverished health care systems, and indirect costs also drain struggling economies. Access to safe, legal abortion is a fundamental right of women. Timely and appropriate management of complications can reduce morbidity and prevent mortality. Treatment delays are dangerous, regardless of their origin. The development of manual vacuum aspiration to empty the uterus, and availability of medical abortion and use of prostaglandin as oxytocic agent, has improved the care of women. While the debate over abortion will continue, the public health record is settled on quote that safe, legal, accessible abortion improves health.

REFERENCES

1. Word Health Organization. The prevention and management of unsafe abortion. Report of a Technical working Group.http://whqlibdoc.who.int/hq/1992/WHO_MSM_92.5.pdf(accessed July 6,2006).
2. Graham WJ, Ahmed S, Stanton C, et al. Measuring maternal mortality: an overview of opportunities and options for developing countries. BMC Med. 2008;6:12. [PMC free article] [PubMed].
3. Okonofua FE, Shittu SO, Oronsaye F, et al. Attitudes and practices of private medical providers towards family planning and abortion services in Nigeria. Acta Obstet Gynecol Scand. 2005;84:270-80.
4. Okonofua FE, Odimegwu C, Ajabor H, et al. Assessing the prevalence and determinants of unwanted pregnancy and induced abortion in Nigeria. Stud Fam Plann. 1999;30:67-77.
5. Hongberg U, Joelsson I. Maternal deaths related to abortions in Sweden,1931-1980. Gynaecol Obstet Invest. 1985;20:169-78.
6. World Health Organization. Unsafe abortion, authors. Global and Regional Estimates of the Incidence of Unsafe Abortion and Associated Mortality in 2003. 5th edn. Geneva: World Health Organization; 2007.http://www.who.int/reproductivehealth/publications/unsafeabortion_2003/ua_estimates03.pdf.
7. Henshaw SK, Singh S, Haas T. The incidence of abortion worldwide. Int Fam Plann Persp. 1999;25:S30-0.
8. Miller S, Billings DL, Clifford B. Midwives and postabortion care: experiences, opinions, and attitudes among participants at the 25th Triennial Congress of the International Confederation of Midwives. J Midwifery Womens Health. 2002;47:247–55.
9. Freedman MA, Jillson DA, Coffin RR, Novick LF. Comparison of complication rates in first trimester abortions performed by physician assistants and physicians. Am J Public Health. 1986;76:550–4.
10. Rogo KO, Aloo-Obunga C, Ombaka C, et al. Maternal mortality in Kenya: the state of health facilities in a rural district. East Afr Med J. 2001;78: 468–72.
11. FOGSI questionnaire on MTP in clinical practice.
12. Berer M. Making abortions safe: a matter of good public health policy and practice. Bull World Health Organ. 2000;78:580–92.
13. Grimes DA, Benson J, Singh S, et al. Unsafe abortion: the preventable pandemic. Lancet. 2006;368:1908–19.
14. Seward PN, Ballard CA, Ulene AL. The effect of legal abortion on the rate of septic abortion at a large county hospital. Am J Obstet Gynecol. 1973;115: 335–8.
15. Cates W Jr. Legal abortion:the public health record. Science. 1982;215: 1586–90.

18

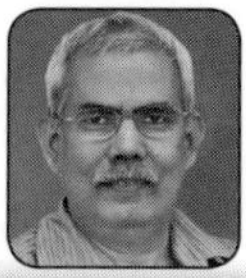

Safe Motherhood Initiatives in Kerala: A Success Story

MK Valsan

INTRODUCTION

Kerala has successfully achieved the health indicator targets when compared to other states in India. The maternal mortality rate (MMR) is one among them. The main reason for these achievements has been the stewardship role of health workers, efficient leadership and the futuristic government initiatives before and after independence.

This chapter deals with the present scenario of MMR in Kerala in comparison with the other Indian states. The medical, socioeconomic and environmental aspects which have contributed to reduction in maternal deaths are highlighted in detail. Though a leader amongst Indian states its MMR is high when compared to the developed world. Hence recommendations at improving this have also been detailed.

Maternal deaths are defined as the number of women who die during pregnancy or within 42 days of the termination of pregnancy. As per the UN data, India recorded around 57,000 maternal deaths in 2010, which translates into 6 deaths per hour and/or one maternal death every 10 minutes. The current MMR of India is 212 per one lakh live births whereas the country's Millennium Development Goal (MDG) set in this regard is 109 by 2015. The 2012 UN report states that although progress has been made on improvements in maternal health, targets remain far from sight. However, India has reduced MMR significantly from 437 in 1999 to 212 as per the latest figures, but needs to hasten the pace under National Rural Health Mission to achieve related MDG. The MMR recorded a 38 percent decline between 1999 and 2009.[1]

Table 1 gives the MMR in major states in India during 2004 to 2006 (SRS 2011).[2] During 2006 in Kerala MMR were 95 while all India average was 254 where as in 2010 the MMR in Kerala became 81. All India average is 212.

Table 1 Maternal mortality rate in major states of India

State	MMR
• Assam	312
• Madhya Pradesh/Chhattisgarh	335
• Odisha	303
• Rajasthan	388
• Uttar Pradesh/Uttarakhand	440
• East and Assam subtotal	375
• Andhra Pradesh	154
• Karnataka	213
• Kerala	95
• Tamil Nadu	111
• South subtotal	149
• Total (India)	254

Millennium development goal aims to reduce MMR to109 by year 2015. Other states realizing MDG target of 109 have gone up to 3 with Tamil Nadu and Maharashtra (new entrants) joining with Kerala. Andhra Pradesh, West Bengal, Gujarat and Haryana are in closer proximity to achieving the MDG target.[3]

CAUSES OF MATERNAL DEATH IN KERALA[4] (2006–2009)

- *Obstetric hemorrhage* accounts for 19.38 percent of deaths. The bleeding is commonly due to an atonic uterus or birth related trauma. The ones seen in a setting of obstructed labor has reduced significantly. DIC as a consequence of massive hemorrhage and the issue of delay in referral is still a reality. The incidence of placenta accreta, related bleeding and death is ever increasing because of the alarming increase in cesarean rates.
- *Hypertensive disease:* Pre-eclampsia/Eclampsia complex remains a major killer even in a setting of universal antenatal care, with an incidence as high as 12 percent. Though magnesium-sulfate has announced itself as the drug of choice in eclampsia, up to 45 percent of women might not have received the optimal dose. Contribution of intracranial hemorrhage as the principal cause of death reduced from 35 to 24 percent with extensive use of antihypertensive medications.
- *Sepsis* accounts for 8.5 percent of cases. Once 12th in the list of contributors to maternal death, as per the data analysis of 2004 to 2006, it is now the third most common. This is probably due to the

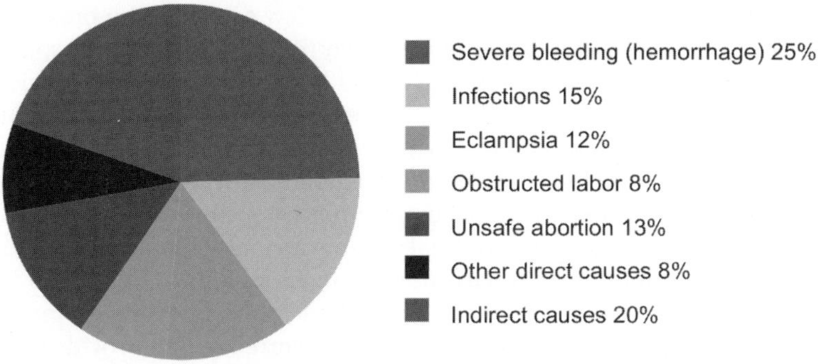

Fig. 1: Causes of meternal death in Kerala *(for color version see Plate 5)*

injudicious and extensive use of antibiotics with the emergence of multidrug resistant strains. It is not surprising that in the recent UK Confidential Enquiry report, incidence of sepsis was found to be more frequent than the previous year's data.

- *Heart disease:* Though still 4th in the list, it is gratifying to see a fall from 9 to 5.13 percent as per the recent data. The variety of heart disease encountered these days' shows a change from rheumatic to congenital. Surgically corrected cases on prosthetic valves are also encountered with the inherent problem of dealing with more women on anticoagulant therapy.
- *Amniotic fluid embolism* ranks 5th in frequency. High dose of prostaglandins at frequent interval was dangerous especially combined with smooth muscle relaxants like drotaverin and valethamate in active labor. It contributes genital tract trauma and PPH.
- *Hepatic diseases:* Acute liver failure due to HEELP or AFLP was the main cause but there were deaths due to viral hepatitis.
- Anesthesia, thromboembolism, suicide due to domestic violence are rare causes
- *Unknown causes:* Due to paucity of investigations or autopsy.

Figure 1 summarizes the incidence of different causes of maternal death in Kerala.

HOSPITAL FACILITIES IN KERALA AND ITS INFLUENCE IN REDUCING MMR[5]

Kerala has many factors which can help it to achieve a much lower MMR. The high female literacy rate, the wide spread availability of transportation and communication facilities and the large number of hospitals spread across the state are only a few of them. The pregnant mother is generally only a few minutes away from a tertiary level hospital. The basis for the state's impressive health standards is the statewide infrastructure at the level of PHCs. There are over 2,700 government medical institutions in the state, with 330 beds per 100,000 populations, the highest in the country. In addition to that the private sector in Kerala grew to meet the demand that was unmet when the government cut back their investment due to fiscal strain. Currently the private sector accounts for more than 70 percent of all facilities and 60 percent of all beds. They vary in sophistication from single doctor hospital to multi-specialty hospitals and have become the preferred health providers for the affluent and middle class.

GENERAL HEALTH INDICATORS AND PREVALENCE OF INFECTIOUS DISEASE IN KERALA

Infectious diseases are under control and infectious complications of peripartum period are rare. The habit of using sanitary latrines, maintenance of body and genital hygiene, use of boiled drinking water, extensive immunization of antenatal mothers and an almost cent percent hospital delivery rate contributes in reducing communicable diseases and hence maternal deaths.

Health development indicators of Kerala in comparison with Indian data-2009[6] are shown in Table 2.

Table 2 Different health indicators of Kerala state vs India

Health indicators	*Kerala*	*India*
• Birth rate (per 1,000 population)	14.60	22.80
• Death rate (per 1,000 population)	6.60	7.40
• Infant mortality rate (per 1,000 population)	6.70	44.00
• Maternal mortality ratio (per 1 lakh live births)	40.00	301.00
• Total fertility rate (per woman)	1.70	2.90
• Couple protection rate (%)	62.30	52.00
• Life expectancy at birth (Male)	71.40	62.60
• Life expectancy at birth (Female)	76.30	64.20
• Life expectancy at birth (Average)	74.00	63.50

In Kerala, the birth rate is 40 percent below the national average and almost 60 percent below that of the underdeveloped countries. In fact, a 1992 survey found that the birth rate had fallen to the replacement level. Kerala's birth rate is 14 per 1,000 females and has a falling trend. India's rate is 25 per 1,000 females and that of the United States is 16. Its adult literacy rate is 94.59 percent compared to India's 65 and 99 of United States. Life expectancy at birth in Kerala is 75 years compared to 64 years in India and 77 years in the United States. Female life expectancy in Kerala exceeds that of the male, just as it does in the developed world.[7] Kerala's maternal mortality rate is 1.3 deaths/1,000 live births (1990), which is the lowest among Indian states.[2]

DIETARY HABITS AND NUTRITIONAL STATUS

Anemia is practically nil except among teenage pregnancies and the tribal population of remote areas. Safe vaginal delivery, lesser operative vaginal deliveries and lesser infective and anesthesia related morbidity at cesarean have helped to improve the status. The tradition of a routine native ayurvedic health care after delivery may also have contributed to a healthy mother and baby. With virtually all mothers being taught and encouraged to breastfeed and a government supported nutrition programme for pregnant mothers, infant mortality in 2011 was found to be 12 compared with 91 per thousand of the under privileged countries.[8,9]

FEMALE LITERACY RATES AND ITS INFLUENCE ON MATERNAL HEALTH

In 1970, despite a low per capita income, the state had high literacy rates and health concerned citizens. The present status of Kerala is comparable to that of the developed world. Kerala ranks highest in India with respect to social development indices such as poverty levels, primary education and health care. This resulted from significant efforts by the erstwhile Cochin and Travancore states from as early as 1911, to boost health care and education among the people. This initiative, unusual in India at that time, was then maintained even in the post independence era.[10] Thus, Kerala attained the highest literacy rate and life expectancy rates amongst Indian states. As per the 2011 census, Kerala and Puducherry are the only states in India with a favorable sex ratio. The ratio for Kerala is 1.084—1084 females per 1000 males—while the national figure is 0.940.[11]

Kerala's unusual socioeconomic and demographic situation was summarized by author and environmentalist Bill McKibben as follows;
"Kerala, a state in India, is a bizarre anomaly among developing nations, a place that offers real hope for the future of the Third World. Though not much larger than Maryland, Kerala has a population as big as California's and an annual per capita income of less than $300 million dollar. But its infant mortality rate is very low, its literacy rate among the highest on Earth, and its birthrate below America's and falling faster.

Kerala's residents live nearly as long as Americans or Europeans. Though mostly a land of paddy covered plains, statistically Kerala stands out in social development; there's truly no place like it."[7]

POLITICAL AWARENESS AND ITS EFFECT ON HEALTH

Political awareness amongst the common man including children is quite high thanks to its social reformers like *Sree Chattambi Swamigal, Sree Narayana Guru* and *Ayyankali*. The Communist activities and the unique political situation that existed in Kerala also helped. Political history in Kerala shows a trend of an alternating Communist and Congress Governments in power, resulting in an increase in public welfare activities, much to the benefit of the common man.

EDUCATION, THE BACKBONE OF PROGRESS IN KERALA

The *Pallikkoodams*, started by Christian Missionaries paved the way for an Educational revolution in Kerala by making education accessible to all, irrespective of caste or religion. Christian missionaries introduced modern education to empower the common man to throw away the yoke of bondage inflicted by themselves in a setting of old customs and practices. Communities such as *Ezvas, Nairs* and *Harijans* were guided by great visionaries and monastic orders (Ashrams)—*Sree Narayana Guru, Sree Chattambi Swamigal* and *Ayyankali*—who exhorted them to educate themselves by starting their own schools. That resulted in numerous Sree Narayana schools and Nair Service Society schools. The teachings of these saints have also empowered the poor and backward classes to organize themselves and claim their rights. Muslim Educational Society (MES) also made significant contributions to education. However, all these would not have been possible unless the 'Aided School' system of the Government of Kerala took up the operating expenses of educational institutions.

Kerala had been a notable center of Vedic learning, having produced one of the most influential Hindu philosophers, *Adi Shankaracharya*. The Vedic learning of the *Nambudiris* is an unaltered tradition that still holds today, and is unique for its orthodox nature, unknown to other Indian communities. However, in feudal Kerala, though only the *Nambudiris* received an education in *Vedam*, other castes and even women were allowed access to sanskrit, mathematics and astronomy.

The upper castes, such as *Nairs*, Tamil Brahmin migrants, *Ambalavasis* as well as backward castes such as *Ezhavas*, had a strong history of Sanskrit learning. In fact many Ayurvedic physicians (such as *Itty Achudan*) were from the backward *Ezhava* community. This level of learning by non-Brahmins was not seen in other parts of India. Also, Kerala had been the site of the notable Kerala school which pioneered principles of mathematics and logic, and cemented Kerala's status as a place of learning.

The right for education was not only restricted to males. In pre-Colonial Kerala, women, especially those belonging to the matrilineal Nair caste, received an education in Sanskrit and other sciences, as well as *Kalaripayattu* (martial arts). This was unique to Kerala and was facilitated by the inherent feeling of equality shown by the society towards both sexes. It became a reality because the society was largely matrilineal, as opposed to the rigid patriarchy in other parts of India which led to loss of women's rights.

The rulers of the Princely state of Travancore (Thiruvithamkoor) were at the forefront in the spread of education. A school for girls was established by the Maharaja in 1859, which was an unprecedented act in the entire Indian subcontinent. In colonial times, Kerala exhibited little defiance against the British Raj. However, they organized mass protests for social causes such as rights for "untouchables" and education for all. Protests to hold public officials accountable became a significant event in the history of emerging Kerala.

In the 1860s, the Government[12] spread the educational programs into Malabar. The northern state that had been ruled directly by the British began granting scholarships to Harijans and the tribal people. By 1981, the general literacy rate in Kerala increased to 70 percent, almost twice the Indian rate of 36 percent. The rural literacy rate was almost identical, and female literacy at 66 percent, was not far behind. The Government continued to press the issue, aiming for "total literacy", usually defined as about 95 percent of the people being able to read and write (Table 3).

A pilot project began in the Ernakulam, with an area of 3 million people that included the city of Kochi. In 1988, 50,000 volunteers fanned

Table 3 Marked rise in literacy rates in Kerala from 1951 to 2011

Year	*Persons*	*Males*	*Females*
1951	47.18	58.35	36.43
1961	55.08	64.89	45.56
1971	69.75	77.13	62.53
1981	78.85	84.56	73.36
1991	89.81	93.62	86.17
2001	90.92	94.20	87.86
2011	94.59	97.10	92.12

out around the district, tracking down 175,000 illiterates between the ages of 5 and 60, two-thirds of them being women. The expectation was that within a year the illiterates would read Malayalam at 30 words a minute, copy a text at 7 words a minute, count and write from 1 to 100, and add and subtract three-digit numbers. On 4th February 1990, 13 months after the initial canvass, Indian Prime Minister VP Singh marked the start of World Literacy Year with a trip to Ernakulam, declaring it the country's first totally literate district. Kerala's literacy rate of 91 percent[11] (2001 survey) is almost as high as in China (93%) or Thailand (93.9%).

LAND REFORM ORDINANCE: AN UNIMAGINABLE FEAT

In 1957, Kerala elected a communist government headed by EMS Namboothiripad who introduced the revolutionary Land Reform Ordinance. The Land reform ordinance was implemented by the subsequent government, which abolished tenancy, benefiting 1.5 million poor households. This achievement was the result of decades of struggle by Kerala's peasant associations. In 1967, in his second term as Chief Minister, Namboothiripad again pushed for reform. The land reform initiative abolished tenancy and landlord exploitation; effective public food distribution that provides subsidized rice to low-income households; protective laws for agricultural workers; pensions for retired agricultural laborers; and a high rate of government employment for members of formerly low-caste communities.

DRAWBACKS IN MATERNAL HEALTH STATUS

Though the maternal mortality rate in Kerala is better than the Indian average, it is unacceptably high compared to the international standards. Government intends to reduce the MMR by 50 percent of the current rate by the end of the 12th five year plan. Almost all deliveries in Kerala take place in institutions and the quality of obstetric care has to be further improved. A strategy to reduce the maternal mortality through a standard framework, developed with the support of the Kerala Federation of Obstetrics and Gynecology (KFOG) and National Institute of Clinical Excellence (NICE) of UK, is being piloted in Kerala. By addressing the most common obstetrical complications like PPH and PIH, this project made a dent in the MMR of the state. For the last one decade, both government and private sector hospitals are reporting a rising trend of cesarean touching an alarming 40 percent, though administrative and technical measures have been taken up at the state level to deal with it. Issues like maternal anemia, early marriage and teenage pregnancy in some of the districts and tribal areas also remain intractable.

INFRASTRUCTURE: A LIMITATION

"Most obstetricians know about these measures but in their clinical practice often there might not be a situation when all emergency measures can come together—could be shortage of staff, drugs or equipment. Once the government adopts these guidelines, the physical infrastructure will also have to be improved to enable its implementation," points out VP Pail, president of KFOG. The guidelines are to be translated into quality measures in selected hospitals.

Recommendations[13]

- All antenatal cases are to be categorized into high risk and low risk and should be monitored accordingly
- Improve the emergency care facilities in labor room to deal with obstetric emergencies
- Obstetrician and nursing staff should be fully equipped with resuscitation of a collapsed patient
- Infrastructure with adequate drug supply, equipment and man power should be available throughout the day
- Early referral to a higher center with a network of ambulance service throughout the state
- Blood and blood components should be freely available round the clock
- Proper sterilization and disinfection is mandatory to all staff in the labor room
- A protocol based management should be practiced for all emergency cases. The doctors and staff should be thorough with the protocol
- Establish obstetric intensive care units in major centers and medical colleges there should be ambulance with transport ventilators attached to such centers
- Documentation of all investigations and procedures is mandatory with date and time. Reporting of maternal death with all details is strictly warranted.

CONCLUSION

Kerala has unique advantages in terms of healthcare indices, accessibility to healthcare, female literacy, educational advantage and empowerment of women compared to other states in India. The state had utilized these advantages to achieve a status at par with the developed world. We believe that the success story from this small State will inspire the other Indian states to improvize and achieve the defined targets in the near future.

REFERENCES

1. Frederica Meijer. India's Representative for United Nations Population Fund, 3rd July 2012.
2. Maternal and Child Mortality and Total Fertility Rates Sample Registration System (SRS) Office of Registrar General, India, 7th July 2011.
3. CIA World Fact book, February 21,2013.
4. Why mothers die in Kerala 2006-2009, 2nd report CRMD Dr VP Paily and others 2012.
5. Kerala model from Wikipedia, the free encyclopedia, 2011.
6. Medical and public health Kerala Govt. retrieved 25th July 2010.
7. Kerala a case study Bill McKibben.
8. State-wise infant mortality rate SRS, 7th July 2011.
9. Morbidity profile of Kerala and All-India. An economic prospective.
10. Medical and Public health Kerala Govt. retrieved 25th July 2010.
11. How almost everyone in Kerala learned to read; 2005.
12. Education. Kerala Government Retrieved, 17 July 2010.
13. Guidelines evolved to reduce MMR.The Hindu. Dec.19,2012.

19

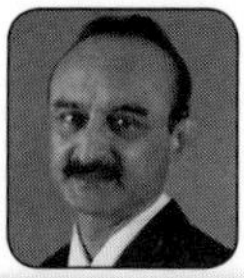

Role of Teaching Institutions for Safe Motherhood Initiative: Beyond the Hospital

Pratap Kumar

INTRODUCTION

The existing system of hospital-oriented obstetric care has failed to serve the majority of the people in the developing countries. In India, about 80 percent of the population reside in the rural areas where hospital facilities are not available. Thus, the obstetric care to the people should be started from the village provided by the major hospital. Moreover, such obstetric care should be integrated with pediatric and social medical care. It has been realized that a very high perinatal and infant mortality rate stand a real threat to the implementation of Family Welfare Program. Hence, an excellent maternal and perinatal health of a region reflects the high quality obstetrical care given by the obstetrician pediatrician and community medicine personnale.

EXPERIENCE OF KASTURBA HOSPITAL, MANIPAL

To serve the rural population, Kasturba Hospital, a private institution, Manipal University, Manipal, Karnataka State, India, maintains seven satellite maternity child health centers to provide obstetricial, pediatric and social medicine care. The area covers a population of 160000. These satellite MCH centers are situated between 6 and 20 km from the main hospital. Regular clinics for obstetrics and gynecology patients, as well as, pediatric patients are carried out by doctors from the main hospital. High-risk cases are picked up and referred to the main hospital. Most of the deliveries are conducted by the postgraduates from the main hospital. The intimation of a case to the main hospital is done through telephones by the Auxiliary Nurse Midwife, who is in-charge of the center. The Flying Squad Ambulance Service is provided to attend any patient or to transport a patient.

In 1985, a total of 6,417 had antenatal care and a total of 1,421 patients had their deliveries in these seven centers. 5,480 children had pediatric care. Those who had intrauterine contraceptive device (IUD), oral contraceptive (OC) or tubal ligation following delivery were 1.54 percent, 10.76 percent and 14.84 percent respectively. Patients who had 3 or more children and who underwent postpartum tubectomy were 211 in number (48.17%). There were 12 perinatal deaths giving a perinatal mortality rate of 8 per 1,000. The existing system of running seven satellite MCH centers by our hospital has served the rural population and helped in the obstetric and pediatric outcome. However, the number has drastically reduced which may be due to small maternity homes which are started by private practitioners. The details are shown in Table 1 and Figure 1 for 2003 to 2012.

The Flying Squad Ambulance Service team consists of one postgraduate of obstetrics and gynecology, one junior house-surgeon and a medical student. The medical equipment required at these centers are supplied by the main hospital.

All the expenditures are met by Manipal University, Manipal, Karnataka, India.

FUNCTION OF THE SATELLITE MATERNITY CHILD HEALTH CENTER ALONG WITH ANALYSIS

To Conduct Regular Antenatal Clinic

Once a week a regular outpatient work is carried out by obstetrics and gynecology and pediatric departments. The patient strength varies in each center, which may be between 20 and 120 obstetric patients per clinic.

Table 1 and Figure 1 show the outpatient strength of antenatal patients. Advice concerned with proper nutrition, hygiene and stress upon common dangers of pregnancy, such as bleeding, anemia, toxemia of pregnancy are explained, antenatal immunization against tetanus is done. High-risk cases are identified and referred to the major hospital for further investigations and care.

Conduct of Deliveries

The ANM in-charge in the center examines and conducts some of the deliveries. All primigravidae in labor are seen by a postgraduate and the delivery also is conducted by the postgraduate who is attending the patient. High-risk obstetrical cases needing further hospital care or surgical interference are brought by the postgraduate to the major hospital for further management. Table 2 and Figure 2 show the number of deliveries in the satellite MCH centers.

Table 1: Antenatal attendance at satellite clinic of Kasturba Medical College, Manipal (2003–2012)

Year	*New*	*Total*
2003	1376	5900
2004	1735	7872
2005	1836	9767
2006	1926	10236
2007	1859	10541
2008	1599	8670
2009	1296	7163
2010	1162	6641
2011	1126	5818
2012	641	3294

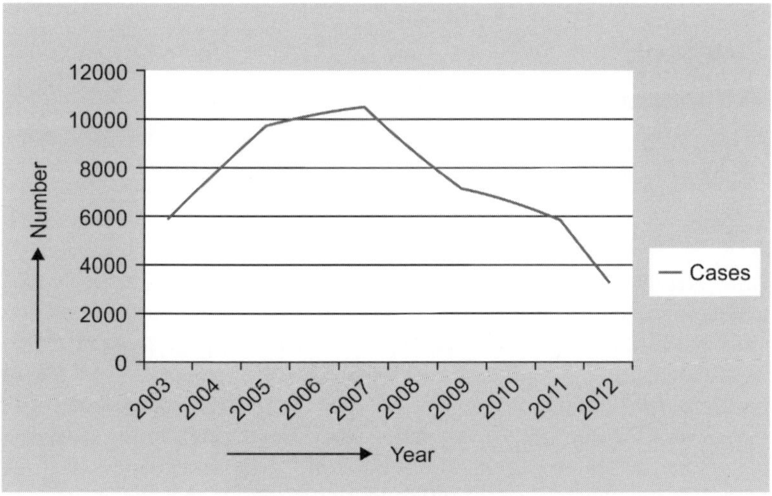

Fig. 1: Antenatal attendance (cases) at satellite clinic of Kasturba Medical College, Manipal (2003–2012)

On an average 29.85 percent of patients are referred to tertiary hospital. All these patients are referred back to the centers.

Other Services Available

Services available in Rural Maternity and Child Welfare (RMCW) homes:

- Antenatal care
- Natal care

Table 2: Institutional delivery conducted at satellite and referral teaching institution from 2003 to 2012

Year	*RMCWH delivery*	*Referred*	*Total delivery*
2003	556	329	885
2004	739	349	1071
2005	795	478	1273
2006	898	440	1335
2007	722	464	1186
2008	485	486	971
2009	332	427	759
2010	229	416	645
2011	140	331	471
2012	122	207	329

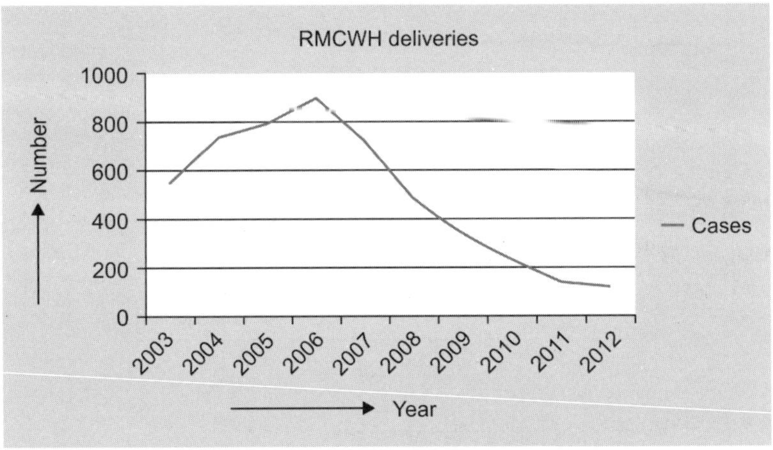

Fig. 2: Institutional delivery (cases) conducted at satellite and referral teaching institution from 2003 to 2012

- Postnatal care
- Postpartum sterilization
- Copper T insertion
- Distribution of oral contraceptions and condoms
- Ultrasonography (through portable ultrasound)
- Counseling by the medical social workers
- Health and nutrition education to mothers
- Referral services to the main hospital

Postpartum/Family Welfare Program

The Kasturba Hospital, Manipal, Karnataka, India, has been performing female sterilizations since 1958 and completed more than 150000 family planning operations. This is the first center which introduced laparoscopic sterilizations in the hospital as a National Family Welfare Program. More than the 30 percent of the female sterilization of undivided Dakshina Kannada district was being done in Kasturba Hospital, Manipal. Several times our hospital was adjudged as the best in the state level for performing highest number of sterilizations under All India Hospital Postpartum Program.

Laparoscopic sterilization camps: We had conducted 929 laparoscopic sterilization camps in different parts of undivided Dakshina Kannada district, covering a population of 25 lakhs (conducted 32,160 laparoscopic sterilization). The same was pioneered and popularized by Late Professor Dr A Padma Rao who was the Head of Department (HOD) at that time.

Other Main Health Education Activities

- Population education
- Reproductive and child health education
- Nutrition education and demonstration
- Education of hygiene on sanitation
- HIV/AIDS/STD awareness program
- Adolescent education
- Education on various communicable diseases
- Education breastfeeding
- Exhibition
- Save the girl child
- Anemia-free India.

The Undergraduate MCH Training

In the satellite MCH centers the undergraduates (pre-final MBBS students) are taught about the integrated maternal and child health care. The whole curriculum is divided into several sessions which are limited to common problems during antenatal, intra- and postnatal periods, normal delivery and common neonatal problems. Each session of 3 hours is attended by the team, each from three departments—obstetrics and gynecology, pediatrics and community medicine. Hence, there will be stress upon the obstetrical care in rural set-up taking into account the meager facilities and personal assistance available, which in the developing country like ours is very important.

The ANM who is posted at the centers is posted in each center permanently so that the people in that particular area get a good contact and confidence with the nurse and there is mutual trust.

Maternal mortality in these centers was nil.

CONCLUSION

The existing system of running seven satellite MCH centers by our hospital has served the rural population and helped in the obstetric and pediatric outcome.

There are many medical colleges and teaching institution which have been built in rural area in last 15 years. Our experience suggest strongly that leaders and workers of these teaching institution can work on such program of satellite maternal and child health clinic, good referral and back up support. It will great help on altering maternal and newborn health statics and health seeking behavior of the community. The need is to look and go beyond the four walls and campus of teaching hospital. Believe it, you are the one, who are going to receive most.

ACKNOWLEDGMENT

Thanks for Dr Veena G Kamath, Head, Department of Community Medicine, Kasturba Medical College, Manipal, Karnataka, India for the statistics.

20

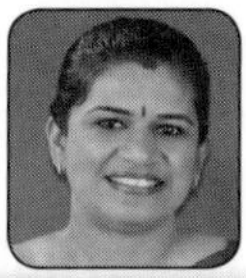

Role of Professional Bodies in Safe Motherhood in Developing Countries

Hema Divakar

INTRODUCTION

The needless death of thousands of women due to pregnancy-related complications casts a shadow over the modern world. The reasons for this in the developing countries is beyond the issues of accessibility and availability of 'technical' care ..... there are social, legal, economical and cultural issues which influence the health seeking behavior, awareness, accessibility and affordability. The article examines the potential roles and responsibilities of professional obstetrical associations in addressing this tolerated tragedy. In light of modern medical advances including the formal organization of many health care professionals, it is important to consider what role professional health care associations might play in reducing maternal mortality. Their roles include lobbying for women's health and rights, setting standards of practice, raising awareness and team building. We will discuss how professional obstetrical associations can be strong stimulants to support change within these countries.

This article will highlight the proactive steps by the professional organizations within the countries where the problem is epidemic, (e.g. India—through FOGSI).

What Professional Associations can do?

Broadly, we agree that professional associations can offer:

- **Technical assistance** which is their core strength by virtue of the qualification of members who are specialists.
- **The human resource** can be harnessed and the members of the professional bodies can audit their own work and set standards and build the capacity of all providers across the country and beyond.

Scope of Professional Bodies in Maternal and Child Health

Setting Standards for Delivering Quality Healthcare

- Consenses on protocols for management of pregnancies—routine and at risk pregnancy and intrapartum and postpartum care.
- Extended also to adolescent and preventive and promotive healthcare.
- Creating centers of excellence as a role model for care and organizational champions to promote and propogate quality standards.

The joint statement by WHO/UNICEF emphasizes the need for co-ordinated long-term efforts to reduce maternal mortality; efforts directed towards the community and family, as well as the health care system. Further, national legislative policies are also urged. The statement goes on to say that medical practice relating to pregnancy care should be regulated with protocols and guidelines for maternal care at each level of the healthcare system. Education and training curricula, along with national standards should be developed for all levels of health care workers. The professional bodies need to act on the recommendations endorsed by the WHO/UNICEF joint statement. FOGSI ICOG is working with Government of India, providing technical assistance for all issues related to Reproductive Maternal, Newborn Child Adolescent Health (RMNCH A+).

CMEs: Dissemination of the Standard Recommendations and Guidelines

- To peer group, postgraduates, medical graduates
- Paramedics and Frontline Healthcare Workers (FHW)
- Sensitizing the peer group for adhering to protocols defined by national bodies and government—emphasizing on uniformity and quality of care.

Professional associations can be active in continuing medical education—emphasizing best practices based on scientific evidence and avoiding harmful practices. The programs address the educational needs of health care providers concerning safe motherhood. It is designed to update the health care providers on labor and high-risk situations during delivery. It includes training of association members as trainers so that the program can be disseminated widely.

Capacity Building Task Shifting, Ensuring Quality and Competency

- Expanding healthcare provision through FHW—training and skill transfer with assessment of competency
- Mentoring, monitoring and supportive supervision
- Implementation partners for healthcare system accreditation process.

The role that professional associations might play in quality assurance is significant. In many developing countries, there is not only a shortage of health care workers, but the quality of services they render is less than adequate thereby adding to an already complex problem. Inadequate care fails not only the individual women but erodes public confidence in the 'system'. This may cause some to seek alternative sources of (potentially riskier) care such as traditional healers or traditional birth attendants.

The FOGSI fast track initiative for *Helping Mothers Survive* is being carried out by the organization in an aggressive manner, recognizing the urgency to prevent needless deaths. Professional associations can stimulate better teamwork within the health care system. The hierarchical structure in many countries fosters a cold and distant relationship between the midwives and doctors. This can be addressed and improved through educational programs for physicians centering on a team approach to care. Professional associations can promote the use of maternal mortality audits to assess barriers and breakdowns within the maternal health care system and recommend changes to improve the access and availability of care for pregnant women.

Advocacy

- At the level of the general public—To generate demand from women themselves promoting and educating the women about the essentials of effective health care for women
- Rights based advocacy for policy making—Unified voice for women's health by lobbying, partnerships with the government and influencing womens healthcare policies by the governments.

GENERATE DEMAND BY MAKING WOMEN AWARE

Professional associations can play a role in public education around women's health issues. They can also liaise between social scientists and health care providers in order to generate an effective outreach to the community. Health care professionals can augment the access to health information for their patients and the general public. This can be done through having patient information booklets in their offices and public places. The association may assist these professionals in both printing and having primary access to literature. The associations can also work with other organizations to produce and update medical publications. In this way, they will support the improvement of both the quality and dissemination of information.

Professional health care organizations targeted at women's health care need to be developed, mentored and motivated into action in order to achieve quality and effective care for women worldwide.

Political Lobbying

The sphere of influence of many professional health care workers is broad and the lobbying audiences are, therefore, similarly broad. Potential targets include National Ministries of Health, their community and international donor programs. Professional associations can both mobilize the community in its collective concern regarding maternal mortality as well as educate the political decision makers that are charged with health resource allocation policy. Internationally, they can draw attention to the unacceptable rates of maternal mortality that might easily be reduced with relatively inexpensive international assistance. Above all, they can demonstrate leadership in ensuring quality care for all women within their country. National associations should be encouraged to carry out a national inventory of emergency obstetrical centers and generate a needs-assessment with the intent to present it to the national government. This needs-assessment will encourage governments to consider the magnitude of the maternal health problem and direct policy-makers to better plan and provide the needed services for delivery as well as upgrading existing facilities.

Partnerships and Collaborations

- With international professional organization of specialists
- With pediatrics and neonatal associations nationally
- Association of midwives and paramedics councils
- Ministry and the NGOs—national and international
- Networking with professional organizations in the neighboring regions to learn and share effective innovations for implementation–making an IMPACT.

These professional associations can both suggest governmental policy and vigorously endorse it. National associations that have international reputations could promote their agenda on an international scene with credibility. Specific deficiencies in the system could receive heightened attention (for example, the three-delay model of maternal mortality: delay in seeking care, delay in reaching care and delay in the provision of care). Maternal mortality is a multifactorial problem and thus the approach must cover the span of factors including women's rights and empowerment, health, and basic education, transportation systems and health care attitudes and systems. As professionals, they can address the human rights issue and lobby their government for action and legislation. 'Safe Maternity' is increasingly being viewed as a basic human right worldwide. It is not a commodity for the privileged only. It has been over 50 years for all people.

It is obvious from the scope listed above that—The role for professional associations might adopt within developing countries are numerous and each has the potential to reduce maternal mortality and ensure safe motherhood.

Section III

Innovations for Safe Motherhood

"This time like all times, is a very good one, if we but to know what to do with it"

Chapters

21

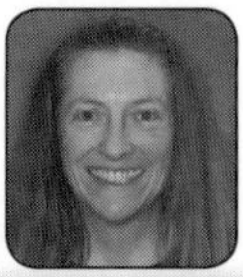

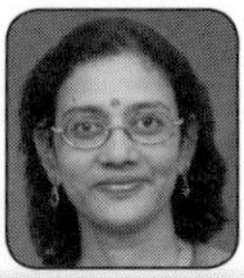

Innovative Simple Technology for Safe Motherhood: An Experience from PATH

Coffey Patricia, W Sita Shankar, Elizabeth Abu-Haydar, Nitya Nand Deepak, Noah Perin, Denise Lionetti

INTRODUCTION

Appropriate technology is generally used to mean a technology that is simple to use, able to withstand environmental and use conditions, culturally sensitive and affordable. Program for appropriate technology in health (PATH) is an international nonprofit organization that transforms global health through innovation. We take an entrepreneurial approach to developing and delivering high-impact, low-cost solutions, from lifesaving vaccines and devices to collaborative programs with communities. Through our work in more than 70 countries, PATH and our partners empower people to achieve their full potential in India and other developing countries. Our approach is to develop technologies that are affordable and acceptable to the communities and cultures that will benefit, and then to make them accessible to the public sector and corollary markets in developing countries. Technology development generally follows the flow described in Figure 1 encompassing the span from research and development through to scale of the product in a market and/or geography.

Although many constraints to the development and scale of appropriate technologies exist, progress is being made towards technology solutions for some aspects of maternal health. In particular, technologies that address postpartum hemorrhage (PPH) have received widespread attention in recent years. This chapter discusses several technologies that are designed to address postpartum hemorrhage in a comprehensive way including both prevention and treatment of this critical experience in the lives of women.

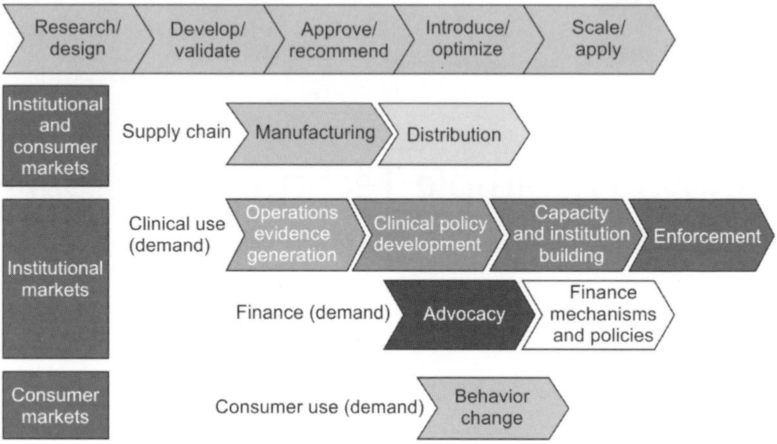

Fig. 1 Technology research design to production

THE BURDEN OF POSTPARTUM HEMORRHAGE

Postpartum hemorrhage is the leading cause of maternal death in India. The majority of these cases are preventable, but due to lack of resources in many settings, maternal death rates in India remain higher than in other developing countries. The current maternal mortality rate (MMR) of India is 212 per 100,000 live births; far away from the Millennium Development Goal (MDG) of 109 per 100,000 live births by 2015. India is on the track, but lagging behind to meet MDG 5 related to maternal health. Currently, one maternal death is being reported every ten minutes in the country.

Every child-bearing woman is potentially at risk for postpartum hemorrhage, but biological and physiological considerations are only a part of the picture. Postpartum hemorrhage prevention and treatment procedures which are well known and proven to be scientifically beneficial are not readily available to health workers and pregnant women. Besides increasing the number of skilled birth attendants and encouraging institutional deliveries, improving quality of care and the availability of simple, easy-to-use, affordable technology can play a vital role in saving maternal lives.

The grim reality is that too often maternal deaths are invisible. They do not leave any trace behind, and their deaths are not accounted for. The aftermath of this tragedy is borne mainly by the children and family of the deceased.

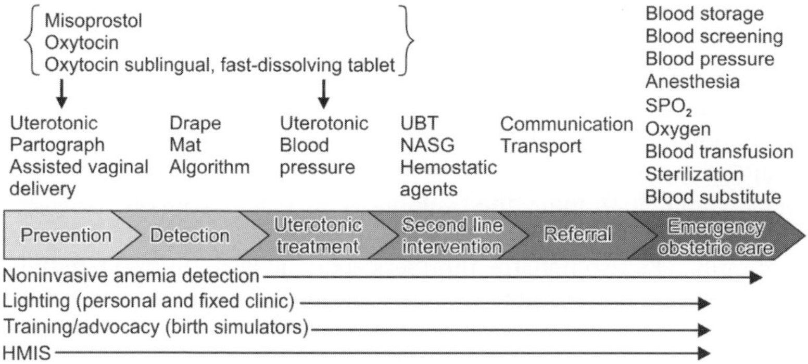

Fig. 2 Postpartum hemorrhage continuum of care

A need based continuum of care approach to improve quality of care such as the current National RMNCH+A (Reproductive Maternal Newborn Child Health + Adolescents) approach in India could help develop and deploy technology innovations. A bundled approach of looking at technology that can help skilled birth attendants handle deliveries safely and provide timely intervention is the need of the hour. The technology innovations discussed in this chapter cover the continuum of care that a pregnant woman and/or a woman who experiences postpartum hemorrhage might encounter. They include screening for anemia, administration of preventive oxytocin as part of active management during the third stage of labor, administration of oxytocin as a first line treatment for management of hemorrhage, stabilization and management of related hypovolemic shock through use of the nonpneumatic antishock garment (NASG), and secondary treatment of bleeding with an uterine balloon tamponade (Fig. 2). The highlighted topics in the figure below are the technologies that are being discussed in this chapter.

NONINVASIVE ANEMIA DETECTION

Anemia can reduce a woman's ability to withstand the adverse effects of blood loss during and after pregnancy. Noninvasive anemia screening devices have been designed to make it easy to monitor a pregnant woman's iron levels to help reduce her risk of potentially life-threatening complications during or shortly after childbirth as well as preventing long-lasting health problems associated with severe anemia.

Anemia continues to be one of the most serious global health problems, with far-reaching consequences for health as well as social and economic development. It is estimated that iron deficiency anemia (IDA) affects more than one billion people worldwide. Anemia particularly affects pregnant women and young children in developing countries. IDA in children has been associated with impaired cognitive performance, motor development, co-ordination, and language development. In developing countries, 42 percent of children less than 5 years of age and 53 percent of children from 5 to 14 years of age are anemic. In India, the National Family Health Survey (NFHS-3) indicated that anemia prevalence was nearly 80 percent in children 6 to 36 months.[1] For women, the numbers are equally alarming: 56 million pregnant women and 468 million nonpregnant women suffer from IDA.[2] The majority of these women live in Africa and Southeast Asia.[3] The same National Family Health Survey indicated that nearly 60 percent of pregnant women in India are anemic. IDA places pregnant women at risk for poor pregnancy outcomes including increased risk of maternal and perinatal mortality and morbidity, preterm births, and low-birth weight babies. Specifically, women who suffer from anemia are less able to withstand the adverse effects of excessive blood loss during pregnancy and are more susceptible to infection, fatigue, and depression.[4] Furthermore, a study conducted by Kavle et al. provides evidence of the link between anemia during pregnancy and increased likelihood of blood loss during and after delivery, thereby increasing the woman's risk of PPH and the subsequent mortality and morbidity risks.[5] A pre-pregnancy store of more than 500 mg of iron is required to avoid iron deficiency during pregnancy, yet these levels of iron are only present in 20 percent of menstruating women in developing countries before the start of their pregnancy.[6] Current World Health Organization guidelines for antenatal care recommend universal iron-folic acid supplementation with a minimum of 90 days of supplementation for pregnant women where anemia is widespread.[7] However, many countries do not meet these standards, many pregnant women do not attend antenatal care in the first trimester, and coverage remains low.[8]

Prevention and early detection, monitoring, and treatment of anemia among pregnant women is critical for appropriate tailoring and targeting of the interventions to serve the population's needs—and to reduce the burden on the health system by targeting interventions and addressing anemia before it becomes an emergency. Effective screening programs for IDA in prenatal and postnatal programs have been hampered by the lack of simple, safe, accurate, low-cost hemoglobin testing tools. The majority of women who suffer from anemia live in low-resource areas where accurate diagnostics are unavailable. In such settings, anemia often goes undetected and untreated. A noninvasive device offers major advantages over current methods and approaches and would expand access to screening and increase early identification and treatment of anemia.

Most IDA point of care screening tests have challenges to their use, especially in rural settings. The most commonly used methods—the Sahli method, the color scale, and clinical assessment—have limited sensitivity and are most commonly used in low-resource health settings to diagnose the most severe cases of anemia. These methods rely on subjective interpretation. Other, more quantitative point-of-care tests such as the HemoCue® require blood samples, maintenance of equipment, and recurrent supplies, limiting their use in resource-poor settings. The commonly used laboratory-based methods are expensive, complex, and necessitate a blood draw, requiring a trained technical person.

Attempts to develop more accurate, easier-to-use, and sustainable anemia screening technologies have been ongoing for many years. Noninvasive technologies have been of special interest, and with recent advances in technology and expertise and continued concern about the risks of blood-borne diseases, there have been renewed efforts among researchers and manufacturers to develop such technologies. Noninvasive devices would reduce the use of costly consumables, and eliminate the need for a blood draw, the disposal of hazardous waste, and the subjective nature of many of the currently available tests. It could potentially improve clinical practice by expanding access to screening among high-risk populations at the periphery and in more remote locations, providing immediate quantifiable measurements to guide and support early treatment and monitoring, and facilitating surveillance and monitoring efforts.

Several promising technologies designed for use at point of care by non-laboratory-trained health care providers in developing countries have emerged, have international regulatory approval, and are commercially available (Table 1).

Nearly all devices use a finger probe and technology analogous to noninvasive pulse oximetry to provide a quick spot check for total hemoglobin. These technologies address many of the problems that faced previous noninvasive devices: they are smaller in size, more compact, simple to use, and provide immediate results. Some have the added advantage of providing simultaneous measurements of hemoglobin, oxygen saturation, and pulse rates, thus increasing the impact and applicability of these tools well beyond anemia screening and control programs to a wider range of programs affecting the health of women.

Table 1 Commercially available technologies designed for use at point of care

Device	*International regulatory approval*	*Commercially available in India*
Pronto™ developed by Masimo Corporation (Irvine, CA)	CE/USFDA	Yes
ToucHb developed by Biosense (Mumbai, India)		Yes
Hemospect® developed by MBR Optical Systems GmbH and Co. KG. (Germany)	CE	No
NBM-200 developed by OrSense (Israel)	CE/USFDA	No

OXYTOCIN—PREVENTION OF POSTPARTUM HEMORRHAGE—INDIAN SCENARIO

Administration of an uterotonic drug immediately following delivery can effectively prevent postpartum hemorrhage, which contributes to nearly two-fifths of maternal mortality in India. However, uses of uterotonics prior to delivery in community and peripheral facilities by low-level health workers is regarded as dangerous, which can lead to uterine rupture, fetal asphyxia and/or fetal demise. Though this is a common practice, there is no documented evidence of inappropriate use of uterotonics in health facilities in India. PATHs oxytocin initiative (OI) project conducted a landscape study to broadly explore how uterotonics are being used and distributed at or around birth in Uttar Pradesh and Karnataka, India.

Key Findings

Augmentation of labor using one or more uterotonic drugs is the norm in three of four districts, with rates ranging from 72 percent to 91 percent (Table 2). Of particular concern, one in three of all deliveries were augmented via IM injection or IV push. There were reports of using multiple (up to 5) uterotonic injections for augmentation. There is also high demand from family members for uterotonic injections to speed up labor, since they are not aware of the disastrous effects such as ruptured uterus, birth asphyxia. Although nearly all women received one or more

Table 2 Percent of deliveries with labor augmentation

	Hassan	*Bagalkot*	*Agra*	*Gorakhpur*
% Augmented	87.7%	73.7%	53.5%	93.0%
Among the Augmented : N = 288				
% using Non-pharm. or Trad. methods	2.0%	1.0%	3.1%	2.6%
% using 1 Pharm. method	42.6%	64.8%	68.7%	76.6%
% using 2 Pharm methods	55.5%	34.2%	22.5%	19.6%
% using 3 Pharm. methods	0.0%	0.0%	4.4%	1.2%
Total	100%	100%	100%	100%

uterotonic drugs after delivery of the baby, none met the criteria in the Government of India Guidelines for Active Management of the 3rd Stage of Labor in three districts and only five percent did so in the 4th district.

A key recommendation based on these findings was the development of strategies to reinforce appropriate use of uterotonics. Changes to this practice require a system-wide top-down approach. The oxytocin initiative (OI) project has partnered with the Federation of Obstetric and Gynecological Societies of India (FOGSI) to improve medical practices around augmentation of labor by obstetricians/gynecologists and auxiliary nurse midwifes. The endeavor is to achieve changes in practice through support for their continuing medical education program and through existing FOGSI mechanisms that advocate for best practices in obstetric care. FOGSI is committed to scaling-up activities in other states.

Drug Quality Work

The study also found the percent of active pharmaceutical ingredient was outside of manufacturer's specification in 36 percent of oxytocin ampoules and 72 percent of methylergometrine ampoules, although none of the ampoules were expired (Fig. 3). While there may be issues with the actual quality of manufactured products, it is more likely that issues exist with transport and storage of products.

SUBLINGUAL, HEAT STABLE OXYTOCIN FAST DISSOLVING TABLETS

The most common cause of postpartum hemorrhage (PPH) is uterine atony, or failure of the uterus to contract after delivery. Uterotonic drugs cause the uterus to contract thus reducing or arresting bleeding. The

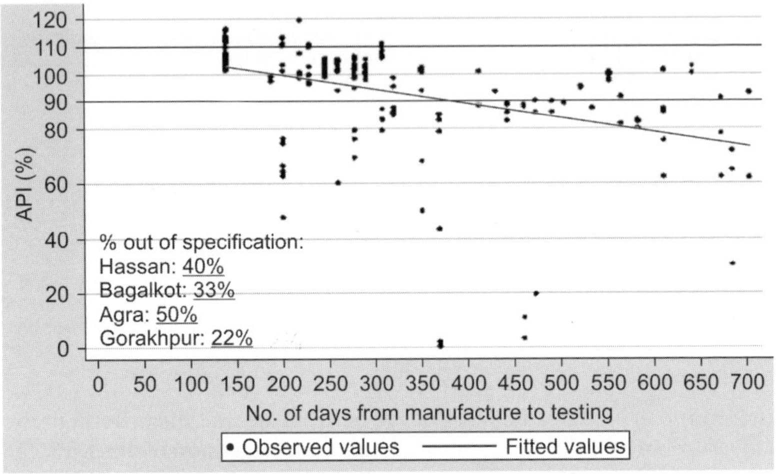

Fig. 3 Active pharmaceutical gradient of oxytocic

gold-standard, and WHO preferred uterotonic for first line prevention and treatment of PPH is oxytocin. Currently oxytocin requires refrigeration, intravenous (IV) or intramuscular (IM) infusion, and administration by skilled providers. These factors can hinder the use of this lifesaving drug. Building on the oxytocin initiative work being carried out in India, PATH is developing heat-stable, Fast dissolving tablets (FDTs) of oxytocin for sublingual administration. The sublingual route of administration bypasses the stomach and goes directly into the blood stream. It is a promising route of delivery that promotes rapid absorption and high bioavailability with subsequent almost immediate onset of pharmacological effect. Placed in the woman's mouth, under the tongue, the tablet dissolves in less than thirty seconds, inducing rapid onset of action required for oxytocin (Figs 4A and B).

This novel approach to the administration of oxytocin will provide an easy and effective way to prevent and treat PPH in rural settings, especially in health facilities lacking emergency obstetric care, and reliable cold chain systems. The sublingual FDT is designed to be heat stable and easy to administer, requiring minimal training of midwives and auxiliary nurse midwifes. A sublingual delivery format for oxytocin has quite a few advantages over the current modes of delivery: transport, storage, and administration of oxytocin FDTs will not require refrigeration, a skilled health worker, a supply of needles and syringes, a painful injection, or disposal of sharps. Additionally, the compact foil blister packaging of the tablets will simplify shipping, storage and

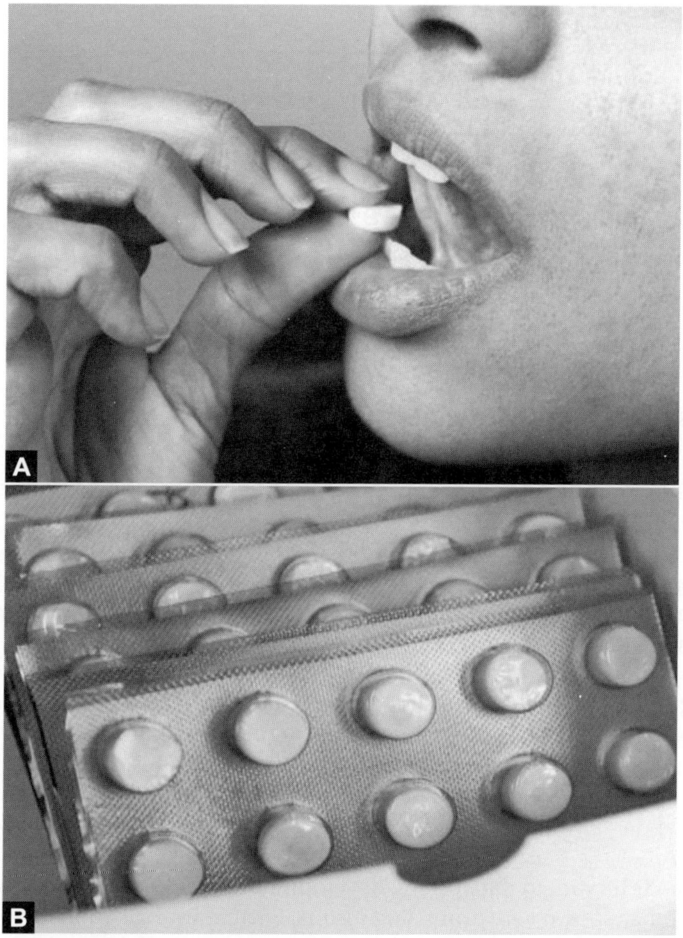

Figs 4A and B Program for appropriate technology in health (PATH) (*Source:* Patrick McKern) Sublingual oxytocin—new technology in development

distribution logistics and decrease waste. The sublingual FDTs are expected to cost less than the conventional ampoule presentation.

Sublingual Fast-disintegrating Tablets

One of the possible challenges associated with the sublingual route is the potential for a patient to swallow parts of the dose thereby requiring higher dose for sublingual uptake. To minimize loss in delivery due to swallowing, PATH formulated the tablets to form a mucoadhesive gel at

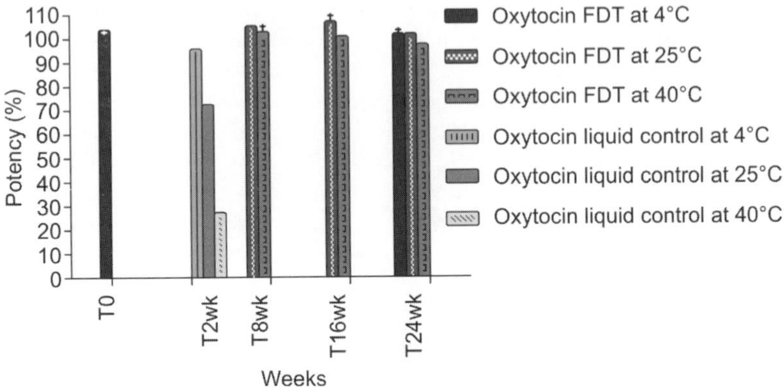

Fig. 5 Four weeks stability data on oxytocin fast dis-integrating tablets (FDTs) stored at 37°C

the site of administration for optimal retention, absorption and uptake. The formulation was tested to assess the efficacy and the safety of the sublingual formulation. Rapid dissolution is critical for release and absorption of oxytocin. PATH conducted a feasibility study in animals that demonstrated rapid onset (5–7 minutes) via sublingually administered oxytocin similar to IM administered oxytocin. Oxytocin is very temperature sensitive. Heat stability studies have reported oxytocin to lose effectiveness after 3 months of being stored at temperatures above 30°C. This is a critical issue and one that has limited the access to the use of the drug especially at peripheral facilities. The sublingual oxytocin FDTs demonstrated elevated heat stability with minimum loss in potency for tablets stored at 40°C for up to 6 months as shown in Figure 5.

PATHs work to date on the development of the sublingual oxytocin FDTs, has shown very promising results. Further investigation involving the systemic bioavailability studies in an animal model having similar oral tissue histology as humans will be conducted to demonstrate response time and oxytocin levels following sublingual administration. The systemic levels obtained via sublingual administration will be compared with levels obtained via standard intramuscular (IM) route of administration to identify effective sublingual dose of oxytocin for PPH treatment.

NONPNEUMATIC ANTISHOCK GARMENT

If a woman with obstetric hemorrhage progresses into shock, she is likely to suffer serious injury or die without advance treatment. In low-resource settings, where specialized care may be hours or even days away, health providers need a reliable, inexpensive way to stabilize patients until help is available. The nonpnetumatic antishock garment (NASG) is gaining acceptance as a simple and effective option.

Active management of the third stage of labor (AMTSL) is recommended by the World Health Organization (WHO) and is endorsed by the International Federation of Obstetricians and Gynecologists (FIGO) and the International Congress of Midwives for the prevention of PPH.[9] Also the recent 'WHO Recommendations for Prevention and Treatment of PPH' guidelines published by WHO in 2012 clearly articulates the recent evidence related to AMSTAL.

Although the effectiveness of AMTSL has been well documented,[10] it poses some challenges and limitations in low-resource settings.[11] Even when it is performed exactly, AMTSL prevents only 40 to 50 percent of PPH caused by uterine atony. Also, AMTSL does not treat shock, a dangerous progression of PPH. If PPH-related shock is not treated immediately, the woman can die of hypovolemic shock or suffer irreparable damage to vital organs. Over the last decade, new research, funded by the Bill and Melinda Gates Foundation, the John D and Catherine T MacArthur Foundation, and the National Institutes of Health, has indicated that the NASG can reverse shock, and stabilize patients experiencing PPH so that they can be safely transported for further medical care.

The NASG is a lightweight neoprene garment that resembles the bottom half of a wetsuit.[12] The design of the NASG permits complete perineal access, allowing health providers to place urinary catheters, suture genital lacerations, perform speculum or bimanual examinations, and provide manual vacuum aspiration or uterine exploration or curettage (Fig. 6). Thus, the source of much obstetrical bleeding can be located and repaired while the garment remains in place, stabilizing vital signs.[13,14] The NASG functions by providing circumferential counter pressure to the lower body in order to shunt blood from the lower extremities and abdominal area to the essential core organs: heart, lungs, and brain. The garment's five neoprene segments close tightly with Velcro around the legs, pelvis, and abdomen to supply from 20 to 40 mm Hg of circumferential pressure. The abdominal segment incorporates a small foam pressure ball to provide uterine compression. In addition to reversing shock and stabilizing the patient, circumferential pressure decreases both the transmural pressure and the radius of uterine, abdominal, and other lower body arteries.[15] The NASG is ideal for low-resource settings because it can be washed and reused at least 40 times. Additional attributes that make

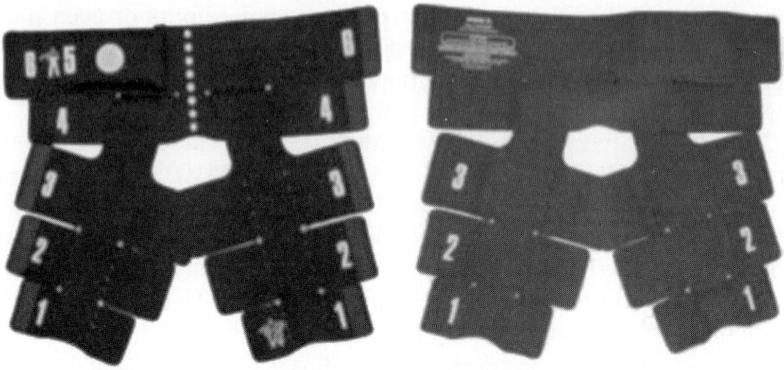

Fig. 6 NASG manufactured in India (*Source:* PATH/VISCO)
(for color version see Plate 6)

this an appropriate technology for developing countries are ease of use, minimal required training, and portability—it can be easily carried to outlying areas.

Pilot studies have shown that the NASG can decrease obstetric hemorrhage and stabilize a patient until proper medical treatment is available.[16–18] Use of the NASG has been reported in a study of 634 women with obstetric hemorrhage (43% with uterine atony) in Egypt.

Women treated with a NASG had a median blood loss that was on average 200 mL lower (range 300–100 mL lower) than women who received standard treatment. However, there have been no completed randomized controlled trials (RCTs) on the use of the NASG in the treatment of PPH. A randomized cluster trial is under way in Zambia and Zimbabwe to examine whether early application of a NASG by midwives prior to transfer to a referral hospital can decrease death and injury.[19] Additional recent 'hemodynamic flow and pressure studies' suggest a significant increase in internal iliac artery flow resistance with NASG application and provide a physiological explanation of how the NASG might reduce PPH.[20]

To introduce a more affordable model in low-resource settings, PATH recently negotiated affordable, high-quality NASG manufacturing with qualified manufacturers and distributors in China (Blue Fusion Group, Hong Kong) and India (Vissco Rehabilitation Aids Pvt. Ltd., Mumbai; Website: www.visscoindia.com), The NASG is not a one-size-fits-all garment. Three sizes (small, medium, and large) have been developed to accommodate differences in women's bodies worldwide (population-dependent anthropomorphic variation). The Indian manufacturer is producing the small size for use in India.

UTERINE BALLOON TAMPONADE FOR THE MANAGEMENT AND TREATMENT OF UNCONTROLLABLE POSTPARTUM HEMORRHAGE

Postpartum hemorrhage (PPH) is the leading cause of maternal mortality worldwide, accounting for approximately 130,000 deaths each year.[21,22] The risk of death is greatest for women who are anemic or have other underlying health problems that make them less able to deal with blood loss. Among women who do survive a PPH, approximately 12 percent will have severe anemia.[23] Also, women who survive severe PPH (greater than 1,000 mL of blood loss) are significantly more likely to die during the following year.[24] In India, it is estimated that 117,000 women die from pregnancy-related causes each year with approximately 30 percent of deaths due to hemorrhage and 19 percent of deaths attributable to anemia.[25,26]

Most cases of severe PPH can be prevented if the bleeding is controlled and managed immediately with uterotonic drugs. Although the use of drugs such as oxytocin, can reduce PPH rates by up to 62 percent,[27] some women will still experience excessive bleeding following delivery. In such cases, uterine balloon tamponade (UBT) provides a simple, rapid, and effective method to manage PPH. While long used in resource-rich settings, UBT as a second line intervention is now also recommended by many organizations (WHO, FIGO) as the standard of care for PPH when uterotonics fail or are unavailable.[28,29]

Uterine balloon tamponade is a minimally invasive intervention that involves inserting a balloon device into the uterus and filling it with liquid, which slowly applies pressure to the uterus until the bleeding stops (Figs 7A and B). Fluid amounts are determined by the health care provider based on how fast the bleeding stops. The balloon is inflated incrementally until the bleeding is controlled—this is often referred to as the 'tamponade test'. On average, from 250 to 350 mL of fluid are needed to control bleeding. UBT can stop the bleeding in as little as 5 to 15 minutes. UBT devices can be kept in place for up to 24 hours after insertion, if needed. If the balloon tamponade is effective in stopping the hemorrhage, the patient is less likely to require surgical interventions and blood transfusions, with their related risks and costs. Even when UBT cannot completely control severe PPH, it still serves a critical role by reducing blood loss until the woman can be referred.

Several types of UBTs are available and have been successfully used to manage and treat PPH (Figs 8A to C). Although they differ slightly from each other, they all generally follow the same principle and have the same indications and contraindications for use. Commercially available UBTs (Fig. 8C) are prohibitively expensive and some countries

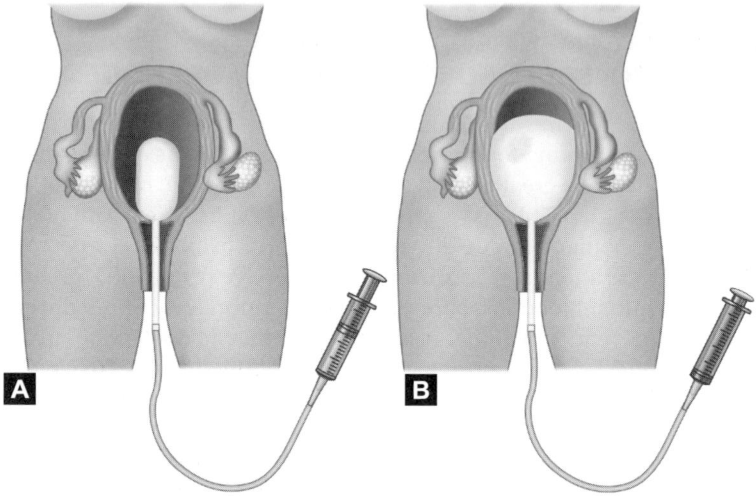

Figs 7A and B Uterine balloon tamponade in the uterine cavity (*Source:* Illustration by PATH/Patrick McKern)

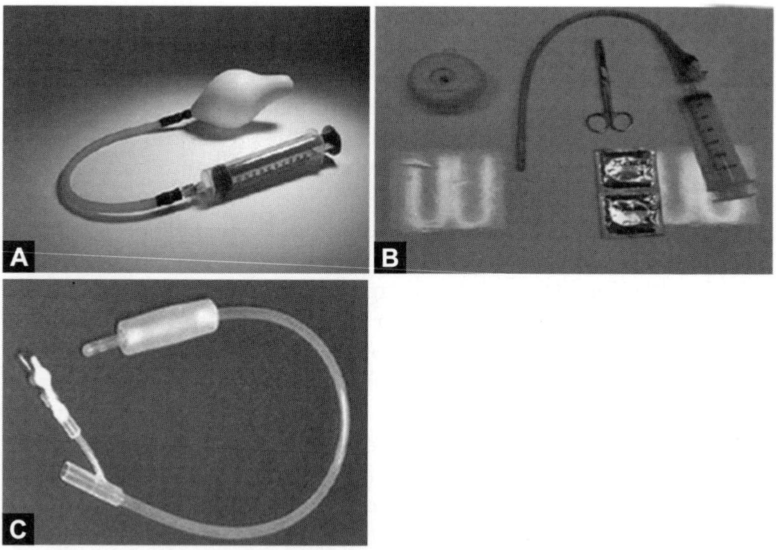

Figs 8A to C (A) Simple low-cost PATH uterine balloon tamponade (*Source:* PATH/Patrick McKern); (B) Akhter Condom Catheter balloon-components (*Source:* Thomas Burke/Massachusetts General Hospital); (C) Bakri balloon (*Source:* PATH/Patrick McKern)

have adopted use of the condom catheter balloon that is assembled from readily available components; a catheter and a condom tied around the catheter at time of use (Fig. 8B). Although UBT devices are most commonly used for PPH caused by uterine atony,[30,31] they have also been used for bleeding following cesarean sections, in cases of placenta previa and accrete, and for post-abortion care. The woman should be monitored for continued or renewed bleeding and her vital signs checked regularly.

Uterine balloon tamponade (UBT) may have the greatest impact on lives saved at peripheral health facilities when bleeding continues despite initial management. A recent systematic review of the effectiveness of UBT in resource-poor settings found that UBT successfully treated severe PPH in 234 out of 241 cases reviewed.[32] UBTs are not currently in common use in rural India, mainly due to their high cost. In India, PATH proposes to develop and commercialize a simple affordable UBT specifically designed for use beyond tertiary facilities (Fig. 8A). In low-resource facilities in India, the UBT could act as a definitive treatment or a temporizing one, buying the health care providers more time to transfer the patient to a facility where she can get the emergency care she needs.

POTENTIAL IMPACT IN INDIA AND THE REGION

The work by PATH to make pregnancy, labor, and delivery safer, and to improve newborn health, has reached an estimated 24.5 million people in India alone. The potential health impact of the technologies we discuss in this paper are great. For example, in the year 2020 an estimated 15,000 maternal deaths due to postpartum hemorrhage uterine atony and 940,000 cases of postpartum hemorrhage will occur in India. Heat stable oxytocin that is delivered by an alternative route such as sublingual has the potential to save 1881 (13%) of these lives and avert 115,479 cases of postpartum hemorrhage in India alone. The potential for global impact is even greater. Increasing access to these types of lifesaving technologies will enhance the safe motherhood experience for women and India and elsewhere.

REFERENCES

1. Government of India. National Family Health Survey-3. Delhi: Government of India; 2007.
2. De Benoist B, McLean E, Egli I, Cogswell M (Eds). WHO and CDC worldwide prevalence of anemia 1993-2005. Geneva: WHO; 2008.
3. World Health Organization, UNICEF, United Nations Population Fund, and The World Bank. Trends in Maternal Mortality: 1990 to 2008. Geneva: WHO; 2010.

4. Sanghvi T, Harvey P, Wainwright, E. Maternal iron-folate acid supplementation on programs: evidence of impact and implementation. Food and Nutrition Bulletin. 2010;31(2):S100-7
5. Kavle JA, Stoltzfus RJ, Witter F, Tielsch JM, Khalfan SS, Caulfield LE. Association between anemia during pregnancy and blood loss at and after delivery among women with vaginal births in Pemba Island, Zanzibar, Tanzania. Journal of Health Population and Nutrition. 2008;26(2):232-40.
6. Breymann C, Bian X, Blanco-Capito L, et al. Expert recommendations for the diagnosis and treatment of iron-deficiency anemia during pregnancy and the postpartum period in the Asia-Pacific region. Journal of Perinatal Medicine. 2011; 39(2):113-21.
7. Stoltzfus RJ, Dreyfuss ML. Guidelines for the Use of Iron Supplements to Prevent and Treat Iron Deficiency Anemia. Washington, DC: International Nutritional Anemia Consultative Group; 1998.
8. Girard AW. Maternal undernutrition: Evidence, links, and solutions. Presented at: Maternal Health Policy Series, December 15, 2010; Washington, DC.
9. International Confederation of Midwives (ICM), International Federation of Gynaecology and Obstetrics (FIGO). Prevention and Treatment of Post-partum Haemorrhage New Advances for Low Resource Settings: Joint Statement. London, UK: FIGO and The Hague, Netherlands: ICM; 2006. Available at: http://www.pphprevention.org/files/FIGO-ICM_Statement_November2006_Final.pdf. Accessed February 6, 2012.
10. Prendiville WJ, Elbourne D, McDonald S. Active versus expectant management in the third stage of labour. Cochrane Database of Systemic Reviews. 2000;3.
11. WHO. WHO Recommendations for the Prevention of Postpartum Haemorrhage. WHO/MPS/07.06. Geneva: WHO; 2006.
12. Miller S, Turan JM, Dau K, et al. Use of the non-pneumatic anti-shock garment (NASG) to reduce blood loss and time to recovery from shock for women with obstetric haemorrhage in Egypt. Global Public Health. 2007;2(2):110-24.
13. Miller S, Ojengbede A, Turan JM, Ojengbede O, Butrick E, Hensleigh P. Anti-shock garments for obstetric haemorrhage. Current Women's Health Reviews. 2007;3(1):3-11.
14. Miller S, Hensleigh P. Non-pneumatic anti-shock garment for obstetric haemorrhage. In: B-Lynch C, Keith L, LaLonde A, Karoshi M (Eds). An International Federation of Obstetrics and Gynecology (FIGO) Book, Postpartum Haemorrhage: New Thoughts, New Approaches. London, UK: Sapiens Publications; 2006.pp.136-146.
15. McSwain NE Jr. Pneumatic anti-shock garment: state of the art 1988. Annals of Emergency Medicine. 1988;17(5):506-25.
16. Miller S, Hamza S, Bray E, et al. First aid for obstetrical haemorrhage: the pilot study of the non-pneumatic anti-shock garment in Egypt. BJOG: An International Journal of Obstetrics and Gynaeocology. 2006;113(4):424-9.
17. Miller S, Turan JM, Ojengbede A, et al. The pilot study of the non-pneumatic anti-shock garment (NASG) in women with severe obstetric

haemorrhage: combined results from Egypt and Nigeria. Proceedings of the International Congress on Evidence Based Interventions to Prevent Post Partum Haemorrhage: Translating Research into Practice. July 12-15, 2006; Goa, India.

18. Miller S, Turan JM, Dau K, et al. Decreasing maternal mortality from hypovolemic shock in low resource settings: The non-pneumatic anti-shock garment (NASG). Global Public Health. 2007;2(2):110-24.
19. Page on Safe Motherhood. UCSF Bixby Center for Global Reproductive Health website. Available at: http://bixbycenter.ucsf.edu/research/safe_motherhood.html. Accessed January 8, 2012.
20. Lester F, Stenson A, Meyer C, Morris J, Vargas J, Miller S. Impact of the non-pneumatic antishock garment on pelvic blood flow in healthy postpartum women. American Journal of Obstetrics and Gynecology. 2011;204(5):409.e1-409.e5.
21. AbouZahr C. Global burden of maternal death and disability. British Medical Bulletin.2003;67:1-11.
22. Khan KS, Wojdyla D, Say L, Gülmezoglu AM, Van Look PFA. WHO analysis of causes of maternal death: a systematic review. The Lancet. 2006;367(9516):1066-74.
23. Karoshi M, Keith L. Challenges in managing postpartum haemorrhage in resource-poor countries. ClinObstet Gynecol.2009;52(2):285-98.
24. Immpact International. Measuring and Addressing Outcomes After Pregnancy: A Holistic Approach to Maternal Health. Aberdeen, UK: Immpact International; 2007.
25. Millenium Development Goals; India Country Report 2006.
26. Chatterjee A, Paily VP. Achieving Millennium Development Goals 4 and 5 in India. BJOG. 2011.118(Suppl 2):47-59.
27. Prendiville WJ, Elbourne D, McDonald S. Active versus expectant management in the third stage of labour. Cochrane Database Syst Rev. 2000;(2): CD000007.
28. Arulkumaran S, Karoshi M, Keith LG, Lalonde AB, B-Lynch C (Eds). A comprehensive textbook of postpartum haemorrhage: An essential clinical reference for effective management. Sapiens Publishing; 2nd Revised edition. 2012.
29. WHO- WHO Recommendations for the Prevention and Treatment - WHO 2012http://www.who.int/reproductivehealth/publications/maternal_perinatal_health/9789241548502/en/.
30. Arulkumaran S, Karoshi M, Keith LG, Lalonde AB, B-Lynch C (Eds). A comprehensive textbook of postpartum haemorrhage: An essential clinical reference for effective management. Sapiens Publishing; 2nd Revised edition. 2012
31. Doumouchtsis SK, Papageorghiou AT, Arulkumaran S. Systematic review of conservative management of postpartum haemorrhage: what to do when medical treatment fails. Obstet Gynecol Surv. 2007;62(8):540-47.
32. Tindell K, Garfinkel R, Abu-Haydar E, et al. Uterine balloon tamponade for the treatment of postpartum haemorrhage in resource-poor settings: a systematic review. BJOG. 2013;120(1):5-14.

22

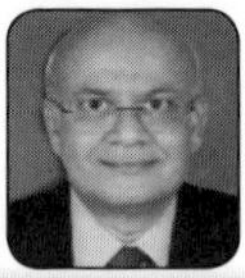

Some Indian Innovative Tool in Obstetric Care

AK Debdas

INTRODUCTION

Essential obstetric care as well initial emergency obstetric care is often given by middle level health care provider or nonspecialist doctor in periphery, rural area. They are not skilled as well not trained to use sophisticated instruments. More ever they are not available due to financial constraint. This chapter discusses few very simple innovative tools, which can be understood and used by any level of health care- giver. All these innovative tools are useful in antenatal care as well obstetric emergencies like postpartum hemorrhage, obstructed labor. The another valuable aspect of all these tools are that they not only give qualitative but also quantitative values, which can help a lot in decision-making.

GROWTH TAPE—A TAPE FOR MONITORING ANTENATAL FETAL GROWTH

It is a specially designed simple measuring tape for objective assessment (instead of guessing) of antenatal fetal growth from week-to-week—from visit-to-visit (Fig. 1). The special thing about this tape is—it is calibrated in weeks of pregnancy so that matching with the calculated week of pregnancy is easy and instant (Fig. 2). Just lay the tape on the uterus in the midline from symphysis to fundus and see whether say 34 weeks of amenorrhea tallies with the 34 weeks mark on the tape or not—if more (it is a case of 'big for date' or if less (it is 'small for date').

Scope

- To spot the intrauterine growth restriction (IUGR) early and more objectively, so that they may be treated early.

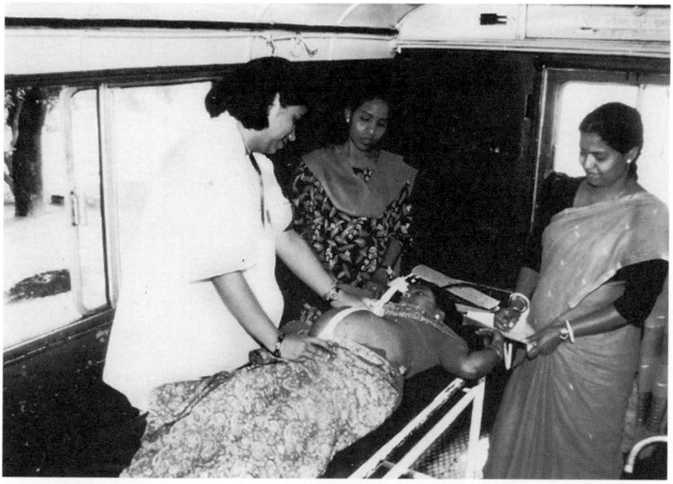

Fig. 1 Growth tape in use in mobile ANC

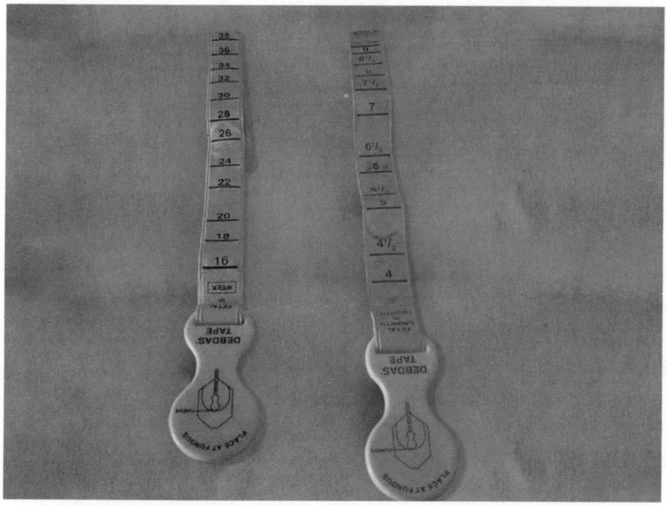

Fig. 2 Growth tape calibrated in week of pregnancy

- It effects standardization of assessment fetal growth—like using the BP instrument for checking BP.
- It is a 'Nomogram' of antenatal fetal growth for Indian fetus.
- It serves as a simple customized one step 'Gravidogram' for Indian fetus in place of complex, time comsuming multistep gravidogram designed in Sweden. No wonder its use have died down (Fig. 3).

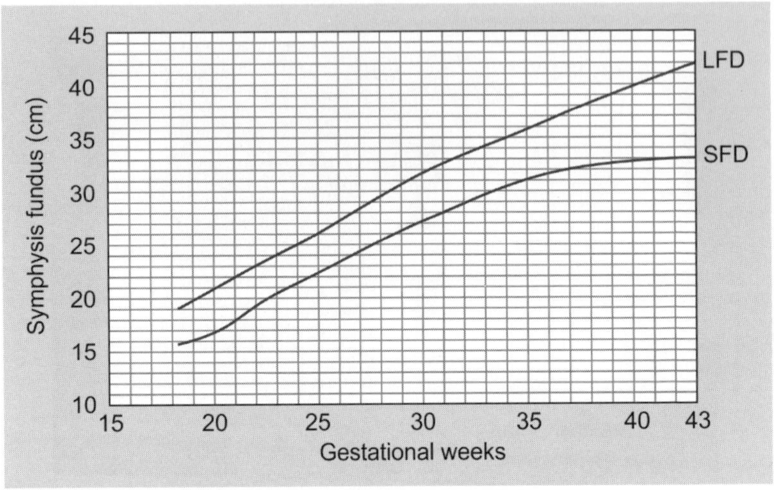

Fig. 3 Conventional complex gravidogram

Practical Advantages

- A very low skill method and can be effectively used by ANMs, health visitors, etc. as in rural obstetrics.
- Very cheap, almost no cost is involved.
- It saves money and trouble of having to do frequent ultrasound examination.
- Reliability—75 to 80 percent correlation with ultrasound growth findings. It has been widely tested in several institutes of Medical Sciences and Teaching Hospitals in India.

STEROID TAPE

Steroid Administration 'Guide Tape' for Premature Labor Cases (Fig. 4)

It is a specially designed 'Growth Tape (Debdas)' which helps to determine whether to give steroid or not in the uncertain cases of premature labor with 'unknown or doubtful dates' specially in Rural Obstetrics without USG facility or USG is not affordable.

Ideal Time for Giving Steroid Injection

To be effective it should be given in the maturity window of 24 to 34 weeks.

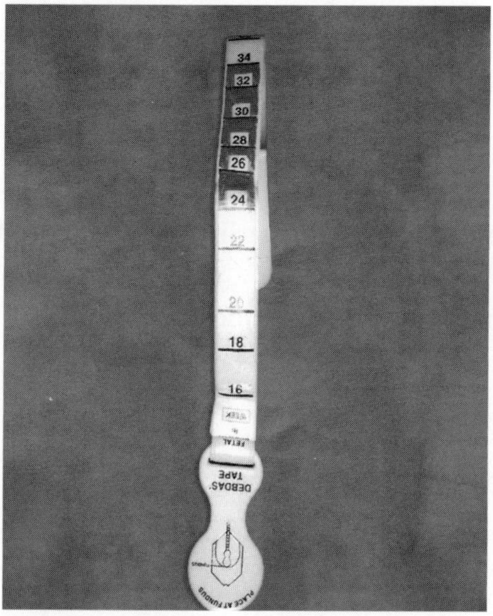

Fig. 4 Steroid tape—give steroid if fundal height falls in red zone

Unique Advantage of the Steroid Tape

The tape gives rough fetal maturity instantly avoiding confusion and delay even abstination.

Many mothers are not given the steroid injection at all because of uncertain maturity.

Dose of Steroid Injection

Betamethasone 12 mg IM—two doses—24 hours apart. For it to be effective, the delivery is to be delayed for 48 hours from the first dose if the clinical situation permits.

Method of Steroid Injection

Give steroid injection to mother prophylactically if fundal height falls in the red zone (24–34 weeks zone) of this tape. Simple principle and simple instruction—no confusion.

The Vital Purpose of Giving the Steroid Injection

For inducing fetal lung maturation and thereby prevent neonatal death from RDS to which these babies are particularly prone.

Special Place of Use of the Steroid Tape

It is ideal low resource and low skill areas like—ANM manned birthing places.

DESCENTMETER (FIG. 5)

New Simple Scale for Measuring Progressive Descent of Fetus in Labor

Descent of fetus is labor all about because it is the final result of the whole mechanism of labor. But it is surprising that, to date, there is no truly objective method available to assess this vital parameter of progress of labor.

How is Descent Measured Today?

By clinical guess estimation in relation to the level of ischial spines.

Disadvantages of the Present Method

- Ischial spines, being very deeply placed structures, are not easy to locate.
- It needs a lot of pocking and prodding which is very uncomfortable and also painful specially in primis.
- The method needs a lot of skill and experience.
- It gives wide (30%) individual variation in findings between observers.

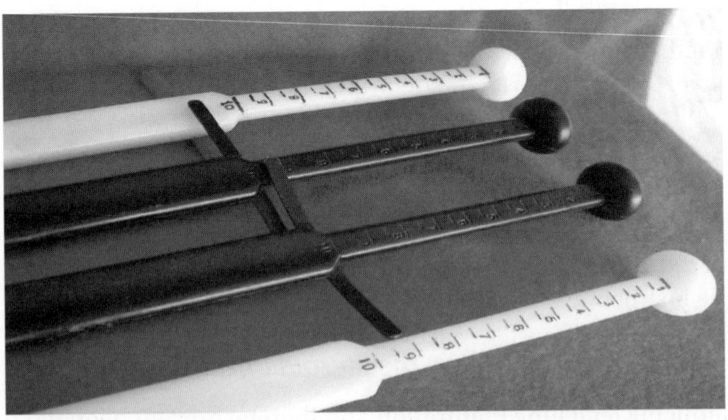

Fig. 5 Descentmeter calibrated up to 10 cm

Introduction of a New 'Reference Point' in Female Pelvis (Debdas)

The Hymen—or Often the Broken Circular Ridge of It

Hither to ignored and neglected (Debdas, FIGO Journal Supplement, 2003)

Few Facts about the Hymen Line in the Context of 'Reference Point'

- It is invariably present—in all women two-thirds even in multi with damaged perineum at least on the anterior two-third of introital opening.
- It is very superficial—can be seen from outside and hence can be very conveniently used for visual correlation and measurement without invading the vagina and also doing strong pocking.
- It is an anatomically fixed line for any particular woman
- Gives "Midpoint-to-midpoint" Correlation, i.e. between midpoint of the head and that of the midpoint/'AXIS' of lower pelvic strait which is approximately 5 cm for all the diameters of this region— allowing easy correlation (Fig. 6).

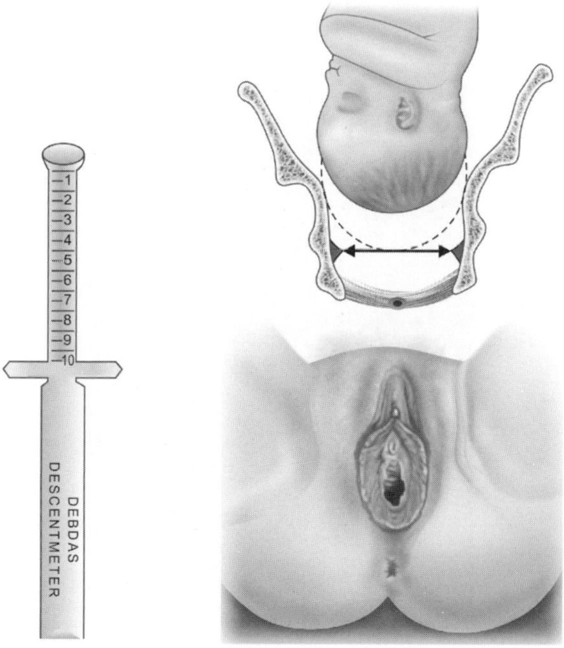

Fig. 6 Descentmeter (DM) measures head-hymen distance

- It happens to be the final exit point for the presenting part from the birth canal.

It is surprising that this very useful anatomical landmark situated right in the area where real intrapartum obstetrics is going on has so far been ignored.

The Descentmeter Introducing a New Scale (Fig. 7)

The descentmeter, which actually objectively measures the descend using the above landmark.

It is a 25 cm long autoclavable polypropylene rod one end (the vaginal end) of which has been calibrated up to 10 cm in 0.5 cm steps—10 cm because the length of both vagina and sacrum is 10 cm. There is a guard on the scale at the end of 10 cm mark so that it cannot be introduced beyond this point. The very top of the vaginal end of the scale is slightly brodened and cupped, so that it sits better on fetal head. The other end works as a handle.

What does it Measure?

It measures the 'head—hymen' distance.

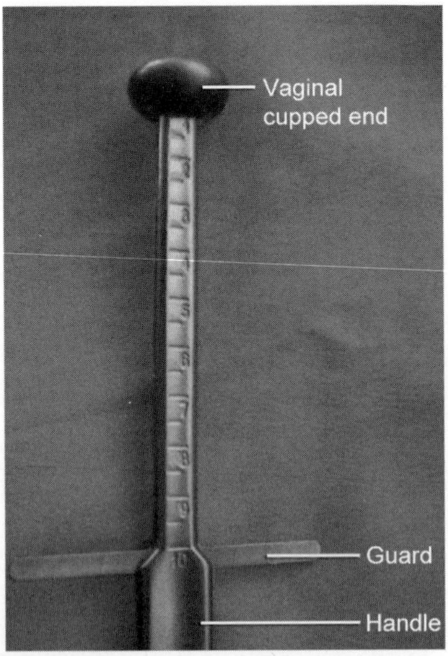

Fig. 7 Descentmeter + Guard + broad head

What does it Communicate for Clinical Purpose?

How far above/inside the final exit point the 'Actual' head is situated.

How to Use it?

After explaining to the patient, under aseptic precautions, the calibrated end of the scale is to be introduced into the vagina under the guidance of two fingers and gently advanced in downwards and backwards direction just like in normal PV until it goes and rests on the lowest point of fetal head. The handle of the scale is then to be depressed firmly on the perineum roughly 5 cm posterior to the external urethral meatus so that it stands perpendicularly on the head (incidentally, 5 cm happens to be the approximately the center of all the diameters of this region). The cm mark on the scale coinciding with the hymen line *posteriorly* is to be read off and recorded as the station of presenting part at that point of time. The procedure is to be repeated at the end of each vaginal examination to measure the progressive descent. As the head would descend, the cm reading would reduce.

When should Reading be Taken in Relation to Uterine Contraction

The reading should always be taken in between contractions.

How to Deal with Caput?

Express the depth of the caput in cm instead of 1+, 2+, 3+, etc. Take descentmeter reading right on the apex of the caput. Add the value of the depth of the caput (whether 1 or 2 or 3 cm) to this reading and this would give the *true station* of the real head.

When to Start Taking Descentmeter Reading?

In First Stage: From about 7 to 8 cm dilatation.

In Second Stage: For primiparae take reading one hourly, for multiparae every 20 minutes. At this stage the head simply has to be sounded with the tip of the descentmeter. There is no need to do full PV unless some problem is anticipated.

When to Stop Taking the Reading?

When the 'actual' head is visible on separating the labia (discount caput if any) in between uterine contractions or when DM reading has reached

3 cm or less. At this stage the head is lying only in the soft tissue of the perineum.

Sterilization

The scale is autoclable. But it may be sterilized by keeping it dipped in CIDEX solution as is done for laparoscope.

Advantages of the Use of Descentmeter

- A truely objective method—gives actual measurement
- Removes the compulsion of guessing
- It would greatly reduce individual variation in findings between observers.
- It can be used by the less skilled "First liners" of labor room like—trainees, doctors and nurses working in remote rural centers.
- Unlike the ischial spine method, the procedure is neither painful nor uncomfortable for the mother.
- Effects standardization of the technique of measuring descend (just like BP instrument for taking BP).

DEBDAS POSTPARTUM HEMORRHAGE BAG

Description of the Bag

The bag has an anterior or front wall (the printed side of the bag) which is split in the middle up to half of its length and a posterior or back wall which is intact and is just like a sheet and is meant to go under the buttock of the patient high up—up to her loin (Fig. 8).

When to Spread the Bag?

After clamping the cord and handing over the baby by which time all liquor would have drained away which would avoid volume dilution effect by the liquor on the blood collection.

How to Spread the Bag?

- Ask the patient to lift her buttock.
- Hold the two lateral margins of the bag by two hands and slip the posterior leaf/wall of the bag upwards under the buttock of the patient to reach to the level of the *waist/loin* which would correspond to the level of the umbilicus anteriorly. Fix it there with two small

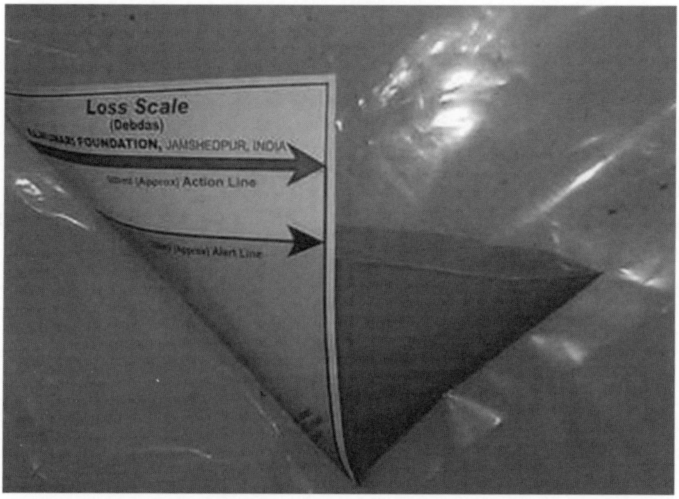

Fig. 8 Postpartum hemorrhage (PPH) bag traffic light model *(for color version see Plate 6)*

pieces of adhesive tapes—one on each side on the antrolateral aspect of the trunk so that the bag sticks to the skin there and also a little elevated too so that there is no chance of leakage due to gravity.

As one does this, the split in the anterior wall of the bag opens up automatically to accommodate the buttocks but leaving the vulva and perineum uncovered and well exposed giving excellent perineal access for—the delivery of the placenta, stitching of the perineum, etc. If necessary, this slit may be increased further by cutting a little more for more space.

- The two triangular anterior/front flaps of the bag are to be fixed with two more adhesive tapes on to the medial side of the thighs a little high up so as to promote gravity for the accumulation of the blood). The wide V shaped gap created by this lateral fixing the anterior flaps allows excellent abdominal access for massaging the uterus. It also allows bimanual compression, even aortic compression for the cases of intractable PPH while efficiently collecting all the lost blood.

Note: With the use of this bag, no linen or draping is required to be put directly on the lower half of the trunk as this part is already encased in the bag. Use of any of these materials and their soakage would affect the estimation of blood loss.

Postures of Delivery in which it can be Used

This bag may be used for delivering mothers in any of the conventional postures of delivery:

- In dorsal position
- In semireclining position
- In lithotomy position

It may also be used for cesarean section where it has to be spread under the patient before draping her. This captures all bleeding that come out through the vagina during and after the operation.

CONCLUSION

The above mentioned simple innovative tools are easy to practice, give clear guidelines for action in obstetric care. The need is to popularize these innovative tools and make them commercially available. It is ironical that while on Hi-tech technology, equipment, a lot of money is invested, the simple tools does not get their due recognition and presence. Wisdom lies in simplicity and common sense. Science only observes nature, nature is always simple.

BIBLIOGRAPHY

1. Debdas AK: Growth Tape (Debdas)—An Indian nomogram for fetal growth, J Obst and Gynae of India, 1996,46:479-500.
2. Debdas AK. Standardisation of clinical assessment of fetal growth—as urgent need, Indian Journal of Perinatology and Reproductive Biology, 1996, pp. 16-21.
3. Debdas AK. Designing a new scale named "Descentmeter" (DM) for measuring the progressive descect of fetus in labour, International Journal of Obs and Gyne, FIGO World Congress 2000, Supplement, Washington DC, Elsevier, 82.
4. Debdas AK. Descentmeter (DM)—a new scale for measuring the progressive descent of fetus in labour, International Journal of Obs and Gyne, FIGO World Congress 2003, Supplement, Sandaigo, Chile, Elsevier, 111-2.

23

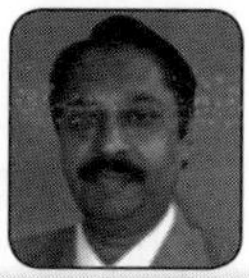

Role of High Dependency Unit for Safe Motherhood: Future Vision

Alpesh Gandhi

GENESIS OF THE CONCEPT

Women are not dying because of a disease we cannot treat. They are dying because societies have yet to make the decision that their lives are worth saving. This was declared by the President, International Federation of Gynecology and Obstetrics (FIGO) during World Congress, 1997 at Copenhagen.

Maternal mortality rate (MMR) in developed countries is < 30. In India, it is 212 and in some of the states even > 300. MMR in India is even worse than its neighboring countries like Sri Lanka and Bangladesh.

Every year 500000 pregnant women die in the world. If quality obstetric health care is provided in time, then we could save 80 percent of these pregnant women, i.e. 400000 women in the world.

Maternal mortality is "just the tip of the iceberg". There is a vast base to this iceberg, which is maternal morbidity (Near-Miss), which remains largely undescribed.

There is no published survey or official data of MMR at institutes in India but in unpublished data, the rate of maternal mortality rate at hospital may be between 70 to 90 which is nearly 3 times more than the MMR in developed world. There is a big gap in MMR between developing and western world in institutional deliveries.

An article was published in the May 2013 publication in the Lancet on implementation of essential obstetric health services and outcome. It showed that the immediate interventions with prophylactic uterotonics and treatment with oxytocics were given in low and high resourced countries to the same magnitude in teaching institutions. The same applied for the use of magnesium sulphate. However, the maternal mortality was high in countries which have already high mortality and it was low in countries which has already low mortality. Several explanations were given to this observation such as late interventions but the most likely explanation is the lack of appropriate level of care, team work and the absence of critical care after the life-threatening incident has happened.

Maternal near-miss case means a woman (in pregnancy/labor/puerperium) who almost died due to any life-threatening complications but survived. For every maternal death that occurs, between 11 to 223 women experience a 'near-miss' event in pregnancy. Recent WHO systematic review, global prevalence of SAMM (defined as severe life-threatening obstetric complication necessitating an urgent medical intervention in order to prevent likely death of mother) varies from 0.01 to 8.23 percent. The case fatality ratio is 0.02 to 37 percent.

The majority of women during their pregnancy, labor and postnatal period require care that can be met through routine obstetric care. A small but significant number, however, require critical care related to the pregnancy itself, aggravation of a pre-existing illness or complications of the delivery. Any pregnant woman can develop life-threatening complications with little or no advance warning which can lead to physical, social, economic and psychological consequences of complications. All such women need access to quality maternal health services that can detect and manage life-threatening complications.

In Europe and US, about 0.1 to 0.9 percent of women during pregnancy or labor require intensive care. In India, it varies from 8 to 16 percent.

Quality maternal health care means facility for invasive monitoring, skill-based services, skilled and experienced persons and 24 hours monitoring. All these can be best accomplished in an obstetric ICU set-up where services from expert and trained medical, nursing and technical staff is available. They use sophisticated State-of-the-art equipment and technology for intensive monitoring and immediate life-saving interventions and organ support that may be necessary.

There is an agreement in the developed world on the need for intensive care facilities for the obstetric patient. This level of care may not be attainable for the pregnant in the developing world as lack of access to quality health facilities and its cost. It is not viable to have a separate ICU only for obstetrics purpose in smaller hospitals and smaller towns.

It is interesting to know that in developed countries nearly 30 percent of big institutes are having facility of Obstetric HDUs. Specialized certified fellowship courses in the name of maternal-fetal medicine or critical care in obstetrics are available. Whereas in developing countries like us, it is still a dream. This is the genesis for the concept of high dependacy unit (HDU).

About the HDU Concept

It is also called step-up, step-down, progressive and intermediate care units. HDUs are wards for people who need more intensive observation, treatment and nursing care than is possible in a routine ward but slightly less than that given in intensive care. The ratio of nurses to patients is 2:1 which is slightly lower than in intensive care but higher than in general wards. It has some its own limitations and advantages. HDU would not normally accept patients requiring mechanical ventilation, but could manage those receiving invasive monitoring. Patients with multiorgan failure cannot be kept in HDU. HDU will suffice when organ support is not vital. It can be established in most obstetric unit in a room which is equipped for it. HDU is an option in terms of efficacy and fulfils the need of tertiary care center. It reduces need of ICU with continuity of care. Risk of getting hospital acquired infection is less with HDU compare to ICU. HDU care is cheaper as compared to ICU care. Psychologically, patient will be more comfortable as her relatives can attend her and in many cases, her baby can be kept with her. It allows continuity of antenatal, intrapartum and postnatal care provided by the same team at the same place. A dedicated obstetric HDU with the knowledge, familiarity, expertise of an obstetrician and a specialist team would be the best place to monitor and treat the critically ill obstetric patients.

Studies

A study was conducted on role of high dependency unit (HDU) in critical care obstetrics at Santokba Durlabhji Memorial Hospital, Jaipur, Rajasthan. Women admitted in HDU/ICU were studied over 3 years (2009–2012). HDU admissions included high-risk pregnancies (APH, PPH, PIH), sepsis, acute fatty liver of pregnancy, pulmonary thromboembolism and DVT, complications of pre-existing medical disorders, peripartum cardiomyopathy, postcesarean complications, anesthesia complications, uterine rupture and other genital tract injuries. Women requiring respiratory/inotropic support shifted to ICU. Outcomes studied in terms of final outcome of women, burden status of ICU, women shifted to ICU from HDU, monetary expenditure to hospital and cost of treatment to the patient.

Result

Out of 594 high-risk women, 427 (72%) were managed in HDU and 167 (28%) required ICU. Out of 167 women in ICU, 109 (65%) were shifted from HDU and 58 (35%) were admitted directly. Out of 427 women in

HDU, 400 (93.6%) discharged in good condition, none expired and 27 (6%) LAMA. Out of 167 in ICU, 106 discharged in good condition, 35 (21%) expired and 26 (15.6%) LAMA. Burden of ICU reduced to 1/3rd in comparison to last 5 years. Expenditure of hospital in maintenance of ICU decreased by 41 percent. Total treatment cost to the patient decreased by 38 percent.

In another study, objective was to establish the utilization of high dependency care in a tertiary referral obstetric unit. Data of pregnant or recently pregnant women admitted to the obstetric high dependency unit from 1984 to 2007 were included to evaluate the admission rate. Four years' information of an ongoing prospective audit was collated to identify the indications for admission, maternal monitoring, transfers to intensive care unit, and location of the baby.

The result was, the overall HDU admission rate is 2.67 percent, but increased to 5.01 percent in the most recent 4 years. Massive obstetric hemorrhage is now the most common reason for admission. Invasive monitoring was undertaken in 30 percent of women. Two-thirds of neonates (66.3%) stayed with their critically ill mothers in the HDU. Transfer to the intensive care unit was needed in 1.4 per 1000 deliveries conducted. Study concluded that obstetric high dependency care provides holistic care from midwives, obstetricians and anesthetists while retaining the opportunity of early bonding with babies for critically ill mothers.

Study was also conducted at Institute of Postgraduate Medical Education and Research (IPGMER), Kolkata—one of the biggest tertiary care and referral institutes in Eastern India. Retrospective cohort study was conducted from May 2007 to May 2011. Relevant data regarding obstetric events, indications for HDU transfer/admission, interventions required, length of stay, eventual outcomes were collected, reviewed, tabulated and analyzed.

Antenatal mothers were monitored clinically along with CTG, biophysical profile and Doppler study. All patients were individualized and managed with invasive or noninvasive measures as and when required. During the 4 year study period, 5052 mothers delivered and 57 patients required HDU admission. Thus obstetric admission in HDU was 11.2 per 1000 deliveries. This data from Eastern India differed from the other parts. The ICU utilization by obstetric patients was 10.2 in 4 years in Dublin (Ireland) and 26.7 in 23 years in UK. Unfortunately, data from other developing nations is lacking. Limited accessibility and higher mortality prior receiving medical attention may help explain this low utilization of HDU services in eastern India. This incidence of HDU utilization reveals just the tip of the iceberg. The indications leading to

HDU admission were analyzed among the patients. Sepsis accounted for the majority (35.08%) of admissions, followed by PPH (29.82%) and severe hypertensive disorders (BP 160/100 mm of Hg) of pregnancy (21.05%).

Another study was conducted in the Rotunda Hospital, Dublin with 121 beds. It incorporates a two-bedded HDU, established in June 1996. Patients were also subdivided into those transferred to ICU in the period January 1994 to June 1996 (before on-site HDU facilities were available) and those transferred to ICU between June 1996 and June 1998 (after the HDU was established).

The total number of deliveries was 14096 before the establishment of the HDU and 12070 after. 123 patients were admitted to the HDU during the study period June 1996 to June 1998, representing 1.02 percent of all deliveries. This includes three patients who were admitted to the HDU from other obstetric centres for further management, but excludes 5 patients transferred to ICU and then admitted back to the HDU for 'step-down' care. The 18 patients were admitted before delivery: 9 with antepartum hemorrhage, 9 with pre-eclampsia, 2 with epilepsy, 2 with appendicitis, 2 with pulmonary embolism, 1 with ischemic heart disease and 1 with renal impairment. Mean age was 30 years and gestation was 34.8 weeks. Median length of stay in HDU was 3 days. The 17 patients were transferred to a general ICU, 12 before the HDU was established (representing 0.08% of all deliveries) and 5 after (0.04%). Before the HDU was established, length of stay in ICU was 3 days and 2 days after HDU. Prior to development of on-site HDU facilities at the hospital, ICU utilization rate was 0.08 percent which decreased to 0.04 percent following the establishment of this facility. Although not statistically significant, there is an apparent trend toward decreased ICU admission rates following the establishment of the HDU. Transfer to ICU in the group before HDU, was necessitated predominantly by obstetric complications, with hemodynamic instability as a result of hemorrhage being the most common ICU admission diagnosis. Following the advent of the HDU, the need for mechanical ventilation became the major indication for maternal ICU admission with an increasing number of patients with hemodynamic instability being managed within the HDU. Duration of ICU stay was short in both groups; interestingly, although not statistically significant, there is a trend toward reduced duration of ICU stay perhaps reflecting the availability of HDU care on discharge to the referring center.

Wheatley et al. suggested that early intervention and treatment of the critically ill obstetric patient might prevent serious complications and avoid the need for ICU. In their study, almost 60 percent of the patients admitted to ICU could have been managed appropriately within the HDU setting. Study concluded that a population of critically ill obstetric patients can be managed successfully in an obstetric HDU with the advantage of concurrent expert obstetric and critical care management.

In another study conducted at Liverpool Women's NHS Foundation Trust, Liverpool, UK. In England, the Critical Care Minimum Data Set (CCMDS) was used to assess critical care activity. This uses the number of organs supported to define level of care. One organ is level 2 (high dependency), two or more level 3 (intensive care). Admissions over a 7-month period was studied to determine rates of admissions and level of care as defined by the CCMDS. 4608 women were delivered and 239 (5.18%) were admitted to the HDU. Average length of stay was 1.97 days. 137 (57%) were CCMDS level 2 and 52 (22%) level 3. An admission rate of 1 to 2 percent quoted in the literature. This predates the publication of the MAGPIE study. Magnesium sulphate treatment constitutes a significant proportion of their HDU admissions, which may account for this increase.

Scope of HDU

When things go wrong in obstetrics, they go wrong very fast. Care of critically ill patients is a unique challenge in obstetrics because of medical conditions which might present risk to the pregnancy and pregnancy may modify the disease state. Drug therapy may be affected by altered pharmacokinetics of pregnancy or it may have impact on the developing fetus. Obstetric patients are generally young and healthy and they do recover rapidly. However, the potential for catastrophic complications is real. Box 1 summarizes the potential situation of management at HDU.

PLANNING AN OBSTETRIC HIGH DEPENDENCY UNIT

It includes cost of initial capital expenditure, purchase of new technology, recruitment of staff and rolling annual cost and other indirect costs like training, consumables, IT facility, etc. Early proper referrals can make it a viable unit.

Setting Up of HDU

Location, space, equipment, personnel, protocols, audit, education and training are important issues to be taken care.

Box 1 Potential situation of management at HDU

- Pregnancy/labor pain with severe anemia
- Accidental hemorrhage—placental abruption, couvelaire uterus
- Severe PET
- Eclampsia
- Placenta previa (PPH)
- Postpartum hemorrhage (HELLP)
- Hemolysis, elevated lever enzymes, low platelets
- Disseninated intravascular coagulation (DIC)
- Multiple gestation with complications
- Pregnancy with uterine anomaly and pathologies
- Adherent placenta and other placental abnormalities
- Obstetric hysterectomy
- Hydatidiform mole
- Ruptured ectopic
- Sepsis
- Ruptured uterus
- Burns during pregnancy
- Perforation during abortion
- Pregnancy with gestational diabetes
- Pregnancy with cardiac diseases
- Pregnancy with jaundice
- Postoperative ARF and other renal problems
- Leukemia and other hemolytic disorders
- Pregnancy with dengue, malaria, etc.
- Asthma and other respiratory problems
- Others.

Space

It will be ideal to have adequate space of at least 120 sq feet for per bed.

Location

It should be near ICU or OT or both. There should be at least one fully equipped obstetric theater within the delivery suite. Where this is not possible, a lift, for the rapid transfer of women to theater must be available. It should have nearby facility of blood bank, fully equipped laboratory and nearby NICU care.

Furniture and Equipment

Along with all routine equipment required in routine ward, following furniture and equipment are necessary for setting up of an HDU.

Maternity coat with electronically manoeuvred with all positions, glucometer, infusion pump, syringe pump, ultrasound machine with color Doppler and echo facility, CTG machine, cardiac monitor with CVP monitor, intubation kit, baby resuscitation kit/cart, Crash cart fully loaded with BCLS medications, stock of all emergency drugs and if possible O-negative blood, CNS tray with torch, hammer, etc. central oxygen supply, wall mount suction, pulse oxymeter, anesthesia apparatus, cautery machine, defibrillator, ventilator (It is ideal for obstetric ICU), biphasic intermittent positive airway pressure (BIPAP), refrigerator with deep freeze facility, X-ray view box, separate Eclampsia box, partogram, input/output chart, generator or inverter, intercom and emergency bell facility with a phone list of helpline and all other required facility, trays for procedures for putting central lines, ICD, catheters, etc. are required for setting up of an HDU.

Personnel

An HDU working team consists of obstetricians, support staff, obstetric anesthetists, neonatologists, support staff experienced with HDU nursing care provides continuous observation—including accurate recording of fluid intake, urine output, blood pressure (via arterial line in some cases), central venous pressure monitoring and pulse-oxymetry, etc., whenever required.

Guidelines and Protocols

As HDU care involves management of critically ill obstetric patients, Protocols should be kept ready in place to ensure appropriate and immediate responses to these critical situations and to justify actions that are sufficient and efficient. Protocols should include protocol for admission and discharge criteria to/from HDU, counseling and for all those conditions being taken care at HDU.

Management

It includes an initial assessment of the condition and resuscitation of the patient, whenever required. Maternal organ function monitoring of cardiovascular, renal, pulmonary, hepatic, cerebral is done. Baseline and specific investigations as indicated are advised. Primary condition (severe pre-eclampsia, hemorrhage, sepsis) is treated. Fetal condition is checked by Clinical trail group (CTG) Fluid therapy in the form of Crystalloid/Colloid/Blood is given. Uteroplacental oxygen delivery is maintained. Noninvasive and invasive monitoring like BP, RR, HR,

Pulse, SPO_2, ABP, CVP, ABGs, hourly UOP, lungs functions and others is done. Proper care for nutrition is taken. Enteral and parenteral nutrition is given. If required, inotropes are given. Fluid balance and electrolytes correction is taken care. Pain management is done. Appropriate clinicians from relevant specialties are involved. Final management is individualized and depends on the underlying clinical condition.

Discharging the Patient from HDU to Ward

When patient is hemodynamically stable, no further continuous intravenous medication or frequent blood tests required, no invasive monitoring is required, no active bleeding, no supplementary oxygen is required and patient is mobilized, then the patient is discharged from HDU and transferred to a ward. When transferring a woman from HDU to the postnatal ward, a personal and detailed handover of care should be given.

Indications of Transfer from HDU to ICU

When patient needs for advanced respiratory support, further inotropic support is required, patient develops DIC, multiorgan failure, adult respiratory distress syndrome (ARDS), she is transferred to ICU for further care and support.

Patient Needs Transfer to ICU

- When RR is outside the range 7 to 35 breaths/minute
- Pulse is outside the range 40 to 140 beats/minute
- BP < 80 mm Hg or 30 mm Hg below patient's usual BP
- U/O < 400 mL in 24 hour, or < 160 mL in 8 hours and unresponsive to simple measures
- GCS < 8 in the context of non-traumatic coma
- Unarousable patient
- S. sodium outside the range 110 to 160 mmol L
- S. potassium outside the range 2.0 to 7.0 mmol L
- pH outside the range 7.1 to 7.7
- PaO_2 < 6.6 kPa
- $PaCO_2$ more than 8.0 kPa
- SaO_2 < 90 percent on supplemental oxygen.

CONCLUSION

HDU provides a level of care in between general ward and ICU set-up. Women not requiring ventilator support can be managed in HDU, reducing the burden of ICUs. Treatment cost reduces, increasing the affordability to all classes of society and above all, it requires less expenditure to establish and manage HDU. A dedicated obstetric HDU with the knowledge, familiarity, experience and expertise of an obstetrician and a specialist team would be the best place to monitor and treat the critically ill obstetric patients. It allows continuity of antenatal, intrapartum and postnatal care by the same team. Delivery of the baby takes place in a more familiar and better-equipped environment with minimal disruption of mother-to-baby bonding. Obstetric HDU allows lactation support.

Care in an obstetric HDU may avoid exposure of the critically ill pregnant mother to a potentially hazardous ICU environment with the risk of hospital-acquired infection. Patient satisfaction may be increased, since it has more liberal family visitation policies. HDU care is less costly than ICU. Care in an ICU sometimes becomes focused on the machines, rather than on the patient whereas in HDU, humanizing aspects of critical care be addressed in caring for a patient and her family. Patients with high-risk pregnancy and critical ill patients can be managed better which ultimately reduce MMR and morbidity.

BIBLIOGRAPHY

1. Critical care in obstetric guidelines; Northern Health and Social Care Trust.
2. Dattaray C, Mandal D, Shanker W, Bhattacharya P, Mandal S. Obstetric patients requiring high-dependency unit admission in a tertiary referral centre; Obstetric patients requiring high-dependency unit admission in a tertiary referral centre. International Journal of Critical Illness and Injury Science.
3. ICU Planning and Designing in India, Guidelines 2010 Guidelines Committee ISCCM; Role of High Dependency Unit (HDU) in critical care Obstetrics: a practical approach, At Santokba Durlabhji Memorial Hospital, Jaipur, Rajasthan.
4. Ryan M, Hamilton V, Bowen M, Mc Kenna P. The role of a high-dependency unit in a regional obstetric hospital; Article first published online: 7 JUL 2008; DOI: 10.1046/ j.13652044.2000.01627. Anaesthesia; Volume 55, Issue 12, pages 1155–1158, December 2000.
5. The May 2013 publication in the Lancet.

24

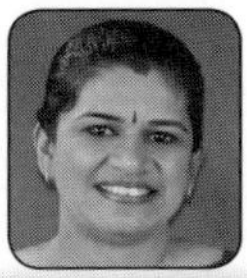

Helping Mothers Survive—FOGSI Jhpiego Program: An Innovative Learning and Teaching Program

Hema Divakar

INTRODUCTION

The Federation of Obstetric and Gynecological Societies of India (FOGSI) is the professional organization representing practitioners of obstetrics and gynecology in India. With 223 member societies and over 29000 individual members spread over the length and breadth of the country, FOGSI is probably one of the largest membership based organizations of specialized professionals. FOGSI came into formal existence in Madras on January 6, 1950 at the sixth All India Congress of Obstetrics and Gynecology, when the obstetric and gynecological societies of Ahmedabad, Bengal, Bombay, Madras and Punjab resolved to form themselves into the Federation of Obstetric and Gynecological Societies of India. Presently, it is the largest professional organization of specialists with member societies—223 and a membership of 29310 specialists. It has numerous committees that address women's health issues (e.g. Practical Obstetrics Committee, Safe Motherhood Committee, Medical Education Committee, Young Talent Promotion Committee). FOGSI also brings out the *Journal of Obstetrics and Gynecology* of India and has an academic wing in the form of Indian College of Obstetrics and Gynecology. Over the years, the organization has established high credibility with the government and is consulted on reproductive health issues.

While South Asian countries currently experience relatively high levels of maternal mortality (MMR), there are also stunning pockets of success. Sites successful in reducing maternal mortality or in increasing the use of skilled birth attendance or emergency obstetric care—Kerala, Tamil Nadu and Gujarat in India; Matlab and Khulna in Bangladesh—and those not as successful—northeast Bangladesh (Sylhet) and

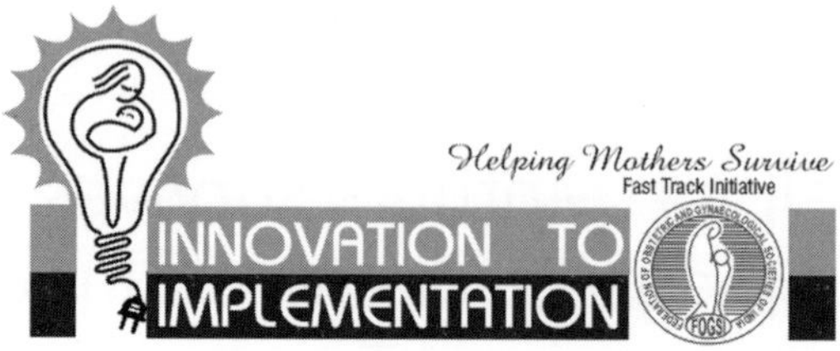

Fig. 1 You cannot have a better tomorrow, if you are thinking about yesterday all the time !–Chareles F Kettering

Rajasthan in India—were studied during 2004 to 2007. Major challenges are typically the lack of available skilled care at birth and referral support, poor quality of care at birth, and lack of use of such care due to costs, distance, and other traditional barriers. Transitioning to use of skilled and referral care and the lowering of the maternal mortality ratio (MMR) can take years: halving the MMR in developed countries, for example, typically took a decade during the mid-20th century.

The most recent example and experience is with the Helping Mothers Survive (HMS) program, which spans through all the points mentioned about what a professional organization like FOGSI can do, we also realize that we need to move on a fast track (Fig. 1).

In keeping with the theme for FOGSI 2013—innovation to implementation, we hope to create an impact through the organization by a focused activity to fulfill its mission of reducing maternal mortality.

We in India are racing against time to achieve the Millennium Development goals 5 (MDG 5). The most pressing need of the hour is to save the mothers. Postpartum hemorrhage (PPH) and pre-eclampsia, eclampsia (PE/E) continue to remain the two major causes of maternal mortality. In keeping with the theme of innovation to implementation, we have embarked on a new journey.

THE FOGSI JHPIEGO FAST TRACK INITIATIVE FOR HELPING MOTHERS SURVIVE

This initiative offers focused training and capacity building of frontline health care providers to handle prevent and manage postpartum hemorrhage, pre-eclampsia and eclampsia with an innovative simulator called **Mammanatalle (Box 1) Jhpiego** has been kind enough to impart the training to our master trainers. These master trainers formed **HMS fast track teams** to conduct the hands on workshop in the PPH/PE/E modules; low dose–high intensity training offered to the teams of healthcare providers at medical colleges, large public sector institutions, private hospitals and at conlinual medical education (CMEs) at various ObGyn Societies and Postgraduate program. It has also been successful in identify two YUVA leaders in house to continue the same program at every 6 monthly by the college itself at least for next 5 years—to commit to continue to train and retrain all health care providers. We hope this would ensure prevention, early recognition and treatment of PPH and PE/E and timely management.

Source-Innovative Module—Mammanatalle

FOGSI invested for 100 modules for 100 master trainers.

Study/Print Material/Certificates

FOGSI manual for HMS includes:

- Facilitators guide
- Participants guide
- Flip charts
- Posters
- Certificates.

Training of Trainer (ToT) Workshop by Jhpiego

Master trainers from all zones had an overview in August 2012 at Bengaluru (Figs 2A and B).

Retraining for smaller batches of master trainers—zone wise (south zone and west zone trainings and then the east and north zone) with consenseus on protocols (Figs 3A and B).

Training Programs—Implementation

"Helping mothers survive" implementation was decided to be spearheaded in medical colleges. Master trainers were spotted, trained at Bengaluru in 2012 October-November by the Jhpiego team. It was followed by Zonal Training of Trainer program in all the four zones of India, in which 150 master trainers were imparted direction, skills presentations for the program. All master trainers were also given simulator Mammanatalle and Neonatalle (Figs 4A and B).

Ongoing Helping Mothers Survive program were organized at the fast pace from the beginning. The key target area were the medical colleges and teaching institution, target participants were resident doctors, faculties in medical colleges. At many places member societies organized the program with enthusiastic participation of practicing gynecologist. Learning capability and impact on change in practice was encouraging all over. We also encouraged involvement of labor room staff nurses for sharing their practices, their concerns and conveying the right messages and skills with rationality (Box 1).

As per feedback it improved a lot in labor room practices and work atmosphere.

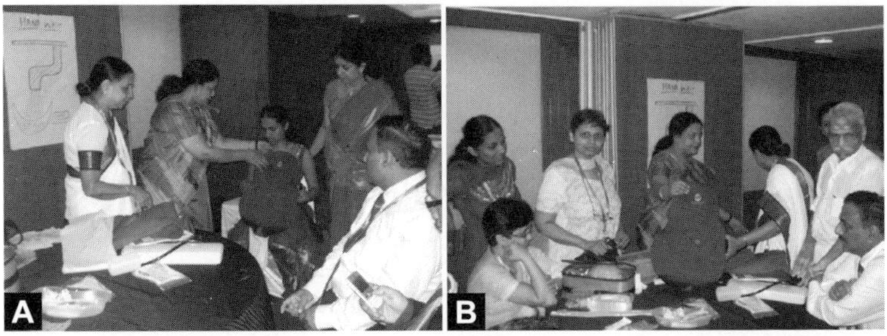

Figs 2A and B Orientation program for helping mothers survive at Bengaluru

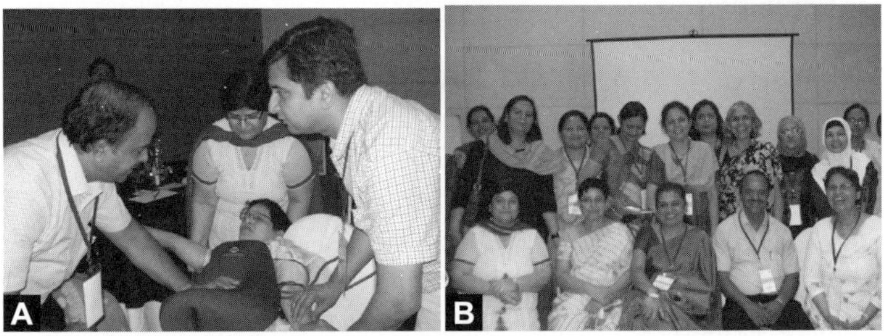

Figs 3A and B Zonal training of trainer program for helping mothers survive

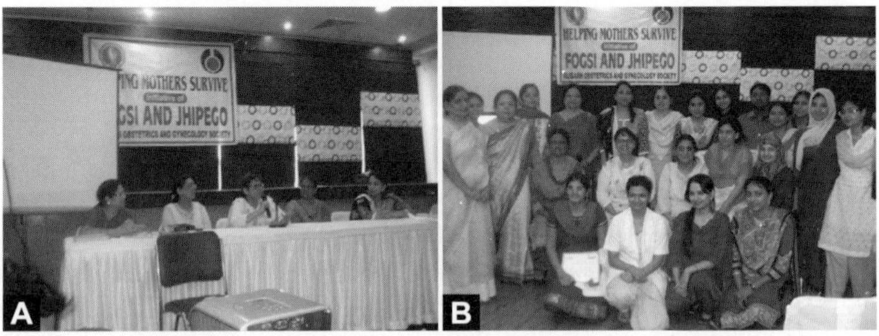

Figs 4A and B Helping mothers survive programs organized at different places pan India

Box 1 HMS-fast track initiative FOGSI Jhpiego project

Innovation—What is New? Helping Mothers Survive: Fast Track Initiative

HMS training is modular, with each module focusing on a manageable set of competencies

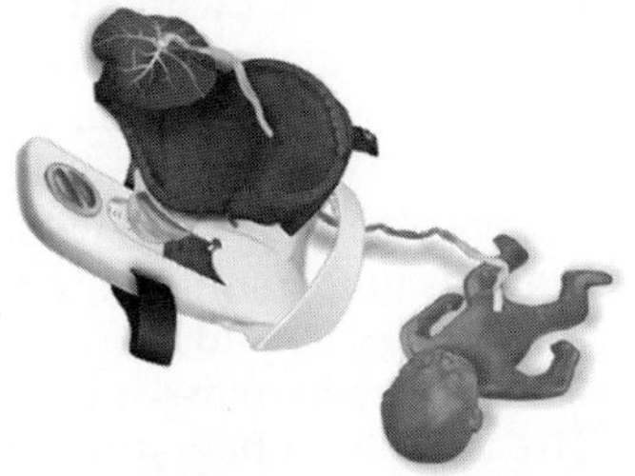

Exciting drills on an interesting and innovative model Mammanetalle.......
A birth simulator with uterus, blood, fetal heart sounds, baby (neonatalle), placenta, cord, retained placental tissue, urethra, cervical rim, drain, and more ......

Implementation—What to Expect during the Workshop?

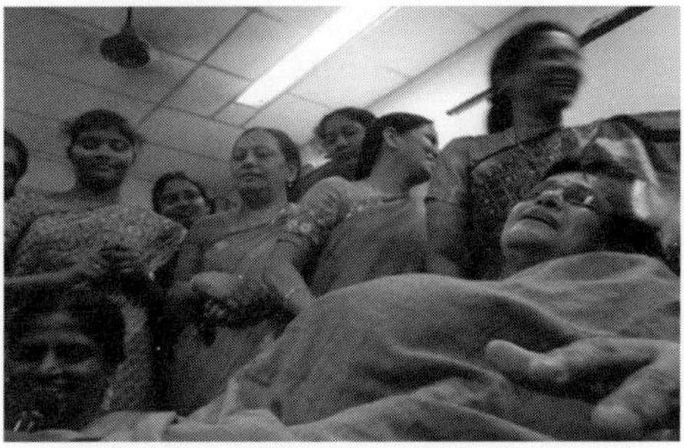

Emergency obstetrics drills on AMTSL and PPH. Introduction, pretest evaluation, role play, conducting the drills, distribution of trainers to different stations, hands on training, blood loss estimation, post-test evaluation, distribution of check lists and interactions competency based-low threshold high impact training.

Helping Mothers Survive program includes:

- Short explanation of third stage of labor, as a serious preventable cause of maternal mortality
- Demonstration of AMSTL, active management of third stage of labor in all deliveries
- Demonstration of management of atonic PPH, blood loss assessment
- Demonstration of management of retained placenta/placental bits management
- Demonstration of management of tissue tears
- Short explanation about PET and eclampsia
- How to administer magnesium sulfate.

Training evaluation includes pretest and post-test questionnaire for objective assessment of impact of program instantly. We propose to have follow up assessment in the institutions to monitor and ensure continued adherence to correct universal protocol.

MONITORING/EVALUATION

FOGSI is preparing data documentation and presenting it to the government. We are negotiating with the government for a PPP module (Public Private Partnership) so that the place for setting this up will be provided by them. The professional association can assist with quality of care assessments. Resources for evaluating quality of care have been published by the Ministry of Health and Family Welfare in India and other South Asian countries and also, the RCOG. These are available to national associations. The Making Pregnancy Safer Initiative, led by the WHO, is committed to national organizations in the annual review of progress made towards reducing maternal morbidity and mortality. Monitoring and assessment tools have been developed to assist in the objective analysis for quality standards. The team members from the professional organizations who are trained to perform the audits and assesments would be very helpful for influencing outcome.

The members of the professional associations would be a part of quality assurance team at the level of central ministry, at the state level, district level and also the facility level.

CHAMPIONS FOR HELPING MOTHERS SURVIVE

Regional awards for the next five years for continued motivation and recognition. The champions in the professional organization could lead by example by creating centers of excellence as a role model for care to promote and propogate quality standards.

SETTING UP OF SKILLS LABS

Setting up of skills labs at eight places across the country; such zonal skills lab will be of immense help not only for our members but also for task shifting with actual impact on the maternal morbidity as well as mortality across our country. The cost of the skill labs needs to be worked out.

2013-FOGSI has taken up implementation of innovations at a fast track pace, FOGSI is to be credited for the speed and effeciency.

COLLABORATING WITH RCOG AND SAFOG—BEYOND THE BOUNDARIES OF INDIA

FOGSI RCOG Satellite Workshop on PPH Management

RCOG World Congress—lead trainers Drs Jayam Kannan, Sheela Mane, and Sadhana Gupta.

IMPACT—Workshop will Enable Task Shifting to Frontline Healthcare Workers

This training would ensure prevention, early recognition and treatment of PPH and timely management. Improved skills rates and confidence in all areas which include provision of AMTSL, management of retained placenta and performance of bimanual uterine compression for severe PPH due to atony, monitoring and transfer alerts, understanding the principles of medical and surgical management.

Likewise it will enable the front level health care provider as well senior and skilled person to provide essential primary care in cases of eclampsia, magnesium sulfate dosage preparation and administration. It also gives message of behavior change communication, universal work precaution, infection prevention and good referral practice.

HMS fast track initiative is a mainly for postgraduates, interns, clinicians, primary health care providers, staff nurses, teaching staff and supportive staff.

CONCLUSION

"*Getting on with what works*"—the Lancet subtitle of an article on strategies for reduction of maternal mortality—states that we know what works to reduce the number of maternal deaths.

The champions to the campaign, such as, the youth leaders and thought leaders from FOGSI will map out the strategies of effective implementation of protocols. *"We will show the world, the impact of what one billion Indians can do—saving mothers preventing needless deaths of mothers,"* so far more than 10,000 frontline healthcare workers have been trained on the FOGSI Fast Track Initiative.

The international community resolved in 1987 to reduce maternal mortality around the world. This resolution was strengthened in 2001 when 189 countries signed the Millennium Declaration, committing themselves to Millennium Development Goal (MDG) 5 towards improvement of maternal health. To accelerate national progress towards achievement of MDG 5, a deeper understanding of what works at scale is needed. This demands a common framework for measuring progress within and across countries and learning processes that engage national stakeholders in using local evidence for programmatic decision-making, identifying critical bottlenecks in scaling up, and generating context-specific implementation solutions. The recommended priority strategy is quality intrapartum care where women deliver in health facilities staffed with a team of midwives available 24 hours a day, with a medical team at a referral hospital for back-up support in the case of life-threatening complications. This strategy has the potential to impact not only to reduce the number of maternal deaths but also mortality of newborns.

The time is right to shift the focus of the global maternal health community to the challenges of effective implementation of services within districts. In this article, FOGSI maternal health initiatives draw on their complementary experiences to identify a set of the central lessons on which to build a new, collaborative effort to implement equitable, sustainable maternal health services at scale. This implementation effort should focus on specific steps for strengthening the capacity of the district health system to convert inputs into functioning services that are accessible to and used by all segments of the population.

Section IV

Safe Motherhood: to Conclude

"The higher order of logic and understanding that is capable of reflecting the soul from the heart"

Chapter

25. Safe Motherhood Initiatives: Where do we Stand Today
Sadhana Gupta

25

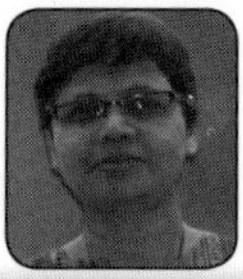

Safe Motherhood Initiatives: Where do we Stand Today

Sadhana Gupta

We have gone through in this book for many aspects, issues, data, programs, and innovations for Safe Motherhood at global and national level of many countries, with special context of India. We seem to be on right track and in the right frame as well. With this we can pat on our back with comfort and contentment or there are few basic and crucially important things which we fail to observe or do not wish to observe.

As the privilege of inceptor and editor of book, at the end of the book I will like to draw everybody's attention to deep cracks in foundation of our global systems and society, which come as big rocks in the way of assuring safe motherhood for each and every women, and naturally it encompasses the unempowered, poor, uneducated, most probably rural women residing in developing and poor world.

Now we think of the basic question—what are the factors and forces which make these women vulnerable to death and sickness, and what is making them poor, uneducated, marginalized, and unable to access health care.

Oh! We may squirm and say—at least not we. They have been like that since ages. These countries, towns and villages are responsible for it.

This chapter is intended to feel—that it is us who are responsible for it. It is also with the aim to feel extremely accountable to every body's basic right to live and live healthy in our personal and professional life.

Let us walk over through major, can say radical changes in world order and ways in this century.

POSITIVE CHANGES IN 20TH CENTURY

End of Colonial Imperialism and Racialism

It was an important era when many countries in the world, became politically independent. Discrimination due to race, religion, class and caste at least principally was not accepted and approved.

These neo independent countries though inherited bankruptcy, debt and instability with independence, yet their people and leaders were free to make program and policy for weaker section which constitute mother, women and children as well. In many countries like Sri Lanka, India, Bangladesh, Nepal, China it really helped as we go through their experience and statistics in this book.

Advances in Medicine

In this century understanding of human physiology, different disease, and the management modalities developed at a very fast pace. It holds true of obstetric care also. Today we have evidence based protocol for management of all major killers of mother like hemorrhage, pre-eclampsia, sepsis and safe abortion. If those simple protocol are universally adhered, it itself can contribute to marked reduction in maternal sickness and death.

Information Technology

There was steep up rise in information technology from very rapid change from Television sets to Computer to freely available and acceptable mobile phones. Optimum use of these techniques is yet to be utilized by health care system. Yet it has been started for data collection, dissemination of data, mobile tracking for pregnant women and promises the positive outcome.

Loud Voices for Women Empowerment and Universal Health Care for Women

It is an important era when many political, professional, and social platforms raised loudly the issue of women education, empowerment and health. From 1987 when WHO and UNFPA first organized Safe Motherhood Conference in Nairobi, Kenya to today's MDG goals of urgent call to reduce maternal mortality by 75 percent by 2015, the scenario changed very fast. Marginalized and neglected mother's health and safety was placed in main frame of nation's development. Many groups and organization were formed and acted in field of safe Motherhood Initiative.

GRAY SHADES OF THE CENTURY FOR UNIVERSAL HEALTH FOR ALL

Now the question arises when we have medical treatment available, we have fastest information technology to spread right messages to masses, we approve every body's right to live, how come we have the widest disparity in maternal death ratio in rich and poor world?

If we do not answer and solve this question, we cannot ensure safety and health to our underprivileged women and families. Let's look into the gray shades of this century. It requires sharp intellect and transparency because the gray is not black and it is in false coat of white.

Colonial Imperialism Changes to Economic Imperialism

This is the most important change in world order which is creating a lot of misery, chaos and confusion in the world. At present it seems that there is no power be it political, social and religious which is not in control of economic imperialism. It causes trapping of people and country in debt pool, cuts the subsidy and investment in education and health, it encourages brain and money drain from poor to riches; it also creates greed and corruption in societies. It is affecting the safe motherhood issues as well with the natural consequences to rob sources of the livelihood of farmers, artisans, skilled workers. In India 5 million farmers have committed suicide in last 5 years due to debt trap, antiagricultural policies, game of multinational companies. When there is no job and food for families, how we can hope for health and health care for rural women?

Kerala and Sri Lanka experiences tells vividly how the pro-people schemes, encouraging local skills and farming can dramatically improve wholesome condition of society, including maternal health.

Hi-tech Medicine

In this era though we had understood very well the simple preventive and promotive measures to improve maternal health, but main highlights and glitter was on Hi-tech medicine and super specialties. It is self-evident fact that health of masses is improved in marked ways by simple interventions and adherence to right simple treatment protocol. Hi-tech medicine can solve the few individualistic situations, besides being expansive and not available easily, its limitations are increased. Offensive advertising and marketing of equipment of business houses forces the already scarce specialist in developing countries to spend a lot of time and money for these and bound to have more scarcity of human resources for health care at periphery.

Medical Tourism and Corporate Health Sector in Developing Countries

India has proudly become a center for medical tourism. Our corporate health sector is fast developing in size and profits. They are not bound to follow any protocol right from management to their fee structure. They are not at all accountable to masses of their own country. They hate poor and poverty and love riches and their sickness. This sector is encouraging brain drain from highest public institution due to sheer money and other hidden advantages.

Energy, money and human resources are limited for every country. Whatever meager we have, we have to decide our priority and concern. It is one of the crucial points to solve, if we wish to achieve Safe Motherhood targets.

Information Technology—Gray Zones

There is everything good or at least nothing bad in technology itself. Whole of wisdom and benefit lies in the fact that it is using for which purpose. To us as citizen of India, it appears that a large number of job have been created by IT industry, but in fact it has robbed the unskilled, semiskilled and artisan from their jobs. It has eroded all the inherent knowledge accumulated through generations of experience and is using to their never satisfying vested interest. So many towns famous for their art work, design have been snatched by IT industry without any information. It has become a most powerful tool for economic imperialism. Again if no job, no food, how any program can deliver the desired results.

Besides, it has also effected medical education badly as on IT technology which are again in hands of big economic corporate are encouraging education and skill which are not required in our own setting. Seed of brain drain from poor to riches is sown at early age.

Question of scarce dedicated human resource in future to face challenge of universal, health care stands before us.

Environmental Safety

Asia and Africa are rich in natural biodiversity. In this century there have been brutal looting of these natural resources be it water, fertile land, forest, minerals.

Sadly the advantage of all dreams of big development projects reaches only rich people, metro cities and big towns. The rural people, schedule tribes, small artisan who depend on the environment for their livings are pushed to wall, only to repercussion inform of instability and violence. Is Safe Motherhood is not the part of whole family, whole socioeconomic cultural scenario?

These are few pertinent hard questions which I'm facing while traveling throughout my and neighboring countries. I don't have any answers, because these seem to be no questions or issues for majority of us.

The truth is always there, you know it you sense it, if we overlook it only we are bound to suffer.

It is a humble attempt to give voices of the weakest among weaker—that is women and children. These mother, children, people are forgiving, not accepting too much from any system. They are source of many comfort and happiness on the Earth.

Please be vigilant, be aware, and Act in righteous way.

It is the most important initiative; you can do for safe motherhood.

Be a part of silent revolution.

Index

Page numbers followed by *f* refer to figure and *t* refer to table

M

N

O

P

Q

R

S

T

U

V

Z